T0302185

Statistical Methods for Dynamic Disease Screening and Spatio-Temporal Disease Surveillance

Disease screening and disease surveillance (DSDS) constitute two critical areas in public health, each presenting distinctive challenges primarily due to their sequential decision-making nature and complex data structures. *Statistical Methods for Dynamic Disease Screening and Spatio-Temporal Disease Surveillance* explores numerous recent analytic methodologies that enhance traditional techniques. The author, a prominent researcher specializing in innovative, sequential decision-making techniques, demonstrates how these novel methods effectively address the challenges of DSDS.

After a concise introduction that lays the groundwork for comprehending the challenges inherent in DSDS, the book delves into fundamental statistical concepts and methods relevant to DSDS. This includes the exploration of statistical process control (SPC) charts specifically crafted for sequential decision-making purposes. The subsequent chapters systematically outline recent advancements in dynamic screening system (DySS) methods, fine-tuned for effective disease screening. Additionally, the text covers both traditional and contemporary analytic methods for disease surveillance. It further introduces two recently developed R packages designed for implementing DySS methods and spatio-temporal disease surveillance techniques pioneered by the author's research team.

Features

- **Presents Recent Analytic Methods for DSDS:** The book introduces analytic methods for DSDS based on SPC charts. These methods effectively utilize all historical data, accommodating the complex data structure inherent in sequential decision-making processes.
- **Introduces Recent R Packages:** Two recent R packages, **DySS** and **SpTe2M**, are introduced. The book not only presents these packages but also demonstrates key DSDS methods using them.
- **Examines Recent Research Results:** The text delves into the latest research findings across various domains, including dynamic disease screening, nonparametric spatio-temporal data modeling and monitoring, and spatio-temporal disease surveillance.
- **Accessible Description of Methods:** Major methods are described in a manner accessible to individuals without advanced knowledge in mathematics and statistics. The goal is to facilitate a clear understanding of ideas and easy implementation.
- **Real-Data Examples:** To aid comprehension, the book provides several real-data examples illustrating key concepts and methods.
- **Hands-on Exercises:** Each chapter includes exercises to encourage hands-on practice, allowing readers to engage directly with the presented methods.

Statistical Methods for Dynamic Disease Screening and Spatio-Temporal Disease Surveillance serves as a primary textbook for a one-semester course focused on disease screening and/or disease surveillance, tailored for graduate students in biostatistics, bioinformatics, health data science, and related disciplines. Additionally, the book can be utilized as a supplementary textbook for courses covering analytic methods and tools relevant to medical and public health studies. Its content is designed to be accessible and beneficial for medical and public health researchers and practitioners.

Chapman & Hall/CRC Biostatistics Series

Recently Published Titles

Quantitative Methods for Precision Medicine
Pharmacogenomics in Action
Rongling Wu

Drug Development for Rare Diseases
Edited by Bo Yang, Yang Song and Yijie Zhou

Case Studies in Bayesian Methods for Biopharmaceutical CMC
Edited by Paul Faya and Tony Pourmohamad

Statistical Analytics for Health Data Science with SAS and R
Jeffrey Wilson, Ding-Geng Chen and Karl E. Peace

Design and Analysis of Pragmatic Trials
Song Zhang, Chul Ahn and Hong Zhu

ROC Analysis for Classification and Prediction in Practice
Christos Nakas, Leonidas Bantis and Constantine Gatsonis

Controlled Epidemiological Studies
Marie Reilly

Statistical Methods in Health Disparity Research
J. Sunil Rao, Ph.D.

Case Studies in Innovative Clinical Trials
Edited by Binbing Yu and Kristine Broglio

Value of Information for Healthcare Decision Making
Edited by Anna Heath, Natalia Kunst, and Christopher Jackson

Probability Modeling and Statistical Inference in Cancer Screening
Dongfeng Wu

Development of Gene Therapies: Strategic, Scientific, Regulatory, and Access Considerations
Edited by Avery McIntosh and Oleksandr Sverdlov

Bayesian Precision Medicine
Peter F. Thall

Statistical Methods for Dynamic Disease Screening and Spatio-Temporal Disease Surveillance
Peihua Qiu

For more information about this series, please visit: https://www.routledge.com/Chapman--Hall-CRC-Biostatistics-Series/book-series/CHBIOSTATIS

Statistical Methods for Dynamic Disease Screening and Spatio-Temporal Disease Surveillance

Peihua Qiu

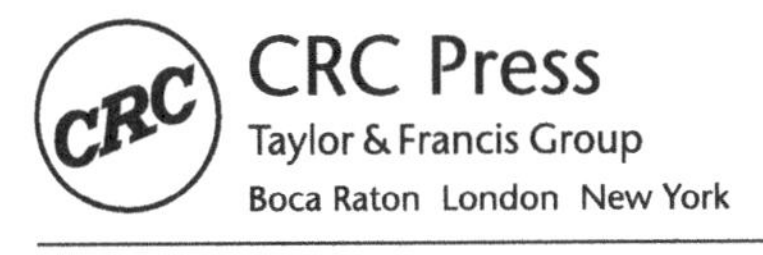

CRC Press is an imprint of the
Taylor & Francis Group, an **informa** business
A CHAPMAN & HALL BOOK

First edition published 2024
by CRC Press
2385 Executive Center Drive, Suite 320, Boca Raton, FL 33431, U.S.A.

and by CRC Press
4 Park Square, Milton Park, Abingdon, Oxon, OX14 4RN

CRC Press is an imprint of Taylor & Francis Group, LLC

Library of Congress Control Number: 2024935314

ISBN: 978-0-367-68580-5 (hbk)
ISBN: 978-0-367-68581-2 (pbk)
ISBN: 978-1-003-13815-0 (ebk)

DOI: 10.1201/9781003138150

Typeset in CMR10 font
by KnowledgeWorks Global Ltd.

Publisher's note: This book has been prepared from camera-ready copy provided by the authors.

To my wife Yan
and our sons Andrew and Alan

Contents

Preface

Early detection and prevention of disease offer numerous benefits to both our health and society. Often, the earlier a disease is detected, the higher the likelihood of successful cure or management. Managing a disease in its early stages can significantly reduce its impact on a patient's quality of life and decrease healthcare costs. To detect a disease early, *disease screening* has become a popular tool. This method aims to determine the likelihood of a given patient having a particular disease by applying medical procedures or tests to check the major risk factors, even in patients without obvious symptoms of the disease. While disease screening primarily focuses on individual patients, disease surveillance is for detecting disease outbreaks early within a given population. For example, our society faces constant threats from bioterrorist attacks and pandemic influenza. It is thus important to monitor the incidence of infectious diseases continuously and detect their outbreaks promptly. This allows governments and individuals to implement timely disease control and prevention measures, minimizing the impact of these diseases. This book introduces some recent analytic methodologies and software packages developed for effective disease screening and disease surveillance.

My exploration into disease screening was motivated by an experience around 2010 when I analyzed a dataset from the Framingham Heart Study (FHS). The FHS primarily aims to identify major risk factors for cardiovascular diseases (CVDs), and numerous CVD risk factors have been recognized since the study's inception in 1948, including smoking, high blood pressure, obesity, high cholesterol levels, physical inactivity and more. During my data analysis, a pivotal question emerged: Could the identified CVD risk factors be utilized to predict the likelihood of a severe CVD, such as stroke, for individual patients? Statistically, this translates into a sequential decision-making problem, where the relevant statistical tool is the statistical process control (SPC) charts. However, traditional SPC charts, developed primarily for monitoring production lines in manufacturing, assume independence and identical distribution of process observations when the process is in-control (IC) and are designed for monitoring a single sequential process. In the context of disease screening, observed data of a patient's disease risk factors would rarely be independent and identically distributed over time, and treating a patient's observed data as a process introduces numerous processes of different patients, making traditional SPC charts unsuitable to use.

Recognizing the importance of the disease screening problem, I dedicated much of the past decade to addressing this issue. This endeavor led to the development of a series of new concepts and methods by my research team. The central methodology, termed the *Dynamic Screening System* (DySS), operates as follows: firstly, the regular longitudinal pattern of disease risk factors is estimated from a pre-collected dataset representing the population without the target disease. Subsequently, a patient's observed pattern of disease risk factors is cross-sectionally compared with the estimated regular longitudinal pattern at each observation time. The cumulative difference between the two patterns up to the current time is then employed to determine the patient's disease status at that time. DySS utilizes all historical data of the patient in its decision-making, and effectively accommodates the complex data structure, including time-varying data distribution.

In the summer of 2013, upon joining the University of Florida (UF), I started to work on the pressing issue of disease surveillance due to its paramount importance in public health. Disease incidence data are typically collected sequentially over time and across multiple locations or regions, constituting spatio-temporal data. Similar to disease screening, disease surveillance is a sequential decision-making problem. However, its complexity arises from the intricate spatio-temporal data structure, encompassing seasonality, temporal/spatial variation, data correlation and intricate data distribution. Common disease reporting and surveillance systems incorporate conventional SPC charts such as the cumulative sum (CUSUM) and exponentially weighted moving average (EWMA) charts. Additionally, retrospective methods like scan tests and generalized linear modeling approaches are employed for routine surveillance. Unfortunately, these methods often prove ineffective or unreliable due to their inability to handle the sequential nature of the problem or their restrictive model assumptions (cf., Section 2.7 and Chapters 7 and 8).

Over the past decade, my research team has devoted significant effort to this domain, resulting in the development of several novel analytic methods for disease surveillance. Our initial method operates as follows: First, a nonparametric spatio-temporal modeling approach is employed to estimate the regular spatio-temporal pattern of disease incidence rates from observed data in a baseline time interval (e.g., a previous year without outbreaks). Second, the new spatial data collected at the current time are compared with the estimated regular pattern and decorrelated with all previous data. Third, an SPC chart is then applied to the decorrelated data to determine the occurrence of a disease outbreak by the current time. Modified versions of this method have been crafted to incorporate covariate information and accommodate specific spatial features of disease outbreaks. These methods adeptly handle the complex structure of observed data and have demonstrated effectiveness in disease surveillance.

As discussed earlier, both disease screening and disease surveillance pose challenges as sequential decision-making problems and traditional SPC charts prove unreliable in addressing them adequately. Consequently, disease screening and disease surveillance emerge as crucial applications of SPC, demanding the development of new methods tailored to their specific requirements.

Fortuitously, my research journey in SPC began in 1998, allowing me to contribute significantly to several key areas within the field. Notable contributions include advancements in nonparametric process monitoring (e.g., Qiu and Hawkins, 2001; Qiu, 2018a), monitoring correlated data (e.g., Qiu et al., 2020a; Xue and Qiu, 2021), dynamic process monitoring (e.g., Qiu and Xiang, 2014; Xie and Qiu, 2023a), profile monitoring (e.g., Qiu et al., 2010; Zhou and Qiu, 2022) and more. For a comprehensive description of SPC and some SPC charts developed by my research group, see Qiu (2014). This extensive experience has proven invaluable in my exploration of disease screening and disease surveillance, providing a robust foundation to innovate and tailor SPC methodologies to the distinctive challenges presented in these critical areas of public health.

The book comprises nine chapters. In Chapter 1, a concise introduction sets the stage for understanding the challenges posed by disease screening and surveillance problems. Chapter 2 delves into fundamental statistical concepts and methods commonly employed in data modeling and analysis. Given that disease screening and surveillance involve sequential decision-making, Chapter 3 is dedicated to introducing essential SPC concepts and methods – a major statistical tool for such problems. Chapters 4–6 focus on recent developments in DySS methods tailored for effective disease screening. Chapter 4 covers univariate and multivariate DySS methods based on direct monitoring of observed disease risk factors, while Chapter 5 introduces methods based on disease risk quantification and sequential monitoring of quantified disease risks. The practical implementation of DySS methods by the R package **DySS** is detailed in Chapter 6. Chapters 7–9 shift the focus to disease surveillance. Chapter 7 explores traditional methods utilizing the Knox test, scan statistics and generalized linear modeling. Chapter 8 presents recent methods developed by my research team based on nonparametric spatio-temporal data modeling and monitoring. The implementation of these methods is demonstrated using the R package **SpTe2M** in Chapter 9.

This book serves as an ideal primary textbook for a one-semester course focused on disease screening and/or disease surveillance, tailored for graduate students in biostatistics, bioinformatics, health data science and related disciplines. Additionally, the book can be utilized as a supplementary textbook for courses covering analytic methods and tools relevant to medical and public health studies. Its content is designed to be accessible and beneficial for medical and public health researchers and practitioners. By introducing recent analytic tools for disease screening and surveillance, the book equips readers with valuable insights that can be easily implemented using the accompanying R packages **DySS** and **SpTe2M**.

I extend my sincere gratitude to my current and former students and collaborators, Drs. Jun Li, Dongdong Xiang, Kai Yang, Lu You and Jingnan Zhang, whose dedicated efforts, stimulating discussions, and constructive comments have played an invaluable role in the completion of this book. Their patience and insights have been indispensable. I express my deep appreciation to Dr. Xiulin Xie and Mr. Zibo Tian, who generously dedicated their time to reading the entire manuscript and diligently corrected numerous typos and mistakes. Completing this book has been a three-year journey, and I owe a debt of gratitude to my wife, Yan, for providing unwavering help and support. Her efforts in managing household responsibilities and caring for our two sons, Andrew and Alan, allowed me to focus on this project. I extend my heartfelt thanks to my family for their love and constant support throughout this endeavor.

PEIHUA QIU
Gainesville, Florida
November 2023

About the Author

Peihua Qiu is the Dean's Professor and Founding Chair of the Department of Biostatistics at the University of Florida. He received his PhD in statistics from the Department of Statistics at the University of Wisconsin at Madison in 1996. He then worked as a senior research consulting statistician for the Biostatistics Center at the Ohio State University (1996–1998), and as an assistant professor (1998–2002), associate professor (2002–2007), and full professor (2007–2013) of the School of Statistics at the University of Minnesota. He was recruited to the University of Florida to develop its new Department of Biostatistics in 2013. Dr. Qiu has made substantial contributions in the research areas of jump regression analysis, image processing, statistical process control, survival analysis, dynamic disease screening, and spatio-temporal disease surveillance. So far, he has published two research monographs and over 160 research papers in refereed journals in these areas. He is an elected fellow of the American Association for the Advancement of Science (AAAS), American Statistical Association (ASA), American Society for Quality (ASQ), and Institute of Mathematical Statistics (IMS), and an elected member of International Statistical Institute (ISI). He served as an associate editor for several top statistical journals, including *Journal of the American Statistical Association*, *Biometrics*, and *Technometrics*. He was the editor-in-chief of the flagship statistical journal *Technometrics* from 2014–2016. Dr. Qiu was the recipient of the 2024 Shewhart Medal.

1

Introduction

Disease is inarguably a major challenge in our daily lives. They impact mortality, quality of life, healthcare cost and many other important aspects of society. To fight against diseases, a tremendous effort has been made in human history. Much effort is in developing or finding effective methods for medical diagnosis and/or disease treatment. In recent years, more and more effort has been put into *disease early detection and prevention* (DEDAP) because of our realization of their benefits. Often, the earlier a disease is detected, the more likely it can be cured or successfully managed. Managing a disease early in its course can lower its impact on a patient's life and prevent or delay complications. Early detection of diseases has not only clinical benefits for patients but also economic benefits for healthcare providers. It often leads to shorter, less invasive treatment regimes, and thus reduces overall healthcare costs. Many diseases are preventable (or can be delayed) if they can be detected early and people's lifestyles and medical interventions can be adjusted or implemented accordingly. The enormous medical and economic benefits of disease prevention have been documented in some authoritative reports (cf., CDC, 2005; USDOH, 2003).

DEDAP is developed mainly for individual people. Its major goal is to detect or predict the occurrence of a disease early for a given person based on that person's observed disease risk factors. This problem is called *disease screening* in this book. A related but different problem is *disease surveillance*, which is for detecting possible disease outbreaks early within one or more population groups. Thus, disease surveillance focuses mainly on population groups instead of individual people. It is often accomplished by monitoring population-based disease incidence data. The major goal of this book is to introduce some recent statistical methodologies for disease screening and disease surveillance.

This chapter aims to provide a brief background introduction about disease, disease screening and disease surveillance. A concise introduction will also be provided about the statistical methods discussed in later chapters of the book and about their major features in comparison with the alternative methods in the literature. From these introductions, we hope to provide a big picture about the problems of disease screening and disease surveillance and about the major contributions of the statistical methods discussed in the book for solving these problems.

DOI: 10.1201/9781003138150-1

1.1 Disease and Disease Screening

A *disease* refers to any characteristic of anatomy, physiology or behavior that is associated with a high risk of illness or death (Morrison, 1992). Diseases can be classified in several different ways, depending on certain disease characteristics. For instance, they can be classified into infectious diseases or non-infectious diseases, depending on whether they can be passed from person to person through body secretions, insects or other means. Examples of infectious diseases include COVID-19, influenza, common cold, tuberculosis (TB), hepatitis A and B and many more. Diseases can also be classified into acute diseases or chronic diseases, depending on whether a disease starts suddenly or gradually and whether it lasts for a short time or a relatively long time. Examples of chronic diseases include heart disease, cancer, chronic lung disease, Alzheimer's disease, diabetes, chronic kidney disease and more.

A typical disease would experience the following five stages: incubation period, prodromal period, period of illness, period of decline and period of convalescence. During the incubation period, the related pathogens start to enter a patient's body and begin to multiply. Then, during the prodromal period, the pathogens continue to multiply and the patient starts to experience some initial signs and symptoms of illness, such as fever, pain, soreness, swelling or inflammation. These signs and symptoms of illness become most obvious and severe during the period of illness. Then, the disease enters the period of decline when the signs and symptoms of illness begin to decline. Finally, during the period of convalescence, the patient can return to normal life in most cases, although some diseases may cause some permanent damages to the patient's health condition. The length of each period depends on the nature of the disease. For instance, the incubation period usually lasts for one or two days for acute diseases but months or years for chronic diseases.

The process of identifying a disease from its signs and symptoms is often referred to as *disease diagnosis*. In order to make an accurate disease diagnosis, medical doctors often use all helpful information available to them, including medical history, physical exams, lab tests (e.g., blood tests), imaging tests, biopsies and others. However, disease diagnosis is usually performed after some disease signs or symptoms appear. For some deadly diseases like liver cancer, it is often too late to treat them effectively after observing some serious disease signs and/or symptoms. To overcome this limitation of disease diagnosis, *disease screening* becomes popular in recent years, which tries to determine the chance for a given person to have a particular disease, by applying a medical procedure or test to the person who does not have any obvious symptoms of the disease yet (Ahn et al., 2014; Wilson and Jungner, 1968). Examples of common disease screening tests include mammography to detect breast cancer, colonoscopy to detect colorectal cancer, ultrasound scans for pregnant women to detect fetal abnormalities, Beck Depression Inventory to screen for depression and many more.

For an effective screening of a disease in an organ (e.g., heart disease), we can definitely test the organ functioning for a patient. However, many such tests are invasive and harmful for the patient, and they may not be effective in the early stage of a disease when the disease symptoms are absent or weak. To overcome these limitations, an alternative strategy for disease screening is to check some important *disease risk factors*, which refer to factors that would affect the chance of developing the disease in concern. For instance, some important disease risk factors for heart disease include high blood pressure, high cholesterol level, obesity, smoking, drinking too much alcohol, unhealthy diet, lack of physical activity, age, family history and more (Frohlich and Quinlan, 2014; Pencina et al., 2019). Some of these risk factors (e.g., age, family history) cannot be controlled by us, while others can be managed or changed by adjusting our lifestyle or receiving medical interventions.

Traditional disease screening approaches are based on regular clinic visits or medical tests for individual people to find early disease symptoms or check the status of major disease risk factors. For instance, during our annual physical exams, blood pressure, heart rate, respiration rate, cholesterol levels and some other medical indices are routinely checked. These are the major risk factors of cardiovascular diseases, lung diseases and some others. To determine the risk level of a given person to have a particular disease, some threshold values of the related medical indices are often pre-specified. For instance, the systolic blood pressure readings are usually compared with the threshold value of 120 mm Hg, that is determined from the systolic blood pressure readings of a healthy population. A given person would be regarded at a high risk of cardiovascular diseases if that person's systolic blood pressure readings are often above this threshold value. Obviously, such methods for predicting the incidence of a disease are simple and convenient to implement in practice. But, they would not be accurate in many cases because their decisions have not taken into account the longitudinal trajectory of the related medical index, people's personal characteristics and more. To overcome these limitations, more frequent medical exams are usually recommended. Then, a direct consequence of this practice is the more healthcare cost due to the consumption of more medical resources.

To improve the accuracy of disease screening/prediction, many analytic approaches have been developed in the research area of *predictive medicine*. Traditional methods in predictive medicine are confined to the realm of genetics (Ference et al., 2000; Warren, 2018) since people once believed that genetics could revolutionize medicine, and genetics and genomics could improve our ability in predicting the incidence of different diseases. In reality, besides genetic risk factors, most diseases are associated with many other risk factors, including diet, physical exercise, stress, environment and more. For a single disease, there could be many different risk factors involved, and the relationship between the disease and its risk factors and among different risk factors could be complicated. Thus, it is often a challenging task to detect/predict the incidence of a disease accurately.

In recent years, machine learning methods have been under rapid development and are widely used in different applications, including predictive medicine (Aggarwal, 2018; Breiman, 2010; Chen and Asch, 2017; Cortes and Vapnik, 1995; Jiang et al., 2017; Kim et al., 2018). A conventional machine learning method tries to approximate the relationship among different variables in a real-world problem by a computer algorithm after learning the data structure of the problem from a training dataset. Thus, its performance depends heavily on how well the training dataset represents the population of interest. To partially overcome this limitation, a tremendous research effort has been made in several different directions, including reinforcement learning (Francois-Lavet et al., 2018; Mnih et al., 2015), recurrent neural networks (Dupond, 2019), machine learning for analyzing sequential or longitudinal data (Ngufor et al., 2019; Ostmeyer and Cowell, 2019) and more. However, these methods cannot usually provide a quantitative description about the functional relationship among different variables and other aspects of the data structure (e.g., within-subject serial data correlation and time-varying data distribution). Therefore, they have much room to improve for effective disease prediction.

In practice, the observed data of disease risk factors are often collected sequentially over time for a given patient in the sense that a new batch of data is collected every time after a new medical exam. After a new batch of data is collected, we should analyze the data properly and reach a conclusion on whether the related patient is at a high risk of a disease or not. In that sense, disease screening is a sequential data collection and decision-making process. Furthermore, if the longitudinal trajectory of the disease risk factors of a patient is regarded as a process over time, then such a process is usually dynamic in the sense that its distribution would change over time, even for people without the disease in concern. As an example, our mean cholesterol level often changes over time when we age. Thus, the longitudinal trajectory of the disease risk factors in such cases can be regarded as a *dynamic process*, and disease screening can be regarded as a sequential monitoring problem for dynamic processes.

We recently developed a new statistical method, called dynamic screening system (DySS), for effective DEDAP (Qiu and Xiang, 2014, 2015). Compared to the existing disease prediction methods, the DySS method has the following major features. First, it is designed for monitoring dynamic processes and thus appropriate to use for DEDAP. Second, it is based on a flexible predictive model that describes the functional relationship between the incidence of a disease in concern and its major risk factors. The predictive model can accommodate (i) a flexible functional relationship between the disease incidence and disease risk factors, (ii) temporal data correlation and (iii) nonparametric data distribution. Its estimate can be updated periodically over time after more data are collected. Unlike previous machine learning methods for disease prediction, the functional data structure that DySS aims to learn from the observed data is well specified in advance. Third, its decision rule is based on the cumulative difference between the regular longitudinal pattern of the disease risk factors described by the estimated predictive model and the observed longitudinal pattern of the disease risk factors of a given patient under monitoring. Thus, its decision-making process has made use of all historic data of the given patient up to the current observation time. As a comparison, most traditional medical diagnostic methods make their decisions about a patient's disease status based on the observed data of the disease risk factors at the recent observation times only, and the patient's historic data have not been used efficiently by them. In addition, to account for disparities among different population groups, age, gender, race and other demographic characteristics can be included in the predictive model of DySS easily as disease risk factors. Thus, the decision-making process of DySS can account for such disparities properly. Because of these important properties, the DySS method should be able to provide a powerful analytic tool for DEDAP.

1.2 Disease Surveillance

As discussed in Section 2.1, disease screening is mainly for predicting the likelihood of diseases for individual people to improve their health condition. For making proper public health policies, we are also interested in knowing the disease incidence in a defined population and whether the disease incidence changes dramatically over time and space. *Disease surveillance* is a research area to address these issues. It involves the systematic collection, analysis, interpretation and dissemination of information about the disease incidence in a given population.

One major purpose of disease surveillance is to detect disease outbreaks, especially for infectious diseases. A *disease outbreak* refers to the occurrence of disease cases in excess of what would normally be expected. In recent years, we experienced the outbreaks of COVID-19, Zika, Ebola, SARS, H1N5, H7N9, MERS-CoV, chikungunya and many other damaging infectious diseases. Our society is under a constant threat of bioterrorist attacks and pandemic influenza. It is therefore important to effectively monitor the occurrence of infectious diseases constantly and detect their outbreaks as quickly as possible. Early detection of infectious disease outbreaks can help governments and individuals to take proper disease control and prevention measures in a timely manner so that the disease epidemic can be controlled at an early stage and its damage can be minimized. Although infectious diseases are the major focus of many disease surveillance systems, other damaging diseases or medical conditions, including different types of cancer, cardiovascular diseases, obesity and more, are also monitored closely by different disease surveillance systems.

Because of the importance of disease surveillance, some global, national and regional disease reporting and surveillance systems have been developed to collect and analyze data about certain important diseases. A nice survey of these disease reporting and surveillance systems can be found in Chen et al. (2009). Commonly used measures of disease frequency include *prevalence* and *incidence* (Noordzij et al., 2010). The prevalence reflects the total number of existing disease cases, while the incidence refers to the number of newly confirmed cases of a disease. Compared to the prevalence, the incidence is often more helpful in understanding the disease etiology and providing guiding principles for targeting interventions. Thus, it is a major quantity in many disease reporting and surveillance systems. Furthermore, even though the disease incidence within a given time period and a given spatial region can provide us useful information about the current burden of the disease, it suffers a limitation that it cannot distinguish a large population with a low disease rate from a small population with a high disease rate. To overcome this limitation, we can consider using *disease incidence rate*, which is defined to be the disease incidence in a spatial region within a given time interval divided by the population in the region.

Disease incidence or its rate depends on a given spatial region in which it is defined, and the given region often consists of sub-regions that are also of our interest. For instance, the state of Florida consists of 67 counties. While it is important to monitor the incidence rate of a disease (e.g., COVID-19) in the entire state, it is often our interest to monitor the disease incidence rates in the 67 counties jointly so that we can be aware of the spatial variation of the disease incidence rates across different counties and the corresponding health policies and/or interventions can be adapted to such spatial variation accordingly. This is the *spatio-temporal (ST) disease surveillance* problem, in which the observed disease incidence rate data are collected at multiple time points and at multiple spatial locations at a given time point. For the ST disease surveillance problem, one major task is to detect a disease outbreak as soon as possible. Once the disease outbreak is detected, another task is to figure out the specific time at which the observed disease incidence rates start to have an abnormal longitudinal/spatial pattern and the specific sub-regions that contribute to such detected abnormality.

The ST disease surveillance problem is challenging to handle, due mainly to the complex structure of the observed disease incidence data. For instance, the distribution of the disease incidence within a given region and a given time interval cannot usually be approximated well by a Poisson, negative binomial or normal distribution (cf., Zhang et al., 2015) because many confounding risk factors could affect the disease incidence in reality, these confounding risk factors may not be easy to measure, and sometimes it is even difficult for us to notice their existence. In addition, the disease incidence often has complex spatial and temporal patterns, such as spatial clusters, seasonality and day-of-week variation (Zhao et al., 2011), which cannot be described well by parametric models either. Furthermore, the observed disease incidence data at different time points and different spatial locations are usually correlated: the closer the distance between two observation times or locations, the stronger the correlation. Such ST data correlation is often difficult to describe and estimate properly.

In the literature, there are some existing methods for ST disease surveillance. First, in the existing disease reporting and surveillance systems, some conventional process control charts, such as the cumulative sum (CUSUM) and the exponentially weighted moving average (EWMA) charts, are usually included for routine disease surveillance (Chen et al., 2009; Kite-Powell et al., 2010). These charts, however, require the assumption that the observed data are independent and identically distributed at different observation times and locations with a normal distribution in cases when no disease outbreaks are present (Qiu, 2014), which is rarely valid in practice. Consequently, they would not be reliable for ST disease surveillance. There exist some retrospective methods for identifying spatial and/or spatio-temporal disease clusters, including the Knox, local Knox and scan methods (e.g., Knox and Bartlett, 1964; Kulldorff, 1997; Marshall et al., 2007). As pointed out by Marshall et al. (2007), Woodall et al. (2008) and Zhou and Lawson (2008), these methods are ineffective, since they are not designed for prospective disease surveillance and cannot properly accommodate the complicated structure of the observed ST disease incidence rate data.

In recent several years, we have developed a series of new statistical methodologies for estimating the mean and variance structures of ST data and for online monitoring of ST processes (Yang and Qiu, 2020; Qiu and Yang, 2021, 2023). These methods do not require restrictive assumptions on the ST data structure, in the sense that they can accommodate nonparametric ST data variation, nonparametric ST data correlation and nonparametric data distribution. They can also make use of helpful covariate information in an effective and flexible way. Thus, they should be able to provide a powerful analytic tool for ST disease surveillance.

1.3 Organization of the Book

This book focuses on introducing some recent statistical methodologies for disease screening and disease surveillance. It has nine chapters. Chapter 2 introduces some basic statistical concepts and methods that are helpful for understanding the statistical methods introduced in later chapters. Because both disease screening and disease surveillance are related to the online monitoring of sequential processes and statistical process control (SPC), which is a major statistical tool for online process monitoring, some basic SPC concepts and methods are described briefly in Chapter 3. Here, the word "online" implies that decisions about the process status need to be made immediately after each batch of process data is collected in the related sequential process monitoring problem. The remaining six chapters are organized in two blocks. The first block of three chapters is on disease screening. This block starts with Chapter 4 to introduce the conventional DySS methodology and some of its variants for handling different scenarios in disease screening. Then, Chapter 5 introduces a modified version of DySS based on the quantification of *disease risk*. Finally, the R-package **DySS** developed specifically for implementing the disease screening methods introduced in Chapters 4 and 5 is described in Chapter 6, where some demonstrations to use this R-package are also provided. The second block has three chapters on disease surveillance. Chapter 7 introduces some representative retrospective methods developed for detecting ST disease clusters. Chapter 8 describes some recent prospective methodologies developed by our research group on ST disease surveillance with and without using covariate information. Finally, Chapter 9 describes the R-package **SpTe2M** developed for implementing the ST disease surveillance methods described in Chapter 8.

This book is written in such a way that readers with some background in basic linear algebra, calculus through integration and differentiation, and an introductory level of statistics can understand most parts of the book. When discussing a particular method, its major idea is explained intuitively without using much mathematics or statistics content. Thus, for those people who do not have the mathematical/statistical background mentioned above, you should still be able to know the major features of each method described in the book. All datasets and source codes in R that are used in the examples, figures, tables and exercises are posted on the book web page for free download. These materials, together with the two R-packages described in Chapters 6 and 9, should make the major methodologies introduced in the book convenient to use in practice. Finally, at the end of each chapter, some exercises are provided for readers to practice the methods discussed in the chapter.

1.4 Exercises

1.1 Use a cardiovascular disease as an example to discuss the major difference between disease screening and disease surveillance.

1.2 Diseases can be classified in several different ways. In the first paragraph of Section 1.1, it has been discussed to classify diseases into infectious diseases and non-infectious diseases, or acute diseases and chronic diseases. Please provide an alternative approach to classify different diseases.

1.3 Use stroke as an example to discuss the five stages that a typical disease would experience. Discuss possible strategies to reduce the damage of stroke to a patient.

1.4 Discuss the major differences between disease diagnosis and disease screening.

1.5 List some possible risk factors of lung cancer, and discuss which ones can be controlled or intervened by adjusting our lifestyle or receiving medical interventions and which ones are out of our control.

1.6 Discuss the pros and cons of predictive medicine, and think about possible ways to overcome its major limitations.

1.7 Predictive medicine by a conventional machine learning approach aims to approximate the relationship between the incidence of a disease and its major disease risk factors by a computer algorithm, and come up with a decision rule after learning such relationship from a training dataset. The decision rule is then used for disease diagnosis and/or disease screening.

(i) Discuss the major strengths and limitations of a conventional machine learning approach for disease diagnosis and disease screening.

(ii) Based on the discussion in part (i), can the machine learning algorithm replace a medical doctor in disease diagnosis and disease screening? Provide reasons for each answer. If the answer is "No", then discuss which aspects of a medical doctor are hard to be replaced by the machine learning algorithm.

(iii) What are the major features of the new statistical method DySS in comparison with a conventional machine learning algorithm for disease screening?

1.8 Use the COVID-19 infectious disease as an example, and discuss the concepts of disease prevalence, disease incidence, disease incidence rate, disease outbreaks and disease surveillance. Why is disease incidence rate, instead of disease incidence or disease prevalence, commonly used in disease surveillance?

1.9 In disease surveillance, the observed disease incidence rate data are usually spatial at a given time point and have temporal variation as well over time.

(i) Discuss the importance of studying both spatial and temporal data variation in the observed data.

(ii) Provide a possible explanation why the observed disease incidence rate data are often spatially and temporally correlated.

(iii) The traditional process control charts, such as the conventional CUSUM and EWMA charts, require the assumption that the observed data are independent and identically distributed at different observation times and locations with a parametric (e.g., normal) distribution. Based on the discussions in parts (i) and (ii), a) explain why these methods would not be appropriate for ST disease surveillance and b) discuss the possible consequences to use these methods for disease surveillance.

2

Basic Statistical Concepts and Methods

Description of the disease screening and disease surveillance methods in later chapters will use some basic statistical concepts and methods. For the convenience of those readers who do not know them well, some necessary ones are briefly introduced in this chapter. The introduction here is kept to a minimum. For a more complete discussion about statistical theory and inference, see, for example, Casella and Berger (2002), Lehmann and Casella (1998) and Lehmann and Romano (2005). For a more complete introduction about commonly used statistical methods, see. for example, Cressie and Wikle (2011), Diggle et al. (2002), Devore (2011), Fan and Gijbels (1996) and Qiu (2005).

2.1 Population and Population Distribution

In statistics, any statement and conclusion is with respect to a specific *population*, which is the entire collection of members or subjects about which information is desired. For instance, if we want to know the incidence rate of COVID-19 among all K-12 students in US within a specific time period, then the collection of all K-12 students in US is the population. In the case when we study the health condition among all senior people whose ages are 60 years or older, these people constitute the population of the study.

In a particular application, usually we are only interested in one or several specific characteristics of the members in a population, e.g., certain health indices like blood pressures and cholesterol levels in the above example about senior people. These characteristics are often called *variables* because their values can change among different members in the population. By the nature of their values, all variables can be classified into three categories: *categorical variables*, *discrete numerical variables* and *continuous numerical variables.* A variable is called a categorical variable if its values are categories. Some examples of categorical variables are gender, race and smoking status. A variable is discrete numerical if its values are isolated numbers on the number line. It is continuous numerical if the set of all its values is an interval on the number line. Height and weight are examples of continuous numerical variables, while the number of disease cases in a region within a given time period is an example of a discrete numerical variable.

DOI: 10.1201/9781003138150-2

Let us first focus on cases with a single variable. Suppose that a member is randomly selected from a population. After the selection, the variable value of the selected member becomes known. But before the selection, the variable value of the member to be selected could be any possible value in the population. In that sense, the variable is random and thus called a *random variable.* In cases when several random variables are involved, we have a random vector.

For a given population, it is often our interest to know how all the values in the population are distributed, or equivalently, how all the possible values of the related random variable are distributed. This distribution is called the *population distribution.* By the connection between a population and a random variable, the population distribution is the same as the distribution of the related random variable.

To describe the population distribution, if the related random variable takes categorical values, then a table listing all the categories and the corresponding proportions of the population members in these categories is sufficient for describing the population distribution. This table is often called the *probability distribution function* or the *probability mass function* (pmf).

Example 2.1 *According to US Census Bureau, the estimated population in US on July 1, 2019 is 328,239,523 people. In this population, the proportions of people in difference race groups are listed in Table 2.1. Then, this table describes the race distribution for all people on US on July 1, 2019.*

TABLE 2.1
Probability distribution function of race for all people in US on July 1, 2019.

Race Group	White	African American	Hispanic/ Latino	Asian	Native American	Others
Probability	60.1%	13.4%	18.5%	5.9%	1.5%	0.6%

If a random variable X is univariate and numerical, then its distribution can be described by the following *cumulative distribution function* (cdf):

$$F(x) = P(X \leq x), \qquad \text{for } x \in R, \tag{2.1}$$

where $P(X \leq x)$ denotes the probability of the event that X is less than or equal to a given value x on the number line R. From (2.1), $F(x)$ is obviously a non-decreasing function on R with its values in $[0, 1]$. When x gets larger, $F(x)$ is closer to 1; it is closer to 0 when x gets smaller. In the case when there is a nonnegative real-valued function $f(x)$ on R such that

$$F(x) = \int_{-\infty}^{x} f(u)\, du, \qquad \text{for } x \in R, \tag{2.2}$$

the random variable X is said to be *absolutely continuous*, and $f(x)$ is called its *probability density function* (pdf). The corresponding curve of a pdf is called a (probability) density curve. Thus, for an absolutely continuous random variable X, its pdf $f(x)$ can be computed easily from its cdf $F(x)$ by the relationship

$$f(x) = F'(x), \qquad \text{for } x \in R. \tag{2.3}$$

From the definition in (2.2), a pdf must be a nonnegative integrable function, and the area under its entire curve is one. If X has a pdf f, then the area under the density curve and above an interval $[a, b]$ equals $P(a \leq X \leq b)$, for any $-\infty \leq a \leq b \leq \infty$. That is, areas underneath the density curve give probabilities for the random variable X, and the probability for X to be in a unit interval will be larger if the density values in the interval are larger.

If a random variable X is discrete, its possible values are $\{x_j,\ j = 1, 2, \ldots, N\}$, and the corresponding probabilities are $\{p_j,\ j = 1, 2, \ldots, N\}$, then the center of the distribution of X can be measured by

$$\mu_X = \sum_{j=1}^{N} x_j p_j. \tag{2.4}$$

Obviously, μ_X is a weighted average of $\{x_j,\ j = 1, 2, \ldots, N\}$ with the probabilities $\{p_j,\ j = 1, 2, \ldots, N\}$ being the weights. In a special case when the probabilities are all the same, μ_X is just the simple average of $\{x_j,\ j = 1, 2, \ldots, N\}$. In the statistical literature, μ_X is called the *mean* of X or its *expectation*. Another commonly used notation for μ_X is $\mathrm{E}(X)$, where E is the first letter of "expectation". The spread of all possible values of X can be measured by

$$\sigma_X^2 = \sum_{j=1}^{N} (x_j - \mu_X)^2 p_j, \tag{2.5}$$

where σ_X^2 is called the *variance* of X. Sometimes, we also write σ_X^2 as $\mathrm{Var}(X)$, where Var denotes "variance". Its square root σ_X is called the *standard deviation* of X. Because σ_X has the same unit as X, it is often more convenient for measuring the spread; but, mathematically, σ_X^2 is easier to manipulate. From (2.4) and (2.5), it is obvious that

$$\sigma_X^2 = \mathrm{E}(X - \mu_X)^2 = \mathrm{E}\left(X^2\right) - \mu_X^2.$$

Namely, σ_X^2 is the mean squared distance from X to its center μ_X, and it can be computed from $\mathrm{E}(X^2)$ and μ_X.

In cases when X is a continuous numerical random variable with a pdf $f(x)$, its mean is defined by

$$\mu_X = \int_{-\infty}^{\infty} u f(u)\, du, \tag{2.6}$$

and its variance is defined by

$$\sigma_X^2 = \int_{-\infty}^{\infty} (u - \mu_X)^2 f(u)\, du = \mathrm{E}(X - \mu_X)^2 = \mathrm{E}\left(X^2\right) - \mu_X^2. \tag{2.7}$$

Obviously, (2.6) and (2.7) are the continuous versions of (2.4) and (2.5), respectively.

In cases when $p > 1$ characteristics of the members in a population are of our interest (e.g., p risk factors of a specific disease), a p-dimensional random vector $\mathbf{X} = (X_1, X_2, \ldots, X_p)'$ can be used for denoting the p characteristics of a randomly selected member from the population. In such cases, the (joint) cdf of $\mathbf{X}$ can be defined similarly to (2.1) by

$$F(\mathbf{x}) = P\left(X_1 \leq x_1, X_2 \leq x_2, \ldots, X_p \leq x_p\right), \quad \text{for } \mathbf{x} = (x_1, x_2, \ldots, x_p)' \in R^p, \tag{2.8}$$

where R^p denotes the p-dimensional Euclidean space. The (joint) pmf and the (joint) pdf of a p-dimensional random vector can be defined similarly to their univariate counterparts (cf., Example 2.1 and Expression (2.2)).

In cases when the (joint) cdf of $\mathbf{X}$ has the property that

$$F(\mathbf{x}) = P\left(X_1 \leq x_1\right) P\left(X_2 \leq x_2\right) \cdots P\left(X_p \leq x_p\right), \qquad \text{for any } \mathbf{x} \in R^p, \tag{2.9}$$

the p random variables $X_1, X_2, \ldots, X_p$ are said to be *independent*. Intuitively, a sequence of random variables are independent of each other if the values of any subset of the sequence provide no information about the values of the remaining random variables in the sequence. Based on (2.1)–(2.3), (2.8) and (2.9), we can have the following two results: (i) if $\mathbf{X}$ has a (joint) pdf $f_{\mathbf{X}}(\mathbf{x})$, then each of $X_1, X_2, \ldots, X_p$ has a pdf, and (ii) $X_1, X_2, \ldots, X_p$ are independent of each other if and only if

$$f_{\mathbf{X}}(\mathbf{x}) = f_{X_1}(x_1) f_{X_2}(x_2) \cdots f_{X_p}(x_p), \qquad \text{for any } \mathbf{x} \in R^p, \tag{2.10}$$

where $f_{X_j}(x_j)$ denotes the pdf of X_j, for $j = 1, 2, \ldots, p$.

2.2 Important Parametric Distributions

In practice, a number of parametric distribution families are frequently used in describing the distributions of the related random variables. Some important discrete and continuous distribution families are introduced in this section. For a more complete discussion on parametric distribution families, see Johnson et al. (1992), Johnson et al. (1994) and Johnson et al. (1995).

2.2.1 Important Discrete Distributions

In reality, many variables are *binary* in the sense that they only take two possible values. Examples of binary variables include disease status (positive or negative), status of a cancer patient after a five-year period (alive or dead), smoking status (smoker or non-smoker) and so forth. For convenience, in the statistical literature, we usually label the value of a binary variable that we are interested in studying as success (S), and the other value as failure (F). Then, for a binary random variable X, its probability distribution function is determined by

$$P(X = S) = \pi, \qquad P(X = F) = 1 - \pi,$$

where $\pi \in [0, 1]$ is the probability of "$X = S$". This distribution is called the *Bernoulli distribution*, which is uniquely determined by the parameter π. In statistical data analysis, without losing any information, we usually assign the number 1 to S, and the number 0 to F. After these assignments, X becomes a binary numerical random variable, and it can be checked that

$$\mu_X = \pi, \qquad \sigma_X^2 = \pi(1 - \pi).$$

In statistics, we often use the conventional notation $X \sim Bernoulli(\pi)$ to denote "X has a Bernoulli distribution with the parameter π".

Now, let us consider an experiment to flip a coin n times. This experiment meets the following four requirements:

(i) The experiment consists of n trials with n fixed in advance.

(ii) The n trials are independent of each other, in the sense that the result of one trial would not affect the result of any other trials.

(iii) Each trial has only two possible outcomes: S and F. Such a trial is often called a *Bernoulli trial.*

(iv) The probability of S is the same from trial to trial.

An experiment meeting the above four requirements is called a *binomial experiment.* So, flipping a coin n times is a simple example of a binomial experiment. Now, let X denote the number of S's in a binomial experiment with n trials, and π denote the probability of S in each trial. Then, X is a discrete numerical random variable taking the values of $0, 1, 2, \ldots, n$. Its probability distribution can be described by the following formula:

$$P(X = x) = \binom{n}{x} \pi^x (1 - \pi)^{n-x}, \qquad \text{for } x = 0, 1, 2, \ldots, n, \tag{2.11}$$

where

$$\binom{n}{x} = \frac{n!}{x!(n - x)!}$$

is the *binomial coefficient*, denoting the total number of combinations when choosing x subjects from a set of n subjects. The distribution described by (2.11) is called the *binomial distribution.* If $X \sim Binomial(n, \pi)$, then X is often called a binomial random variable, and it can be checked that its mean and variance are

$$\mu_X = n\pi, \qquad \sigma_X^2 = n\pi(1 - \pi). \tag{2.12}$$

Example 2.2 *Consider a population of 100 people, among which 10 people are smokers and the remaining 90 people are non-smokers. Assume that we want to randomly select 10 people from the population with replacement. Let X be the number of selected people who are smokers. Then, the random selection of 10 people is obviously a binomial experiment with $n = 10$ trials. If a smoker is labeled as S, then $\pi = 10/100 = 0.1$, and $X \sim$ Binomial $(10, 0.1)$. By (2.12), $\mu_X = 10 * 0.1 = 1$ and $\sigma_X = \sqrt{10 * 0.1 * (1 - 0.1)} = 0.949$.*

The binomial distribution can be generalized as follows. In an experiment with n trials, assume that each trial has k possible outcomes with $k \geq 2$, the probabilities of the k outcomes are respectively $\{\pi_1, \pi_2, \ldots, \pi_k\}$ in each trial, and the trials are independent of each other. Let X_j be the number of trials having the jth outcome, for $j = 1, 2, \ldots, k$. Then, the distribution of $(X_1, X_2, \ldots, X_k)$ is

$$P(X_1 = x_1, X_2 = x_2, \ldots, X_k = x_k) = \frac{n!}{x_1! x_2! \cdots x_k!} \pi_1^{x_1} \pi_2^{x_2} \cdots \pi_k^{x_k},$$

for any non-negative integers $x_1, x_2, \ldots, x_k$ that satisfy $\sum_{j=1}^k x_j = n$. This distribution is called the *multinomial distribution*, denoted as $Multinomial(n, \pi_1, \pi_2, \ldots, \pi_k)$. Obviously, when $k = 2$, the multinomial distribution is just the binomial distribution. Furthermore, if $(X_1, X_2, \ldots, X_k) \sim Multinomial(n, \pi_1, \pi_2, \ldots, \pi_k)$, then $X_j \sim Binomial(n, \pi_j)$, for any j. Therefore, by (2.12), if $(X_1, X_2, \ldots, X_k) \sim Multinomial(n, \pi_1, \pi_2, \ldots, \pi_k)$, then

$$\mu_{X_j} = n\pi_j, \qquad \sigma_{X_j}^2 = n\pi_j(1 - \pi_j), \qquad \text{for } j = 1, 2, \ldots, k.$$

Let X be the number of independent Bernoulli trials needed to get the first S. Then, X is a discrete numerical random variable taking the values of $\{1, 2, \ldots\}$. Its probability distribution can be described by

$$P(X = x) = (1 - \pi)^{x-1}\pi, \qquad \text{for } x = 1, 2, \ldots$$

This distribution is called the *geometric distribution*, denoted as $Geom(\pi)$. If $X \sim Geom(\pi)$, then it can be checked that

$$\mu_X = \frac{1}{\pi}, \qquad \sigma_X^2 = \frac{1 - \pi}{\pi^2}.$$

The geometric distribution plays an important role in statistical process control (SPC) discussed in Chapter 3, because in SPC we are mainly concerned about the first time when a control chart gives a signal that the process under monitoring is out-of-control.

When describing the distribution of a discrete random variable X whose value is a count (e.g., the number of COVID-19 cases on a specific day in a region), the *Poisson distribution* is often useful. By definition, X has a Poisson distribution if it takes count values in $\{0, 1, 2, \ldots\}$ and

$$P(X = x) = \frac{\lambda^x e^{-\lambda}}{x!}, \qquad \text{for } x = 0, 1, \ldots, \tag{2.13}$$

where $\lambda > 0$ is a parameter. If X has a Poisson distribution with parameter λ, denoted as $X \sim Poisson(\lambda)$, then it can be checked using (2.4), (2.5) and (2.13) that

$$\mu_X = \lambda, \qquad \sigma_X^2 = \lambda. \tag{2.14}$$

From (2.14), we can notice an important property of the Poisson distribution that *its mean and variance are the same.* In practice, people often use this property to verify whether a random variable has a Poisson distribution. Another important property of the Poisson distribution is that, if X_1 and X_2 are two independent random variables, $X_1 \sim Poisson(\lambda_1)$ and $X_2 \sim Poisson(\lambda_2)$, then $X_1 + X_2 \sim Poisson(\lambda_1 + \lambda_2)$.

The four discrete distributions described above are summarized in Table 2.2.

TABLE 2.2
Some important discrete distributions discussed in Subsection 2.2.1.

Distribution of X	Probability Mass Function	Mean and Variance
$Bernoulli(\pi)$	$P(X=1)=\pi$, $P(X=0)=1-\pi$	$\mu_X=\pi$, $\sigma_X^2=\pi(1-\pi)$
$Binomial(n,\pi)$	$P(X=x)=\binom{n}{x}\pi^x(1-\pi)^{n-x}$, for $x=0,1,2,\ldots,n$	$\mu_X=n\pi$, $\sigma_X^2=n\pi(1-\pi)$
$Geom(\pi)$	$P(X=x)=(1-\pi)^{x-1}\pi$, for $x=1,2,\ldots$	$\mu_X=1/\pi$, $\sigma_X^2=(1-\pi)/\pi^2$
$Poisson(\lambda)$	$P(X=x)=\lambda^x e^{-\lambda}/(x!)$, for $x=0,1,\ldots$	$\mu_X=\lambda$, $\sigma_X^2=\lambda$

2.2.2 Important Continuous Distributions

A very important family of continuous parametric distributions is the *normal* (or *Gaussian*) *distribution* family. When a continuous random variable X has the following pdf:

$$f(x) = \frac{1}{\sqrt{2\pi}\sigma}\exp\left[-\frac{(x-\mu)^2}{2\sigma^2}\right], \qquad \text{for } x \in R, \tag{2.15}$$

where μ and σ are two parameters, then its distribution is called a normal distribution. It can be checked using (2.6) and (2.7) that if X has a normal distribution with parameters μ and σ as defined in Equation (2.15), then $\mu_X = \mu$ and $\sigma_X^2 = \sigma^2$. Therefore, a normal distribution is uniquely determined by its mean and variance. We use the conventional notation $X \sim N(\mu, \sigma^2)$ to denote "X has a normal distribution with mean μ and variance σ^2". The normal distribution is important in statistics for two main reasons. One is that distributions of many continuous variables in practice, such as the height or weight of all people in this country, can be described reasonably well by normal distributions. The second main reason is that many statistical theory and methods in the literature are developed under the normality assumption.

Some properties of a normal distribution are discussed as follows. First, its density curve is bell-shaped, symmetric about the mean μ, and its spread is controlled by the standard deviation σ. Thus, μ is a *location parameter* and σ is a *scale parameter.* If $X \sim N(\mu, \sigma^2)$, then the random variable defined by

$$Z = \frac{X - \mu}{\sigma}$$

has a normal distribution with mean zero and variance one. This specific normal distribution is called the *standard normal distribution.* Its pdf $\phi(x)$ is displayed in Figure 2.1. From the figure, the density curve of Z indeed looks bell-shaped. By the way, in the statistical literature, it is a convention to use Z to denote ε [illegible] istribution.

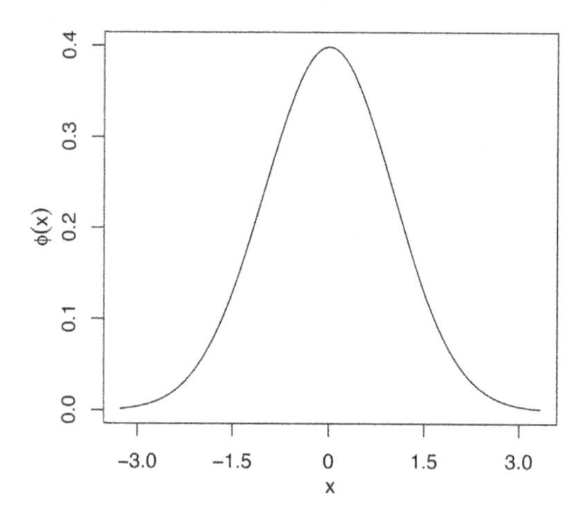

FIGURE 2.1
Probability density function $\phi(x)$ of the standard normal distribution.

If $X_1, X_2, \ldots, X_k$ are independent normal random variables with means $\mu_1, \mu_2, \ldots, \mu_k$, respectively, and with a common variance of 1, then the distribution of

$$Q = X_1^2 + X_2^2 + \cdots + X_k^2$$

is called the non-central *chi-square distribution* with k degrees of freedom (df) and a non-central parameter $\delta = \mu_1^2 + \mu_2^2 + \ldots + \mu_k^2$. By notation, we can write $Q \sim \chi_k^2(\delta)$. In cases when $\delta = 0$ (i.e., all $\mu_1, \mu_2, \ldots, \mu_k$ are 0), the corresponding distribution is called the (central) chi-square distribution with k dfs, which is simply denoted as χ_k^2. The pdf of the χ_k^2 distribution has the expression

$$f(x) = \frac{1}{2^{k/2}\Gamma(k/2)} x^{k/2-1} e^{-x/2}, \qquad \text{for } x \geq 0,$$

where $\Gamma(x) = \int_0^\infty u^{x-1} e^{-u} du$ is the gamma function. If $Q \sim \chi_k^2$, then it can be checked using (2.6) and (2.7) that

$$\mu_Q = k, \qquad \sigma_Q^2 = 2k.$$

One important property of the chi-square distribution is that if Q_1 and Q_2 are two independent random variables, $Q_1 \sim \chi_{k_1}^2$ and $Q_2 \sim \chi_{k_2}^2$, then $Q_1 + Q_2 \sim \chi_{k_1+k_2}^2$.

Another important continuous distribution is the t distribution defined as follows. Assume that Z and V are two independent random variables, Z has the standard normal distribution and V has a chi-square distribution with k dfs. Then, the distribution of

$$T = \frac{Z}{\sqrt{V/k}}$$

is called the t *distribution* with k degrees of freedom. From its definition, the t distribution is uniquely determined by the parameter k. For that reason, the distribution is conventionally denoted as t_k. Its pdf is

$$f(x) = \frac{\Gamma((k+1)/2)}{\sqrt{k\pi}\Gamma(k/2)} \left(1 + \frac{x^2}{k}\right)^{-(k+1)/2}, \qquad \text{for } x \in R.$$

By (2.6) and (2.7), it can be checked that, when $T \sim t_k$, μ_T exists only when $k > 1$ and σ_T^2 exists and is finite only when $k > 2$. In such cases,

$$\mu_T = 0, \text{ when } k > 1, \qquad \sigma_T^2 = \frac{k}{k-2}, \text{ when } k > 2.$$

The t_k distribution has the following properties:

(i) For a given value of k, the density curve of t_k is bell-shaped and symmetric about 0;

(ii) When k increases, the density curve of t_k gets closer and closer to the density curve of the standard normal distribution; and

(iii) For any constant $a > 0$ and any finite positive integer k, it is always true that

$$P(T \geq a) > P(Z \geq a),$$

where $T \sim t_k$ and $Z \sim N(0,1)$. Note that the probabilities $P(T \geq a)$ and $P(Z \geq a)$ equal the areas of the t_k and $N(0,1)$ density curves, respectively, in the right-tail region of $[a, \infty)$. Therefore, this property implies that the density curve of a t distribution has *heavier tails*, compared to the density curve of the standard normal distribution.

If X_1 and X_2 are two independent random variables, $X_1 \sim \chi^2_{k_1}$ and $X_2 \sim \chi^2_{k_2}$, then the distribution of

$$F = \frac{X_1/k_1}{X_2/k_2}$$

is called the F *distribution* with numerator degrees of freedom k_1 and denominator degrees of freedom k_2. It is denoted as $F \sim F_{k_1,k_2}$. The pdf of the F_{k_1,k_2} distribution is

$$f(x) = \frac{1}{xB(k_1/2, k_2/2)} \sqrt{\frac{(k_1 x)^{k_1} k_2^{k_2}}{(k_1 x + k_2)^{k_1+k_2}}}, \qquad \text{for } x \geq 0,$$

where $B(x, y) = \int_0^1 u^{x-1}(1-u)^{y-1} du$ is the beta function. Its mean exists and is finite only when $k_2 > 2$, and its variance exists and is finite only when $k_2 > 4$. In such cases,

$$\mu_F = \frac{k_2}{k_2 - 2}, \text{ when } k_2 > 2, \qquad \sigma_F^2 = \frac{2k_2^2(k_1 + k_2 - 2)}{k_1(k_2 - 2)^2(k_2 - 4)}, \text{ when } k_2 > 4.$$

From the definitions of the t and F distributions, it is obvious that, if $T \sim t_k$, then $T^2 \sim F_{1,k}$.

In medical sciences, the *Weibull distribution* family is widely used for describing the distribution of patients' life times. Its pdf is

$$f(x) = \frac{b}{a}\left(\frac{x}{a}\right)^{b-1} e^{-(x/a)^b}, \qquad \text{for } x \geq 0,$$

where $a > 0$ is a scale parameter, and $b > 0$ is a shape parameter. If a random variable W has a Weibull distribution with the scale parameter a and the shape parameter b, denoted as $W \sim Weibull(a, b)$, then its mean and variance are

$$\mu_W = a\Gamma(1 + 1/b), \qquad \sigma_W^2 = a^2\left[\Gamma(1 + 2/b) - \Gamma^2(1 + 1/b)\right].$$

In the special case when $b = 1$, the Weibull distribution becomes the *exponential distribution*, denoted as $Exp(a)$, which is another important continuous distribution that is widely used in applications. When $X \sim Exp(a)$, it is easy to check that $\mu_X = a$ and $\sigma_X^2 = a^2$.

Another commonly used continuous distribution is described as follows. Assume that the pdf of a random variable X is

$$f(x) = \begin{cases} 1/(b-a), & \text{if } a \leq x \leq b \\ 0, & \text{otherwise,} \end{cases}$$

where $a < b$ are two constants. Then, $f(x)$ defined above is a constant when $a \leq x \leq b$, and 0 otherwise, which implies that the chance for X to take any value in the interval $[a, b]$ is the same. This distribution is called the *uniform distribution* on the interval $[a, b]$, denoted as $X \sim U[a, b]$. It is easy to check that if $X \sim U[a, b]$, then

$$\mu_X = \frac{a+b}{2}, \qquad \sigma_X^2 = \frac{1}{12}(b-a)^2.$$

In the special case when $a = 0$ and $b = 1$, the related uniform distribution is called the standard uniform distribution. An important property of the standard uniform distribution is that if $Y \sim U[0, 1]$ and $F(x)$ is a legitimate cdf, then $X = F^{-1}(Y)$ would be a random variable whose cdf is $F(x)$. A direct conclusion of this result is that if X has the cdf $F(x)$, then $Y = F(X)$ would have the standard uniform distribution.

The seven continuous distributions described above are summarized in Table 2.3.

TABLE 2.3
Some important continuous distributions discussed in Subsection 2.2.2.

Distribution of X	PDF $f_X(x)$	Mean and Variance
$N(\mu, \sigma^2)$	$\frac{1}{\sqrt{2\pi}\sigma} \exp\left[-\frac{(x-\mu)^2}{2\sigma^2}\right]$, for $x \in R$	$\mu_X = \mu$, $\sigma_X^2 = \sigma^2$
χ_k^2	$\frac{1}{2^{k/2}\Gamma(k/2)} x^{k/2-1} e^{-x/2}$, for $x \geq 0$	$\mu_X = k$, $\sigma_X^2 = 2k$
t_k	$\frac{\Gamma((k+1)/2)}{\sqrt{k\pi}\Gamma(k/2)} \left(1 + \frac{x^2}{k}\right)^{-(k+1)/2}$, for $x \in R$	$\mu_X = 0$, if $k > 1$, $\sigma_X^2 = \frac{k}{k-2}$, if $k > 2$
F_{k_1,k_2}	$\frac{1}{xB(k_1/2,k_2/2)} \sqrt{\frac{(k_1 x)^{k_1} k_2^{k_2}}{(k_1 x+k_2)^{k_1+k_2}}}$, for $x \geq 0$	$\mu_X = \frac{k_2}{k_2-2}$, if $k_2 > 2$, $\sigma_X^2 = \frac{2k_2^2(k_1+k_2-2)}{k_1(k_2-2)^2(k_2-4)}$, if $k_2 > 4$
$Weibull(a, b)$	$\frac{b}{a}\left(\frac{x}{a}\right)^{b-1} e^{-(x/a)^b}$, for $x \geq 0$	$\mu_X = a\Gamma(1 + 1/b)$, $\sigma_X^2 = a^2[\Gamma(1 + 2/b) - \Gamma^2(1 + 1/b)]$
$Exp(a)$	$\frac{1}{a} e^{-x/a}$, for $x \geq 0$	$\mu_X = a, \sigma_X^2 = a^2$
$U[a, b]$	$1/(b-a)$, for $a \leq x \leq b$	$\mu_X = (a+b)/2$, $\sigma_X^2 = (b-a)^2/12$

2.3 Data and Data Description

In applications, it is often our interest to know the distribution of a population or some major characteristics of the population distribution (e.g., population mean and population standard deviation). For instance, to know how serious an infectious disease (e.g., COVID-19) is in a given population, we need to know the proportion of all people in the population who have the disease, which is often referred to as disease prevalence rate in the literature (cf., Section 1.2). Because individual people in the population have only two possible disease statuses (i.e., either "have the disease" or "do not have the disease"), the population distribution is uniquely determined by the disease prevalence rate in this example, or the *population proportion* of the diseased people. More generally, when a population distribution has a parametric form, such as those discussed in Sections 2.2, the population parameters appearing in the parametric form uniquely determine the entire population distribution. Therefore, it suffices to know the values of these parameters in order to know the population distribution. In some cases, our major interest is in one or more population parameters, instead of the entire population distribution. As an example, it is often sufficient to know the average exam score of the students in a class in order to have a rough idea about the overall performance of these students in the exam. To know the population distribution or its parameters, we should know variable values for all members in the population. In many applications, however, the related population is large and thus it is time-consuming or even impossible to observe or measure the related variable(s) for all members in the population. To overcome this difficulty, in statistics, we often use the idea to sample the population, which is described below.

A *sample* of the population is a subset of the population, selected in a prescribed manner for study. After a sample is obtained, the population distribution or its parameters can be estimated based on the sample. In practice, most people call the sample selected properly from a population *data*, although the word "data" is also used for some other purposes in our daily life (e.g., representing some generic information that may not necessarily be a sample from a population).

To have a good estimation of the population distribution or its parameters, the sample should represent the population well. In the literature, many different sampling techniques have been proposed to handle different cases. Interested readers can read Cochran (1977) or other textbooks on statistical sampling for a comprehensive discussion on this topic. In this book, if there is no further specification, we assume that all samples are *simple random samples.* A simple random sample of size n is a sample that consists of n selected members, which is generated in a way that the result of one selection has nothing to do with the result of any other selections, and every member in the population has the same chance to be selected to the sample. By this definition, each observation in the sample can be regarded as a random variable whose distribution is the same as the population distribution, because the value of the observation can be any member in the population (i.e., the observation value is random) and each member in the population has the same chance to be selected as the observation value. Of course, after the sample is obtained, observations in the sample are uniquely determined and non-random. To make the distinction, we conventionally use capital letters to denote observations in a sample that are treated as random variables, and little letters to denote observations in a sample that have been obtained and are non-random.

Simple random samples have some nice statistical properties. One property is described as follows. Assume that the characteristic of interest for each member of a population is univariate numerical, the cdf of the population distribution is F, and $\{X_1, X_2, \ldots, X_n\}$ is a simple random sample from the population. Then, by the definition of the simple random sample, $\{X_1, X_2, \ldots, X_n\}$ is a sequence of independent and identically distributed (i.i.d.) random variables with a common cdf F. Thus, by (2.9) in Section 2.1, the joint cdf of $\{X_1, X_2, \ldots, X_n\}$ is

$$P(X_1 \leq x_1, X_2 \leq x_2, \ldots, X_n \leq x_n) = \Pi_{i=1}^n P(X_i \leq x_i) = \Pi_{i=1}^n F(x_i),$$

for any $(x_1, x_2, \ldots, x_n)' \in R^n$. If the population distribution has a pdf f, then by (2.10) in Section 2.1, the joint distribution of $\{X_1, X_2, \ldots, X_n\}$ also has a pdf, and the pdf is

$$\Pi_{i=1}^n f(x_i), \qquad \text{for } (x_1, x_2, \ldots, x_n)' \in R^n.$$

For a sample $\{X_1, X_2, \ldots, X_n\}$, there are several different ways to describe its *center*. One natural way is to use the following *sample mean*:

$$\overline{X} = \frac{1}{n} \sum_{i=1}^{n} X_i,$$

which is a simple average of all n observations in the sample. By using the sample mean, if there are some extremely large or extremely small values in the data, which are often called *outliers*, then these outliers would affect the sample mean quite dramatically, which is demonstrated by the example below.

Example 2.3 *A research project aims to evaluate the weight distribution of college students in Florida. For that purpose, 10 college students are randomly selected and their weights (in pounds) are listed below.*

$$135, 168, 147, 295, 174, 156, 162, 149, 166, 146$$

The value of the sample mean is $\overline{x} = 169.8$. *But, obviously this is not a good measure of the data center, since there are only two observations in the sample that are larger than* $\overline{x}$ *and the remaining 8 observations are all below* $\overline{x}$. *This phenomenon is due to the outlier "295" which pulls the mean weight up quite dramatically.*

From Example 2.3, we can see that in cases when outliers are present, the sample mean may not be a good measure of the data center. In such cases, to remove the impact of outliers, people often use the *sample median* as an alternative measure of the data center. To compute the sample median, the observations in the sample $\{X_1, X_2, \ldots, X_n\}$ are first ordered from the smallest to the largest as follows:

$$X_{(1)} \leq X_{(2)} \leq \cdots \leq X_{(n)}. \tag{2.16}$$

Then, $X_{(1)}$ is the first order statistic, $X_{(2)}$ is the second order statistic and so forth. Roughly speaking, the sample median is defined by the observation at the middle position of the ordered data. So, about half of the observations in the data are smaller than the sample median, and the other half are larger than the sample median. More specifically, the sample median, denoted as $\widetilde{X}$, is defined by

$$\widetilde{X} = \begin{cases} X_{((n+1)/2)}, & \text{if } n \text{ is odd} \\ \left[X_{(n/2)} + X_{(n/2+1)}\right]/2, & \text{if } n \text{ is even.} \end{cases}$$

From its definition, it is obvious that the sample median would not be affected by a small amount of outliers in the sample.

An alternative method to remove the impact of outliers on the sample mean is to use the so-called *trimmed sample mean*, computed as follows. First, we need to choose a trimming percentage $q\%$, where $q \in [0, 50)$. Then, the observed data are ordered, as in (2.16), and the $q\%$ smallest observations and the $q\%$ largest observations are removed. Finally, the $q\%$ trimmed sample mean is computed as the simple average of the remaining observations.

Example 2.3 (continued) *For the data discussed in Example 2.3, the ordered data are*

$$135, 146, 147, 149, 156, 162, 166, 168, 174, 295$$

So, the sample median is $\widetilde{x} = (156 + 162)/2 = 159$, *which is smaller than the sample mean* $\overline{x} = 169.8$ *because the former is not affected by the outlier 295. The* 10% *trimmed sample mean is* $(146 + 147 + 149 + 156 + 162 + 166 + 168 + 174)/8 = 158.5$, *after the* 10% *(i.e., one in this example) smallest observations and the* 10% *largest observations are removed.*

Besides the center of a dataset. another important feature of the dataset is its spread. Consider the following three datasets, each of which has five observations:

Dataset 1: 1, 3, 5, 7, 9

Dataset 2: 1, 4.5, 5, 5.5, 9

Dataset 3: 4, 4.5, 5, 5.5, 6

Obviously, the sample means of the three datasets are all 5. But, their distributions have quite different spreads. The first dataset seems to have the largest spread, while the spread of the third dataset seems to be the smallest.

To describe the spread of a dataset of size n, denoted as $\{X_1, X_2, \ldots, X_n\}$, a conventional measure is *sample variance*, defined by

$$s^2 = \frac{1}{n-1}\sum_{i=1}^{n}(X_i - \overline{X})^2,$$

where $\overline{X}$ is the sample mean. From its definition, the sample variance s^2 is basically the average of the squares of the n deviations $\{X_i - \overline{X},\ i = 1, 2, \ldots, n\}$. Therefore, if its value is large, then the individual observations are generally far away from the sample mean, implying that the data spread is large. The square root of the sample variance, s, is another spread measure, which is called *sample standard deviation.* Regarding the two measures, the sample standard deviation is easier to interpret as a measure of the data spread because it has the same unit as the original observations, but the sample variance is easier to manipulate mathematically.

Similar to the sample mean, the sample variance or the sample standard deviation would be affected in a substantial way by possible outliers in the data. To eliminate such impact, we can once again consider the ordered observations in (2.16). Then, the first sample quartile, denoted as Q_1, is defined as the median of the first half of the ordered data. More specifically,

$$Q_1 = \begin{cases} \text{median of } \{X_{(1)}, \ldots, X_{((n-1)/2)}\}, & \text{if } n \text{ is odd} \\ \text{median of } \{X_{(1)}, \ldots, X_{(n/2)}\}, & \text{if } n \text{ is even.} \end{cases}$$

The third sample quartile, denoted as Q_3, is defined similarly as the median of the second half of the ordered data. In cases when outliers are present in the observed data, we can use the sample *inter-quartile range (IQR)*, defined as $Q_3 - Q_1$, as a measure of the data spread. Obviously, IQR would not be affected by a small number of outliers in the data.

It should be pointed out that all measures of the data center and data spread discussed in this section can be applied to a numerical population to measure the center and spread of the population, although some of these measures of a population distribution are not defined explicitly in this book. For instance, we can define population median in the same way as the sample median, except that all population members should be used in defining the population median. If a sample represents a population well, then the sample version of a given measure should provide a good estimate of the corresponding population version. A related discussion is given in Section 2.4 below.

2.4 Parametric Statistical Inferences

As discussed in the previous section, a sample from a population of interest carries useful information about the population. After a sample is obtained, the next question is how to properly estimate the population distribution or its parameters based on the sample. After an estimator is obtained, we also need to evaluate its performance, so that the best one can be chosen if multiple estimators are available. These are the major goals of statistical inference. In this section, we briefly introduce some basic concepts and methodologies of statistical inference in cases when the population distribution has a parametric form.

2.4.1 Point Estimation and Sampling Distribution

In cases when a population distribution has a parametric form with one or more parameters, the population distribution itself and all of its summary measures (e.g., mean and variance) are uniquely determined by these parameters. In such cases, estimation of the distribution parameters becomes important. Based on a sample $\{X_1, X_2, \ldots, X_n\}$, some commonly used estimators are listed below.

- In cases when the population distribution is $N(\mu, \sigma^2)$, the sample mean $\overline{X}$ is a good estimator of the population mean μ, the sample variance s^2 is a good estimator of the population variance σ^2, and the sample standard deviation s is a reasonable estimator of the population standard deviation σ.

- In cases when the population distribution is Bernoulli with π being the probability of success (S) (cf., Subsection 2.2.1), a good estimator of π is the *sample proportion* of S, defined by

$$\widehat{\pi} = \frac{\text{number of S's in the sample}}{n}.$$

  The parameter π is also called the population proportion of S, as mentioned in Section 2.2. Clearly, if we use 1 to denote S and 0 to denote F, then $\widehat{\pi}$ is just $\overline{X}$.

All estimators mentioned above are calculated from the sample $\{X_1, X_2, \ldots, X_n\}$. In statistics, any quantity calculated from the sample and uniquely determined by the sample is called a *statistic*. Therefore, $\overline{X}$, s^2, s and $\widehat{\pi}$ are all statistics.

To estimate a specific population parameter θ (e.g., the population mean or standard deviation), an appropriate statistic should be chosen as an estimator. It has become a convention in the literature to put a hat above the parameter to denote its estimator. By this convention, $\widehat{\theta}$ is often used to denote an estimator of θ. Although $\widehat{\theta}$ is a function of the sample, this is often not made explicit in its notation for simplicity. To estimate θ by $\widehat{\theta}$, we have used a single-valued statistic calculated from the sample (i.e., $\widehat{\theta}$) for estimating a single-valued parameter of the population (i.e., θ). This parameter estimation method is therefore called *point estimation* in the literature, and the estimator is called a *point estimator*. For instance, $\overline{X}$ is a point estimator of μ, and s^2 is a point estimator of σ^2.

Because the sample is random, any statistic computed from the sample, including all point estimators mentioned above, is also random. Thus, a point estimator has its own distribution, which is called *sampling distribution*. To assess the accuracy of a point estimator for estimating a parameter, we need to study its sampling distribution, especially the mean and variance of the sampling distribution.

In cases when the population distribution is $N(\mu, \sigma^2)$, it can be checked that the sampling distributions of the sample mean and sample variance have the properties summarized in the box below.

Properties of the Sampling Distributions of $\overline{X}$ and s^2

Assume that the population distribution is $N(\mu, \sigma^2)$, and $\overline{X}$ and s^2 are the sample mean and sample variance of a simple random sample $\{X_1, X_2, \ldots, X_n\}$ from the related population. Then, their sampling distributions have the following properties:
(i) $\overline{X} \sim N(\mu, \sigma^2/n)$,
(ii) $(n-1)s^2/\sigma^2 \sim \chi^2_{n-1}$ and
(iii) $\overline{X}$ and s^2 are independent of each other.

By combining all these three properties and by the definition of a t distribution (cf., Subsection 2.2.2), we have

$$T = \frac{\overline{X} - \mu}{s/\sqrt{n}} \sim t_{n-1}. \tag{2.17}$$

In cases when it is unknown whether the population distribution is normal or not, it has been confirmed in the statistical literature (e.g., Lehmann and Casella, 1998) that the sampling distribution of $\overline{X}$ would be asymptotically normal. Namely, it is asymptotically true that

$$\frac{\overline{X} - \mu}{\sigma/\sqrt{n}} \sim N(0, 1),$$

where the words "asymptotically true" mean that the distribution of $(\overline{X} - \mu)/(\sigma/\sqrt{n})$ is closer and closer to $N(0, 1)$ when the sample size n increases. This result plays an important role in statistics, because the population mean is often the population characteristic of interest in applications and this result gives a general conclusion about its point estimator $\overline{X}$ that the sampling distribution of $\overline{X}$ is always asymptotically normal no matter what is the real population distribution. Because of its importance, this result is called the *Central Limit Theorem* (CLT) in the statistical literature, and it is formally stated in the box below.

Central Limit Theorem

Assume that $\{X_1, X_2, \ldots, X_n\}$ is a simple random sample from a population, and $\overline{X}$ is its sample mean. Then, the sampling distribution of $(\overline{X} - \mu)/(\sigma/\sqrt{n})$ converges to $N(0,1)$ when n increases.

The CLT provides an intuitive explanation about the phenomenon that many variables in our daily life, including height, weight, blood pressure readings and more, would roughly follow normal distributions. For instance, our height is affected by our parents' heights, grandparents' heights, our food intake and other nutritional factors, environmental factors and many other factors. Therefore, it is a weighted average of many different factors, similar to $\overline{X}$, which is an average of n observations. By the CLT, our height would roughly have a normal distribution. The CLT also explains why the normal distribution family is important in statistics. As pointed out in the previous paragraph, many statistical inferences involve the sample mean $\overline{X}$ for estimating the population mean μ. By the CLT, the sampling distribution of $\overline{X}$ would be close to normal when the sample size n is reasonably large.

In practice, we need to determine a threshold value for the sample size n, so that n can be regarded as "large" and consequently the sampling distribution of $\overline{X}$ can be treated as a normal distribution. Of course, the asymptotic behavior of the sampling distribution of $\overline{X}$ depends on the true population distribution. Intuitively, if the true population distribution is very skewed, then the sampling distribution of $\overline{X}$ would be slow in converging to a normal distribution. On the other hand, if the true population distribution is already quite close to a normal distribution, then the sampling distribution of $\overline{X}$ would be fast in converging to a normal distribution. However, the true population distribution is usually unknown in practice, making the problem of choosing a threshold value for n complicated. Based on much theoretical and numerical research, a conventional threshold value for n is 30. By this threshold value, the sample size can be regarded as "large" when $n \geq 30$.

Example 2.4 *Assume that $\{X_1, X_2, \ldots, X_n\}$ is a simple random sample from a population with mean 2 and variance 9, and $n = 36$. Then, $\overline{X}$ is asymptotically distributed as $N(2, 1/4)$ by the CLT. So, we can compute different probabilities related to $\overline{X}$ easily. For instance,*

$$\begin{aligned} P(\overline{X} > 2.5) &= P\left(\frac{\overline{X} - 2}{1/2} > \frac{2.5 - 2}{1/2}\right) \\ &\approx P(Z > 1) = 0.1587, \end{aligned}$$

where Z denotes a random variable with the standard normal distribution, and "$\approx$" denotes the asymptotic equality. As a comparison, without the CLT, the exact distribution of $\overline{X}$ would be unknown in most cases, and thus it would *be difficult to compute probabilities related to $\overline{X}$ in such cases. Therefore, the CLT is helpful in practice.*

In cases when the population distribution is Bernoulli with π being the population proportion of S, $\{X_1, X_2, \ldots, X_n\}$ is a simple random sample from the population, and S and F are represented by 1 and 0, respectively. The sampling distribution of $\sum_{i=1}^{n} X_i$ is $Binomial(n, \pi)$, and the sampling distribution of the sample proportion $\widehat{\pi} = \overline{X} = \sum_{i=1}^{n} X_i/n$ can be determined accordingly. When the sample size is large in the sense that both $n\pi$ and $n(1-\pi)$ are large, by the CLT, the distribution of $\widehat{\pi}$ would be asymptotically normal. In other words, when the sample size is large, the distribution of $\widehat{\pi}$ can be regarded as $N(\pi, \pi(1-\pi)/n)$. In practice, the sample size can be regarded as "large" if $n\pi \geq 5$ and $n(1-\pi) \geq 5$.

For a given population parameter, there could be multiple point estimators. Let us revisit Example 2.3, in which a research project aims to estimate the population mean weight μ of all college students in Florida. In that problem, different people can come up with different point estimators of μ. For instance, assume that the following three point estimators have been proposed for estimating μ:

- one person prefers to use the first observation X_1 in the sample to estimate μ,
- another person thinks that $X_1 + 20$ would be a more reasonable estimator of μ and
- the third person has some statistical knowledge and wants to use the sample mean $\overline{X}$ to estimate μ.

To choose among multiple point estimators, or to convince people why one point estimator is better than another one, we need a criterion for evaluating the performance of a point estimator. For estimating a population parameter θ, if a point estimator $\widehat{\theta}$ satisfies the condition that the mean of its sampling distribution, denoted as $\mu_{\widehat{\theta}}$, equals θ, i.e.,

$$\mu_{\widehat{\theta}} = \theta$$

for all values of θ, then $\widehat{\theta}$ is called an *unbiased estimator* of θ. Otherwise, the estimator is biased and the bias is defined to be

$$\text{Bias}\left(\widehat{\theta}, \theta\right) = \mu_{\widehat{\theta}} - \theta.$$

By the above definition, on average, an unbiased estimator equals the parameter to estimate. Therefore, in practice, people often require a point estimator to be unbiased. In the student weight example mentioned in the previous paragraph, both the first and third estimators are unbiased estimators, and the second estimator is biased. So, by the criterion of unbiasedness, the second estimator should be avoided.

To compare two unbiased estimators, the one with a smaller variance is obviously a better estimator, because its sampling distribution would have a smaller spread and consequently that estimator is generally closer to the true value of the population parameter. Therefore, among all unbiased estimators of θ, the one with the smallest variance should be the best unbiased estimator. This estimator is often called the *minimum variance unbiased estimator* (MVUE). It can be checked that, if the population distribution is normal, then $\overline{X}$ is the MVUE for estimating the population mean μ. Therefore, in the student weight example, if it is reasonable to assume that the population distribution of students' weights is normal, then the estimator $\overline{X}$ should be the best unbiased estimator among all unbiased estimators.

Another commonly used criterion for choosing a good point estimator is the following *mean squared error* (MSE):

$$\begin{aligned} \text{MSE}\left(\widehat{\theta}, \theta\right) &= \text{E}\left(\widehat{\theta} - \theta\right)^2 \\ &= \text{E}\left(\widehat{\theta} - \mu_{\widehat{\theta}} + \mu_{\widehat{\theta}} - \theta\right)^2 \\ &= \sigma^2_{\widehat{\theta}} + \text{Bias}^2\left(\widehat{\theta}, \theta\right), \end{aligned}$$

where $\sigma^2_{\widehat{\theta}}$ denotes the variance of $\widehat{\theta}$. The MSE criterion measures the average squared distance between the point estimator $\widehat{\theta}$ and the parameter θ. By this criterion, the best point estimator has the smallest MSE value among all possible point estimators. Obviously, the MSE criterion makes a trade-off between the bias and the variance of a point estimator. The best point estimator by this criterion may not be unbiased, and the MVUE estimator may not be the best point estimator by this criterion either, because the MVUE estimator has the smallest MSE value among all unbiased point estimators only, instead of among all point estimators.

Although it is not explicit in notation, both $\text{Bias}(\widehat{\theta}, \theta)$ and $\text{MSE}(\widehat{\theta}, \theta)$ depend on the sample size n. Generally speaking, when n is larger, the sample carries more information about the population, and thus it is natural to expect that both $\text{Bias}(\widehat{\theta}, \theta)$ and $\text{MSE}(\widehat{\theta}, \theta)$ would be smaller. If a point estimator $\widehat{\theta}$ of θ is biased but the bias converges to zero as n increases, then it is called an *asymptotically unbiased estimator*. If $\widehat{\theta}$ satisfies the condition that

$$\lim_{n \to \infty} \text{MSE}\left(\widehat{\theta}, \theta\right) = 0,$$

then we say that $\widehat{\theta}$ is L_2 *consistent*.

"Consistency" is a kind of large-sample property of a point estimator. There are several different versions of consistency in the literature. If the cdf of $\widehat{\theta}$ converges to the cdf of the constant θ at all continuity points of the latter cdf, then $\widehat{\theta}$ is said to be *consistent in distribution*. If, for any constant $\rho > 0$,

$$\lim_{n \to \infty} P\left(\left|\widehat{\theta} - \theta\right| > \rho\right) = 0,$$

then $\widehat{\theta}$ is said to be *consistent in probability.* Another commonly used consistency is defined as follows: if

$$P\left(\lim_{n\to\infty} \widehat{\theta} = \theta\right) = 1,$$

then $\widehat{\theta}$ is said to be *almost surely (a.s.) consistent.* Based on some routine mathematical manipulations, it is easy to check the following relations among the four types of consistency defined above.

- If $\widehat{\theta}$ is consistent in probability, then it must also be consistent in distribution.
- If $\widehat{\theta}$ is L_2 consistent or a.s. consistent, then it must also be consistent in probability.
- There are L_2 consistent estimators that are not a.s. consistent, and there are a.s. consistent estimators that are not L_2 consistent.

For each type of consistency mentioned above, there is a convergence rate associated with it, which tells us how fast the related convergence is. For example, if $n^{\nu}\text{MSE}(\widehat{\theta}, \theta) = O(1)$ for some positive constant ν, then we say that $\widehat{\theta}$ is L_2 consistent with the convergence rate $O(n^{-\nu})$. Here, the big O notation "$a_n = O(b_n)$" has been used, where $\{a_n\}$ and $\{b_n\}$ are two sequences of nonnegative numbers. Its formal definition is that there exist two positive constants A and B such that $A \leq a_n/b_n \leq B$. Thus, if $a_n = O(b_n)$ and b_n converges to 0 as n tends to infinity, then a_n also converges to 0 with the *same* convergence rate. Sometimes, the small o notation will also be used. By definition, the expression "$a_n = o(b_n)$" means that $\lim_{n\to\infty} a_n/b_n = 0$. So, if $a_n = o(b_n)$ and b_n converges to 0 as n tends to infinity, then a_n also converges to 0 with a *faster* rate. For other types of consistency, the convergence rate can be discussed similarly. More systematic discussions about large-sample properties of point estimators can be found in textbooks such as Ash (1972) and Chung (2001).

2.4.2 Maximum Likelihood Estimation and Least Squares Estimation

In statistics, *maximum likelihood estimation* and *least squares estimation* provide two general methods for constructing point estimators of population parameters, which are briefly introduced in this subsection.

Assume that a population distribution has a pdf with the parametric form $f(x; \theta_1, \theta_2, \ldots, \theta_r)$, where $\theta_1, \theta_2, \ldots, \theta_r$ are r unknown population parameters. To estimate these population parameters based on a simple random sample $\{X_1, X_2, \ldots, X_n\}$, the maximum likelihood estimation procedure is based on the following likelihood function:

$$L(\theta_1, \theta_2, \ldots, \theta_r; X_1, X_2, \ldots, X_n) = \Pi_{i=1}^{n} f(X_i; \theta_1, \ldots, \theta_r). \tag{2.18}$$

The likelihood function $L(\theta_1, \theta_2, \ldots, \theta_r; X_1, X_2, \ldots, X_n)$ is treated as a function of the unknown parameters $\theta_1, \theta_2, \ldots, \theta_r$ only, and the sample $\{X_1, X_2, \ldots, X_n\}$ is assumed to be given in this function. From the discussion about the pdf of a distribution in Section 2.1, the value of $f(x; \theta_1, \theta_2, \ldots, \theta_r)\Delta x$ is roughly equal to $P(X \in [x, x + \Delta x])$, where Δx is a small positive number. So, the likelihood function would be proportional to the likelihood that the random observations in the sample take values around the observed sample $\{X_1, X_2, \ldots, X_n\}$.

The *maximum likelihood estimators* (MLEs) $\widehat{\theta}_1, \widehat{\theta}_2, \ldots, \widehat{\theta}_r$ of $\theta_1, \theta_2, \ldots, \theta_r$ are defined to be the maximizers of the likelihood function $L(\theta_1, \theta_2, \ldots, \theta_r; X_1, X_2, \ldots, X_n)$. So, the likelihood that the observations in the sample take values around $\{X_1, X_2, \ldots, X_n\}$ reaches the maximum when the parameters equal their MLEs, which is intuitively reasonable because the sample $\{X_1, X_2, \ldots, X_n\}$ has been obtained before parameter estimation.

In practice, it is often more convenient to work with the logarithm of the likelihood function because the likelihood function has an exponential form in many cases (e.g., cases with normal or exponential distributions) and it is a product of n terms (cf., Equation (2.18)). Then, the MLEs of $\theta_1, \theta_2, \ldots, \theta_r$ are the solutions to $\tilde{\theta}_1, \tilde{\theta}_2, \ldots, \tilde{\theta}_r$ of the following maximization problem:

$$\max_{\tilde{\theta}_1, \tilde{\theta}_2, \ldots, \tilde{\theta}_r} \sum_{i=1}^{n} \log\left[f(X_i; \tilde{\theta}_1, \tilde{\theta}_2, \ldots, \tilde{\theta}_r)\right]. \tag{2.19}$$

In cases when the population has a normal distribution $N(\mu, \sigma^2)$, the likelihood function is

$$\begin{aligned} L(\mu, \sigma^2; X_1, X_2, \ldots, X_n) &= \Pi_{i=1}^{n}\left[\frac{1}{\sqrt{2\pi}\sigma}\exp\left(-\frac{(X_i-\mu)^2}{2\sigma^2}\right)\right] \\ &= \left(\frac{1}{\sqrt{2\pi}\sigma}\right)^n \exp\left(-\sum_{i=1}^{n}\frac{(X_i-\mu)^2}{2\sigma^2}\right). \end{aligned}$$

The log-likelihood function is

$$\log\left(L(\mu, \sigma^2; X_1, X_2, \ldots, X_n)\right) = -n\log\left(\sqrt{2\pi}\sigma\right) - \sum_{i=1}^{n}\frac{(X_i-\mu)^2}{2\sigma^2}.$$

It is easy to check that the maximization problem (2.19) with the above log-likelihood function gives the following MLEs of μ and σ^2:

$$\widehat{\mu} = \overline{X}, \qquad \widehat{\sigma}^2 = \frac{1}{n}\sum_{i=1}^{n}(X_i - \overline{X})^2.$$

So, $\overline{X}$ is both the MVUE and MLE of μ in the normal-distribution case. The sample variance s^2 is slightly different from the above MLE of σ^2 in that $s^2 = \frac{n}{n-1}\widehat{\sigma}^2$. Because s^2 is an unbiased estimator of σ^2, $\widehat{\sigma}^2$ is biased, although the bias is the small quantity $-\sigma^2/n$, which tends to 0 when n increases. For this reason, in practice, most people prefer to use the unbiased estimator s^2 for estimating σ^2, instead of its MLE $\widehat{\sigma}^2$.

In cases when the population distribution is discrete, the likelihood function can still be defined by (2.18), except that the pdf needs to be replaced by the probability distribution function. For instance, when the probability distribution is Bernoulli with π being the probability of S and we use 1 to denote S and 0 to denote F, the likelihood function is defined to be

$$\begin{aligned} L(\pi; X_1, X_2, \ldots, X_n) &= \Pi_{i=1}^n \left[\pi^{X_i}(1-\pi)^{1-X_i}\right] \\ &= \pi^{\sum_{i=1}^n X_i}(1-\pi)^{n-\sum_{i=1}^n X_i}. \end{aligned}$$

Then, it is easy to check that the MLE of π is $\widehat{\pi} = \overline{X}$, which is also the sample proportion of S.

Besides the MLE, least squares (LS) estimation is another general methodology for estimating population parameters. Usually, the LS estimation is used for parametric regression modeling described below. Assume that there are two variables X and Y, and we are interested in building a numerical relationship between them. Between X and Y, assume that Y is a variable to predict based on the relationship to build, and X is a variable to predict from. Then, Y is often called a *response variable*, and X is often called an *explanatory variable* or *predictor*. We further assume that X and Y follow a linear regression model

$$Y = \beta_0 + \beta_1 x + \varepsilon, \tag{2.20}$$

where $\beta_0+\beta_1 x$ is the *linear regression function* that can be written as $E(Y|X = x) = \beta_0 + \beta_1 x$, denoting the assumption that the mean value of Y when X is given at x is assumed to be a linear function of x. In (2.20), β_0 and β_1 are two regression coefficients, and ε is a random error term. Now, assume that we have n observations of (X, Y), denoted as $\{(x_i, Y_i), i = 1, 2, \ldots, n\}$, and they are all generated from the linear regression model (2.20). Namely,

$$Y_i = \beta_0 + \beta_1 x_i + \varepsilon_i, \ i = 1, 2, \ldots, n,$$

where $\{\varepsilon_i, i = 1, 2, \ldots, n\}$ are random errors at the *design points* $\{x_i, i = 1, 2, \ldots, n\}$. For the error terms, we conventionally assume that they are i.i.d. and normally distributed, so that $\varepsilon_i \sim N(0, \sigma^2)$, for all $i = 1, 2, \cdots, n$, and the common variance σ^2 is usually unknown. All these conventional assumptions can be summarized by the four letters in LINE, where "L" denotes the assumption that the regression function is linear, "I" denotes the assumption that the error terms are independent, "N" denotes the assumption that all error terms are normally distributed, and "E" denotes the assumption that all error terms have equal variance of σ^2.

A widely used criterion for measuring the goodness-of-fit of a candidate estimator $b_0+b_1 x$ of the true linear regression function $\beta_0+\beta_1 x$ is the *residual sum of squares* (RSS), defined by

$$\mathrm{RSS}(b_0, b_1) = \sum_{i=1}^{n} \left[Y_i - (b_0 + b_1 x_i)\right]^2.$$

The LS estimators of β_0 and β_1 are then defined to be the minimizers of $\mathrm{RSS}(b_0, b_1)$. It can be checked that these LS estimators have the following expressions:

$$\begin{aligned} \widehat{\beta}_1 &= \frac{\sum_{i=1}^{n}(x_i - \overline{x})\left(Y_i - \overline{Y}\right)}{\sum_{i=1}^{n}(x_i - \overline{x})^2}, \\ \widehat{\beta}_0 &= \overline{Y} - \widehat{\beta}_1 \overline{x}, \end{aligned} \tag{2.21}$$

where $\overline{x}$ and $\overline{Y}$ are the sample means of the x and Y values, respectively. Then, the estimated regression model is

$$\widehat{Y} = \widehat{\beta}_0 + \widehat{\beta}_1 x.$$

Under the four conventional assumptions (i.e., LINE), it can be checked that

$$\begin{pmatrix} \widehat{\beta}_0 \\ \widehat{\beta}_1 \end{pmatrix} \sim N\left(\begin{pmatrix} \beta_0 \\ \beta_1 \end{pmatrix}, \sigma^2 \begin{pmatrix} \frac{1}{n} + \frac{\overline{x}^2}{sxx}, & -\frac{\overline{x}}{sxx} \\ -\frac{\overline{x}}{sxx}, & \frac{1}{sxx} \end{pmatrix} \right), \tag{2.22}$$

where $sxx = \sum_{i=1}^{n}(x_i - \overline{x})^2$. For the error variance σ^2, it is often estimated by

$$\widehat{\sigma}^2 = \frac{1}{n-2} \sum_{i=1}^{n} \left[Y_i - \left(\widehat{\beta}_0 + \widehat{\beta}_1 x_i\right)\right]^2, \tag{2.23}$$

which is the so-called *residual mean squares (RMS)* of the estimated regression model. For the variance estimator in (2.23), by the results in (2.22), we have

$$\frac{(n-2)\widehat{\sigma}^2}{\sigma^2} \sim \chi^2_{n-2}. \tag{2.24}$$

From the above description, it can be seen that the LS estimation does not use any information about the distribution of Y, which is an advantage, compared to the maximum likelihood estimation. Under the conventional assumptions of LINE, $Y_i \sim N(\beta_0 + \beta_1 x_i, \sigma^2)$, for $i = 1, 2, \ldots, n$. Therefore, β_0, β_1 and σ^2 can also be estimated by their MLEs. As a matter of fact, it can be checked that the LS estimators of β_0 and β_1 given in (2.21) are the same as their MLEs, and the MLE of σ^2 is

$$\frac{n-2}{n}\widehat{\sigma}^2,$$

where $\widehat{\sigma}^2$ is the estimator defined in (2.23). By the way, $\widehat{\sigma}^2$ is an unbiased estimator of σ^2, and the MLE of σ^2 is slightly biased.

2.4.3 Confidence Intervals and Hypothesis Testing

Besides point estimation discussed in the previous subsection, there are two other methods for statistical inference about a population parameter. The first one uses confidence intervals, by which a population parameter θ is estimated by an interval with some specific properties. Suppose that a point estimator $\widehat{\theta}$ of θ has a normal distribution with mean θ and variance $\sigma^2_{\widehat{\theta}}$. Then,

$$Z = \frac{\widehat{\theta} - \theta}{\sigma_{\widehat{\theta}}} \sim N(0,1),$$

and

$$P\left(\widehat{\theta} - Z_{1-\alpha/2}\sigma_{\widehat{\theta}} < \theta < \widehat{\theta} + Z_{1-\alpha/2}\sigma_{\widehat{\theta}}\right) = 1 - \alpha,$$

where α is a given number between 0 and 1, and $Z_{1-\alpha/2}$ is the $(1-\alpha/2)$-th *quantile* of the standard normal distribution (cf. Figure 2.1), defined by $P(Z \leq Z_{1-\alpha/2}) = 1 - \alpha/2$. Therefore, the random interval

$$\left(\widehat{\theta} - Z_{1-\alpha/2}\sigma_{\widehat{\theta}},\ \widehat{\theta} + Z_{1-\alpha/2}\sigma_{\widehat{\theta}}\right)$$

has a $100(1-\alpha)\%$ chance to cover the true value of θ. This interval is called a $100(1-\alpha)\%$ *confidence interval* (CI) for θ, and the number $100(1-\alpha)\%$ is called the *confidence level*. For simplicity, the above CI is often written as

$$\widehat{\theta} \pm Z_{1-\alpha/2}\sigma_{\widehat{\theta}}.$$

Usually, the standard deviation $\sigma_{\widehat{\theta}}$ has some unknown population parameters involved, such as the population standard deviation σ. So, the above CI formula can be used only after these parameters are replaced by their point estimators. In other words, the standard deviation $\sigma_{\widehat{\theta}}$ needs to be estimated by the *standard error* $\widehat{\sigma}_{\widehat{\theta}}$, in which the unknown parameters have been replaced by their point estimators.

In cases when a population distribution is $N(\mu, \sigma^2)$ and $\{X_1, X_2, \ldots, X_n\}$ is a simple random sample from this population, by the discussion in Subsection 2.4.1, $\overline{X} \sim N(\mu, \sigma^2/n)$. Therefore, when σ is known,

$$Z = \frac{\overline{X} - \mu}{\sigma/\sqrt{n}} \sim N(0,1), \tag{2.25}$$

and the $100(1-\alpha)\%$ CI for μ is

$$\overline{X} \pm Z_{1-\alpha/2}\frac{\sigma}{\sqrt{n}}.$$

In cases when σ is unknown, it should be replaced by the sample standard deviation s in (2.25). Because of the extra randomness added by this replacement, the resulting statistic has a t distribution with $n-1$ degrees of freedom. Namely,

$$T = \frac{\overline{X} - \mu}{s/\sqrt{n}} \sim t_{n-1}. \tag{2.26}$$

See (2.17) and the related discussion in Subsection 2.4.1. So, based on (2.26), the $100(1-\alpha)\%$ CI for μ is

$$\overline{X} \pm t_{1-\alpha/2}(n-1)\frac{s}{\sqrt{n}}, \tag{2.27}$$

where $t_{1-\alpha/2}(n-1)$ is the $(1-\alpha/2)$-th quantile of the t_{n-1} distribution.

In applications, the exact distribution of $\widehat{\theta}$ is often unknown for a fixed sample size n. If its *asymptotic distribution*, which is the limit distribution of $\widehat{\theta}$ when n tends to infinity, can be derived, then the CI for θ can be constructed based on this asymptotic distribution. Of course, in such cases it is only asymptotically true that the CI has a $100(1-\alpha)\%$ chance to cover the true value θ. In cases when we are interested in estimating the population mean μ (i.e., $\theta = \mu$), if the population distribution is unknown, or it is known but non-normal, then by the CLT, (2.25) is asymptotically true. Namely, when the sample size n is large (i.e., $n \geq 30$), the CI formula (2.27) can still be used, in which we can use either $t_{1-\alpha/2}(n-1)$ or $Z_{1-\alpha/2}$ because these two quantities should be almost the same in such cases. See a related discussion in Subsection 2.2.2.

In cases when the population distribution is Bernoulli with π being the probability of success and when the sample size is large (i.e., $n\widehat{\pi} \geq 5$ and $n(1-\widehat{\pi}) \geq 5$), by similar arguments to those in the previous two paragraphs, the large-sample $100(1-\alpha)\%$ CI for π is

$$\widehat{\pi} \pm Z_{1-\alpha/2}\sqrt{\frac{\widehat{\pi}(1-\widehat{\pi})}{n}}, \tag{2.28}$$

where $\widehat{\pi}$ is the sample proportion of success.

Another method for statistical inference about a population parameter involves testing hypotheses. In our daily life, we often make a statement or *hypothesis* about a population parameter. For example, some reports claim that smoking would increase the chance of lung cancer in a general circumstance. In this example, all smokers constitute the population. Assume that the prevalence rate of lung cancer in this population is an unknown parameter π, and that the prevalence rate of the same disease among all non-smokers is known to be π_0. Then, the above statement basically says that $\pi > \pi_0$. A major goal of many research projects is to collect data for verifying such a hypothesis. If the hypothesis is supported by the data obtained from one or more repeated experiments, then it becomes a new theory. In statistics, the hypothesis that we want to validate is called an *alternative hypothesis*. Usually, an alternative hypothesis represents a potential new theory, new method, new discovery and so forth. It is a competitor to a so-called *null hypothesis*, which often represents existing theory, existing method, existing knowledge and so forth. Because the null hypothesis is usually verified in the past, it is initially assumed true. It is rejected only in cases when the observed data from the population in question provide a convincing evidence against it.

By convention, the null hypothesis is denoted by H_0, and it usually takes the equality form

$$H_0 : \theta = \theta_0,$$

where θ_0 is the hypothesized value of the population parameter θ. The alternative hypothesis is denoted by H_1 or H_a, and it can take one of the following three forms:

$$\begin{aligned} H_1 : \theta &> \theta_0 \\ H_1 : \theta &< \theta_0 \\ H_1 : \theta &\neq \theta_0. \end{aligned}$$

The first form is called right-sided or right-tailed alternative hypothesis, the second one is called left-sided or left-tailed alternative hypothesis, and the last one is called two-sided or two-tailed alternative hypothesis.

To test whether H_0 should be rejected in favor of H_1, we need a criterion constructed from the observed data. To this end, assume that $\{X_1, X_2, \ldots, X_n\}$ is a simple random sample from the population of interest and $\widehat{\theta}$ is a point estimator of θ. To describe how to construct a hypothesis testing procedure, let us assume that $\widehat{\theta} \sim N(\theta, \sigma^2_{\widehat{\theta}})$ and $\sigma^2_{\widehat{\theta}}$ does not include any unknown parameters. Then, in cases when H_0 is true, we have

$$Z = \frac{\widehat{\theta} - \theta_0}{\sigma_{\widehat{\theta}}} \sim N(0, 1).$$

Let us assume that the alternative hypothesis of interest is right-sided, and the observed value of Z is denoted as Z^*. Then, the probability

$$P_{H_0}(Z \geq Z^*)$$

would tell us the likelihood that we can observe Z^* or values of Z that are more favorable to H_1 when H_0 is assumed true, where P_{H_0} denotes the probability under H_0. The probability $P_{H_0}(Z \geq Z^*)$ is called the *p-value* and the statistic Z is called a *test statistic*. The p-value is defined by $P_{H_0}(Z \leq Z^*)$ when H_1 is left-sided, and by $P_{H_0}(|Z| \geq |Z^*|)$ when H_1 is two-sided.

From the definition of p-value, the data provide more evidence against H_0 if the p-value is smaller. Then, the question becomes: how small is small? To answer this question, we usually compare the calculated p-value with a pre-specified *significance level*, denoted conventionally as α. If the p-value is smaller than or equal to α, then we reject H_0 and conclude that the data have provided significant evidence to support H_1. Otherwise, we fail to reject H_0 and conclude that there is no significant evidence in the data to support H_1. This process of decision making is called *hypothesis testing*.

For a given significance level α, an alternative approach to perform hypothesis testing is to compare the observed value Z^* of the test statistic Z with its *α-critical value*. In the case considered above, when $Z = (\widehat{\theta} - \theta_0)/\sigma_{\widehat{\theta}} \sim N(0, 1)$, its α-critical value is defined by $Z_{1-\alpha}$ if the alternative hypothesis H_1 is right-sided, by Z_α if H_1 is left-sided, and by $Z_{1-\alpha/2}$ if H_1 is two-sided. Then, the null hypothesis H_0 is rejected when $Z^* > Z_{1-\alpha}$, $Z^* < Z_\alpha$, and $|Z^*| > Z_{1-\alpha/2}$, respectively, for the three types of H_1 considered above. It is easy to check that decisions made by the two approaches are actually equivalent to each other. In applications, the p-value approach is often preferred because it provides us decisions regarding whether H_0 should be rejected at a given significance level and a quantitative measure of the strength of evidence against H_0 in the observed data as well.

Decisions by any hypothesis-testing procedure would make mistakes. There are two types of mistakes, or, more conventionally, two types of errors that we can make. *Type I error* refers to the case in which H_0 is rejected when it is actually true. *Type II error* refers to the case in which H_0 fails to be rejected when it is actually false. The probabilities of type I and type II errors are denoted by α and β, respectively. Note that α is used to denote both the significance level and the probability of type I error because these two quantities are the same in most cases.

Intuitively, an ideal hypothesis-testing procedure should have small α and small β. However, in reality, if α is kept small, then β would be large, and vice versa. To handle this situation, a conventional strategy is to control α at a fixed level, and let β be as small as possible. By this strategy, H_0 is protected to a certain degree since the probability to reject it when it is true cannot exceed the fixed level of α. This strategy is reasonable because H_0 often represents existing methods or knowledge, and it has been justified in the past. In practice, selection of α usually depends on the consequence of a type I error in a specific application. If the consequence is serious, then a small α should be preferred. Otherwise, a relatively large value could be chosen. Commonly used α values include 0.1, 0.05, 0.01, 0.005 and 0.001. A default α value adopted by most scientific communities is 0.05.

From the above discussion, it can be seen that a major step for solving a hypothesis-testing problem is to find an appropriate test statistic, which should have the property that its distribution under H_0, or its *null distribution*, is known or can be computed. For a given hypothesis-testing problem, different testing procedures are possible. In statistics, we usually only consider the procedures whose type I error probabilities are below a given level (i.e., α). Among these procedures, the one with the smallest type II error probability β, or equivalently the largest *power*, defined to be $1-\beta$, is the best.

A general methodology for deriving a testing procedure for a hypothesis-testing problem is the *likelihood ratio test (LRT)* described below. Let $L(\theta; X_1, X_2, \ldots, X_n)$ be the likelihood function of the related hypothesis-testing problem, Θ_0 be the set of θ values under H_0, and Θ_1 be the set of θ values under H_1. Consider the following ratio of two maximum likelihoods:

$$\Lambda(X_1, X_2, \ldots, X_n) = \frac{\max_{\theta \in \Theta_0} L(\theta; X_1, X_2, \ldots, X_n)}{\max_{\theta \in \Theta_0 \bigcup \Theta_1} L(\theta; X_1, X_2, \ldots, X_n)}. \tag{2.29}$$

Obviously, it is always true that $0 \leq \Lambda(X_1, X_2, \ldots, X_n) \leq 1$. In cases when H_0 is true, the two maximum likelihoods in (2.29) should be close to each other; consequently, $\Lambda(X_1, X_2, \ldots, X_n)$ is close to 1. Otherwise, $\Lambda(X_1, X_2, \ldots, X_n)$ should be small. Therefore, we can make decisions about the hypotheses H_0 and H_1 using the *LRT statistic* $\Lambda(X_1, X_2, \ldots, X_n)$, and reject H_1 in cases when $\Lambda(X_1, X_2, \ldots, X_n)$ is too small. Wilks (1938) showed that, under some regularity conditions, it was asymptotically true that

$$-2\log(\Lambda(X_1, X_2, \ldots, X_n)) \overset{H_0}{\sim} \chi^2_{df}, \tag{2.30}$$

where the notation $\overset{H_0}{\sim} \chi^2_{df}$ means "has the χ^2_{df} distribution under H_0", and df equals the difference of the dimensions of Θ_0 and Θ_1. Thus, in large sample cases, H_1 can be rejected at the significance level of α if the observed value of $-2\log(\Lambda(X_1, X_2, \ldots, X_n))$ is larger than the $(1-\alpha)$-th quantile of the χ^2_{df} distribution. In cases when multiple parameters are involved in the testing problem, the LRT test can be described in a similar way. It has been demonstrated in the literature that LRT tests have certain desirable statistical properties. For a related discussion, see Casella and Berger (2002) and Lehmann and Romano (2005).

When the population distribution is $N(\mu, \sigma^2)$, the null hypothesis is $H_0 : \mu = \mu_0$, and σ is known, a commonly used test statistic is

$$Z = \frac{\overline{X} - \mu_0}{\sigma/\sqrt{n}} \overset{H_0}{\sim} N(0, 1).$$

In such cases, it can be checked that

$$\begin{aligned} & -2\log(\Lambda(X_1, X_2, \ldots, X_n)) \\ = & \frac{\sum_{i=1}^n (x_i - \mu_0)^2 - \sum_{i=1}^n (x_i - \overline{X})^2}{\sigma^2} \\ = & n\left(\frac{\overline{X} - \mu_0}{\sigma}\right)^2 \\ = & Z^2. \end{aligned}$$

Therefore, the test based on Z and the LRT test are exactly the same when the alternative hypothesis H_1 is two-sided. Also, the result (2.30) is exact in such cases. In cases when σ is unknown, it should be replaced by s when defining the test statistic Z. The resulting test statistic and its null distribution are

$$T = \frac{\overline{X} - \mu_0}{s/\sqrt{n}} \overset{H_0}{\sim} t_{n-1}. \tag{2.31}$$

In cases when the population distribution is non-normal, the test statistic in (2.31) can still be used, as long as the sample size n is large (i.e., $n \geq 30$), because of the Central Limit Theorem discussed in Subsection 2.4.1. In such cases, the asymptotic null distribution of T is $N(0,1)$, to which the t_{n-1} distribution is close. Therefore, either distribution can be used when computing the p-value.

In cases when the population distribution is Bernoulli with π being the probability of success, the null hypothesis is $H_0 : \pi = \pi_0$, and the sample size is large (i.e., $n\pi_0 \geq 5$ and $n(1-\pi_0) \geq 5$), a commonly used test statistic is

$$Z = \frac{\widehat{\pi} - \pi_0}{\sqrt{\pi_0(1-\pi_0)/n}} \overset{H_0}{\sim} N(0,1), \tag{2.32}$$

where π_0 is the hypothesized value of π, and $\widehat{\pi}$ is the sample proportion of success. Of course, the null distribution specified in (2.32) is only asymptotically true in such cases.

In certain applications, we need to compare two populations with regard to a specific population characteristic (e.g., the population mean). To this end, assume that $\{X_{11}, X_{12}, \ldots, X_{1n_1}\}$ and $\{X_{21}, X_{22}, \ldots, X_{2n_2}\}$ are two samples from the two populations, respectively, and that the two samples are independent of each other. The sample means and the sample variances of the two samples are denoted as $\overline{X}_1, \overline{X}_2, s_1^2$, and s_2^2. If we are interested in comparing the two population means μ_1 and μ_2, then the null and alternative hypotheses would be

$$H_0 : \mu_1 - \mu_2 = \delta_0 \qquad \text{versus} \qquad H_1 : \mu_1 - \mu_2 \neq \delta_0 (> \delta_0, < \delta_0), \tag{2.33}$$

where δ_0 is a given number, and $\mu_1 - \mu_2 \neq \delta_0 (> \delta_0, < \delta_0)$ denotes one of the three forms: $\mu_1 - \mu_2 \neq \delta_0$, $\mu_1 - \mu_2 > \delta_0$, and $\mu_1 - \mu_2 < \delta_0$. In most cases, we are interested in the case when $\delta_0 = 0$. In such cases, H_0 in (2.33) says that the two population means are the same. To test the above hypotheses, it is natural to use $\overline{X}_1 - \overline{X}_2$, which is a good point estimator of $\mu_1 - \mu_2$, according to the related discussion about the sample mean in one-population cases (cf., Subsections 2.4.1 and 2.4.2).

In cases when the two population distributions are $N(\mu_1, \sigma_1^2)$ and $N(\mu_2, \sigma_2^2)$, it is easy to check that

$$Z = \frac{(\overline{X}_1 - \overline{X}_2) - (\mu_1 - \mu_2)}{\sqrt{\sigma_1^2/n_1 + \sigma_2^2/n_2}} \sim N(0,1).$$

In such cases, if both σ_1^2 and σ_2^2 are known, then a $100(1-\alpha)\%$ CI for $\mu_1 - \mu_2$ is

$$(\overline{X}_1 - \overline{X}_2) \pm Z_{1-\alpha/2}\sqrt{\sigma_1^2/n_1 + \sigma_2^2/n_2},$$

and a good test statistic for the hypotheses in (2.33) is

$$Z = \frac{(\overline{X}_1 - \overline{X}_2) - \delta_0}{\sqrt{\sigma_1^2/n_1 + \sigma_2^2/n_2}} \overset{H_0}{\sim} N(0,1).$$

Of course, in practice, the two population variances σ_1^2 and σ_2^2 are often unknown. If the two population distributions are still $N(\mu_1, \sigma_1^2)$ and $N(\mu_2, \sigma_2^2)$ and both σ_1^2 and σ_2^2 are unknown, then we have

$$T = \frac{(\overline{X}_1 - \overline{X}_2) - (\mu_1 - \mu_2)}{\sqrt{s_1^2/n_1 + s_2^2/n_2}} \sim t_{\text{df}}, \tag{2.34}$$

where

$$\text{df} = \frac{(V_1 + V_2)^2}{V_1^2/(n_1 - 1) + V_2^2/(n_2 - 1)}, \tag{2.35}$$

$V_1 = s_1^2/n_1$, and $V_2 = s_2^2/n_2$. Based on the statistic T in (2.34), the $100(1-\alpha)\%$ CI for $\mu_1 - \mu_2$ is

$$(\overline{X}_1 - \overline{X}_2) \pm t_{1-\alpha/2}(df)\sqrt{s_1^2/n_1 + s_2^2/n_2},$$

where $t_{1-\alpha/2}(df)$ is the $(1 - \alpha/2)$-th quantile of the t_{df} distribution with df defined in (2.35). For testing hypotheses in (2.33), a good test statistic is

$$T = \frac{(\overline{X}_1 - \overline{X}_2) - \delta_0}{\sqrt{s_1^2/n_1 + s_2^2/n_2}} \overset{H_0}{\sim} t_{\text{df}}. \tag{2.36}$$

The test using the test statistic in (2.36) is often called the *two independent sample t-test*. In certain cases, it is reasonable to assume that $\sigma_1^2 = \sigma_2^2 = \sigma^2$. In such cases, we can estimate σ^2 by the following *pooled sample variance*:

$$s_p^2 = \frac{(n_1 - 1)s_1^2 + (n_2 - 1)s_2^2}{n_1 + n_2 - 2}.$$

Then, the statistic in (2.34) can be replaced by

$$T = \frac{(\overline{X}_1 - \overline{X}_2) - (\mu_1 - \mu_2)}{s_p\sqrt{1/n_1 + 1/n_2}} \sim t_{n_1+n_2-2}. \tag{2.37}$$

The CI formula and the test statistic for testing the hypotheses in (2.33) can be modified accordingly, using the statistic in (2.37).

In cases when the two population distributions are unknown, but both n_1 and n_2 are large (i.e., $n_1 \geq 30$ and $n_2 \geq 30$), it is asymptotically true that

$$Z = \frac{(\overline{X}_1 - \overline{X}_2) - (\mu_1 - \mu_2)}{\sqrt{s_1^2/n_1 + s_2^2/n_2}} \sim N(0, 1). \tag{2.38}$$

In such cases, the large sample CI for $\mu_1 - \mu_2$ and the large sample testing procedure for testing the hypotheses in (2.33) can be constructed using the statistic in (2.38). For instance, for testing the hypotheses in (2.33), the test statistic would be the same as that in (2.36), except that its null distribution could be approximated well by either t_{df} or $N(0, 1)$.

If we are interested in comparing two population proportions π_1 and π_2 using two independent samples from the two populations, then in large sample cases,

$$Z = \frac{(\widehat{\pi}_1 - \widehat{\pi}_2) - (\pi_1 - \pi_2)}{\sqrt{\widehat{\pi}_1(1-\widehat{\pi}_1)/n_1 + \widehat{\pi}_2(1-\widehat{\pi}_2)/n_2}} \sim N(0,1),$$

where $\widehat{\pi}_1$ and $\widehat{\pi}_2$ are the two sample proportions. Therefore, a $100(1-\alpha)\%$ CI for $\pi_1 - \pi_2$ would be

$$(\widehat{\pi}_1 - \widehat{\pi}_2) \pm Z_{1-\alpha/2}\sqrt{\widehat{\pi}_1(1-\widehat{\pi}_1)/n_1 + \widehat{\pi}_2(1-\widehat{\pi}_2)/n_2}.$$

The large sample condition is satisfied if $n_1\widehat{\pi}_1 \geq 5$, $n_1(1-\widehat{\pi}_1) \geq 5$, $n_2\widehat{\pi}_2 \geq 5$, and $n_2(1-\widehat{\pi}_2) \geq 5$. To test the hypotheses

$$H_0: \pi_1 - \pi_2 = 0 \qquad \text{versus} \qquad H_1: \pi_1 - \pi_2 \neq 0 (> 0, < 0),$$

a good test statistic is

$$Z = \frac{\widehat{\pi}_1 - \widehat{\pi}_2}{\sqrt{\widehat{\pi}_p(1-\widehat{\pi}_p)}\sqrt{1/n_1 + 1/n_2}} \overset{H_0}{\sim} N(0,1),$$

where

$$\widehat{\pi}_p = \frac{n_1\widehat{\pi}_1 + n_2\widehat{\pi}_2}{n_1 + n_2}$$

is the pooled sample proportion.

When we compare two populations, sometimes certain variables that may affect the variable of interest should be taken into account. For instance, if we are interested in studying whether physical exercise can significantly affect our weight, then one possible approach is as follows. First, we specify two populations. For example, one population could be all adults aged 20 and above who go to gym regularly (e.g., at least two times a week), and the other population includes all adults aged 20 and above who do not go to gym regularly. Second, we randomly select a group of people from each population and record their weights. Finally, we can use the two independent sample t-test to compare the mean weights of the two populations. This approach seems appropriate. But, it can happen that, in the two selected groups, one group includes more males than the other group. So, in the case a significant difference between the two population means of weight is found by the t-test, the significant difference could be due to the gender difference between the two samples, instead of the difference in physical exercise. Therefore, to make a more appropriate comparison, we should take into account the variables that are not our major interest but may affect the result, such as gender, age, profession and so forth. These variables are often called *confounding risk factors*. To avoid the impact of the confounding risk factors on the testing result, we can collect data in an alternative way as follows. First, we list all major confounding risk factors that we can think of. Second, for each randomly selected member from the first population, we randomly select a member from all members in the second population who match the selected member in the first population by all the confounding risk factors. In that way, the two resulting samples from the two populations are *paired* with respect to all confounding risk factors. Let the two samples be $\{X_{11}, X_{12}, \ldots, X_{1n}\}$ and $\{X_{21}, X_{22}, \ldots, X_{2n}\}$. Then, X_{11} is paired with X_{21}, X_{12} is paired with X_{22}, and so forth. So, the sample sizes of the two samples must be the same in such cases. To test the hypotheses in (2.33), we can use the difference between the two paired samples, by defining $D_i = X_{1i} - X_{2i}$, for $i = 1, 2, \ldots, n$. Then, $\{D_1, D_2, \ldots, D_n\}$ can be regarded as a simple random sample from a "difference" population with the mean $\mu_d = \mu_1 - \mu_2$. Therefore, the original two-population problem becomes a one-population problem with the hypotheses

$$H_0 : \mu_d = \delta_0 \qquad \text{versus} \qquad H_1 : \mu_d \neq \delta_0 (> \delta_0, < \delta_0).$$

And, most statistical inference methods for the one-population problem can be used here. For instance, if it is reasonable to assume that the "difference" population has a normal distribution with an unknown variance, then a good test statistic for the above hypotheses would be

$$T = \frac{\overline{D} - \delta_0}{s_d/\sqrt{n}} \overset{H_0}{\sim} t_{n-1}, \tag{2.39}$$

where $\overline{D}$ and s_d are the sample mean and sample standard deviation of the "difference" sample $\{D_1, D_2, \ldots, D_n\}$. The test based on (2.39) is often called the *two paired sample t-test.* By the way, the $100(1-\alpha)\%$ CI for μ_d can be derived accordingly, to be

$$\overline{D} \pm t_{1-\alpha/2}(n-1)\frac{s_d}{\sqrt{n}}.$$

2.4.4 The Delta Method and the Bootstrap Method

In the previous subsection, we discussed how to construct a CI or perform a hypothesis test for a population parameter θ using the exact or asymptotic distribution of its point estimator $\widehat{\theta}$. In some cases, we are interested in statistical inferences about a function of θ, denoted as $g(\theta)$. In such cases, it is natural to estimate $g(\theta)$ by $g(\widehat{\theta})$. If the exact distribution of $g(\widehat{\theta})$ is available, then the related inferences can be made accordingly. Otherwise, the method described below can be considered for deriving the asymptotic distribution of $g(\widehat{\theta})$.

Assume that the function g has the second-order derivative at θ, and $\sqrt{n}(\widehat{\theta} - \theta)$ converges in distribution to $N(0, \sigma^2)$, written in notation as

$$\sqrt{n}\left(\widehat{\theta} - \theta\right) \xrightarrow{D} N(0, \sigma^2). \tag{2.40}$$

Then, by the Taylor's expansion, we have

$$g(\widehat{\theta}) = g(\theta) + g'(\theta)\left(\widehat{\theta} - \theta\right) + O\left(\left(\widehat{\theta} - \theta\right)^2\right).$$

So,

$$\sqrt{n}\left(g(\widehat{\theta})-g(\theta)\right)=g'(\theta)\sqrt{n}\left(\widehat{\theta}-\theta\right)+O\left(\sqrt{n}\left(\widehat{\theta}-\theta\right)^2\right).$$

The second term on the right-hand side of the above expression would converge to 0 in distribution, and by (2.40) the first term would converge to a normal distribution. Therefore, we have

$$\sqrt{n}\left(g(\widehat{\theta})-g(\theta)\right)\xrightarrow{D}N\left(0,\sigma^2\left[g'(\theta)\right]^2\right). \tag{2.41}$$

Then, statistical inferences about $g(\theta)$ can proceed using the result in (2.41). This general approach for statistical inferences about $g(\theta)$ based on the Taylor's expansion is often called the *delta method.*

Example 2.5 *Assume that $\{X_1, X_2, \ldots, X_n\}$ is a simple random sample from a population of interest, and that we are interested in estimating $g(\mu) = \mu(\mu+1)$, where μ is the population mean. Then, a reasonable point estimator of $g(\mu)$ is $g(\overline{X})$, where $\overline{X}$ is the sample mean. By the CLT, we have*

$$\sqrt{n}\left(\overline{X}-\mu\right)\xrightarrow{D}N(0,\sigma^2),$$

where σ^2 is the population variance. By (2.41), we have

$$\sqrt{n}\left(g(\overline{X})-g(\mu)\right)\xrightarrow{D}N\left(0,\sigma^2\left[g'(\mu)\right]^2\right).$$

So, a large-sample $100(1-\alpha)\%$ CI for $g(\mu)$ would be

$$g(\overline{X})\pm Z_{1-\alpha/2}g'(\overline{X})s/\sqrt{n},$$

where $g'(\overline{X}) = 2\overline{X}+1$ and s is the sample standard deviation.

In some cases, when making statistical inferences about a population parameter θ, the exact distribution of its point estimator $\widehat{\theta}$ is difficult to derive. Furthermore, the asymptotic distribution of $\widehat{\theta}$ is also difficult to derive, or it is inappropriate to use the asymptotic distribution because the sample size n in a given application is not large enough. In all such cases, the *bootstrap* method (cf., Efron (1979), Efron and Tibshirani (1993)) is often useful. A typical bootstrap procedure works in several steps as follows.

Step 1 Draw a random sample of size n from the observed data $\{X_1, X_2, \ldots, X_n\}$ with replacement. The new sample, which is called the *bootstrap sample*, is denoted as $\{X_1^*, X_2^*, \ldots, X_n^*\}$. Compute the estimate of θ from the bootstrap sample, and the estimate is denoted as $\widehat{\theta}^*$.

Step 2 Repeat step 1 for B times, and the estimates of θ from the B bootstrap samples are denoted as $\{\widehat{\theta}_j^*,\ j=1,2,\ldots,B\}$, where B is often called the *bootstrap sample size.*

Step 3 The empirical distribution of $\{\widehat{\theta}_j^*,\ j = 1, 2, \ldots, B\}$ (cf., the related discussion in Subsection 2.5.1 below), denoted as $\widehat{F}_{\widehat{\theta}}$, is used as an estimate of the true distribution of $\widehat{\theta}$, denoted as $F_{\widehat{\theta}}$, for statistical inferences.

For instance, in the case when $B = 10{,}000$, we can use the interval $(\widehat{\theta}_{(251)}^*, \widehat{\theta}_{(9750)}^*)$ as the 95% CI for θ, where $\widehat{\theta}_{(251)}^*$ and $\widehat{\theta}_{(9750)}^*$ are the 251th and 9750th order statistics (cf., Subsection 2.5.1 below for their definitions) of $\{\widehat{\theta}_j^*,\ j = 1, 2, \ldots, 10{,}000\}$.

2.5 Nonparametric Statistical Inferences

Statistical methods introduced in the previous section are appropriate to use in cases when the parametric model imposed on the population distribution (e.g., the normal distribution) is valid. In practice, however, the assumed parametric model is often invalid. Statistical inferences without a parametric model of the population distribution are often called *nonparametric statistical inferences.* In this section, we briefly introduce some basic concepts and methodologies in this area. More comprehensive discussions on this topic can be found in text books, such as Gibbons and Chakraborti (2003), Hollander and Wolfe (1999) and Kvam and Vidakovic (2007).

2.5.1 Order Statistics and Their Properties

When a population characteristic of interest is numeric and a parametric form of the population distribution is unavailable, statistical inferences about the population distribution are often based on the ordering (or *ranking*) information of the observations in a sample. So, in such cases, the order statistics play an important role. In this subsection, we briefly discuss some basic properties of the order statistics.

Let $\{X_1, X_2, \ldots, X_n\}$ be a simple random sample from a population with the cdf F, and $X_{(1)} \leq X_{(2)} \leq \cdots \leq X_{(n)}$ be the order statistics. Then, $\{X_{(1)}, X_{(2)}, \ldots, X_{(n)}\}$ is an ordered version of $\{X_1, X_2, \ldots, X_n\}$. If X_i is the R_i-th order statistic, for $i = 1, 2, \ldots, n$, then R_i takes its value in $\{1, 2, \ldots, n\}$ and $\{R_1, R_2, \ldots, R_n\}$ is a permutation of $\{1, 2, \ldots, n\}$. In the literature, R_i is often called the *rank* of X_i. On the other hand, if $X_{(i)}$ is the A_i-th observation in the sample, for $i = 1, 2, \ldots, n$, then A_i is often called the ith *inverse rank*, or the ith *antirank*. Obviously, $\{A_1, A_2, \ldots, A_n\}$ is also a permutation of $\{1, 2, \ldots, n\}$. Regarding the ranks and antiranks, they are all random variables because they are uniquely determined by the random sample. The sampling distribution of $\{R_1, R_2, \ldots, R_n\}$ is that it takes any permutation of $\{1, 2, \ldots, n\}$ with the probability of $1/n!$, and the sampling distribution of $\{A_1, A_2, \ldots, A_n\}$ is the same.

In the above discussion, we have assumed that there are no ties in the observed data, which is often true in cases with a continuous population distribution. When there are one or more ties in the observed data, the ranks and antiranks can also be defined properly, which is demonstrated by the following example.

Example 2.6 *Assume that an observed sample consists of the following 10 numbers*

$$2.3, 1.5, 3.4, 1.5, 0.9, 1.7, 1.5, 1.7, 2.1, 0.7.$$

In this sample, the number 1.7 is observed twice, and the number 1.5 is observed three times. The ordered observations are

$$0.7, 0.9, 1.5, 1.5, 1.5, 1.7, 1.7, 2.1, 2.3, 3.4.$$

So, $R_1 = 9, R_3 = 10, R_5 = 2, R_9 = 7$ *and* $R_{10} = 1$*. However, each of* R_2, R_4 *and* R_7 *can be defined to be 3, 4 or 5, because* (X_2, X_4, X_7) *is a tie. In such a case, we can define* $R_2 = R_4 = R_7 = (3+4+5)/3 = 4$*. Similarly, we can define* $R_6 = R_8 = 6.5$*. The antiranks can be handled similarly. Of course, other solutions for handling the ties are possible. For instance, to break the tie of* (X_6, X_8) *when defining* R_6 *and* R_8*, we can draw a random number from the uniform distribution on* $[0, 1]$*, which has the same chance to be any number in the interval* $[0, 1]$*. If the random number is smaller than or equal to 0.5, then we define* $R_6 = 6$ *and* $R_8 = 7$*. Otherwise, we define* $R_6 = 7$ *and* $R_8 = 6$*.*

For the last order statistic $X_{(n)}$, its cdf $F_{X_{(n)}}$ can be derived easily as follows:

$$\begin{aligned} F_{X_{(n)}}(x) &= P(X_{(n)} \leq x) \\ &= P(X_1 \leq x, X_2 \leq x, \ldots, X_n \leq x) \\ &= P(X_1 \leq x)P(X_2 \leq x)\cdots P(X_n \leq x) \\ &= F^n(x). \end{aligned}$$

Similarly, the cdf of the first order statistic $X_{(1)}$, denoted as $F_{X_{(1)}}$, can be derived to be

$$F_{X_{(1)}}(x) = 1 - [1 - F(x)]^n.$$

For a general $1 \leq i \leq n$, the cdf of the ith order statistic $X_{(i)}$ is

$$F_{X_{(i)}}(x) = \sum_{j=i}^{n} \binom{n}{j} F^j(x)[1 - F(x)]^{n-j}.$$

In cases when the population distribution has a pdf f, the pdf of the ith order statistic $X_{(i)}$, denoted as $f_{X_{(i)}}$, is

$$f_{X_{(i)}}(x) = i \binom{n}{i} F^{i-1}(x)[1 - F(x)]^{n-i} f(x),$$

for $1 \le i \le n$. When $i = n$, the pdf of $X_{(n)}$ is

$$f_{X_{(n)}}(x) = nF^{n-1}(x)f(x).$$

When $i = 1$, the pdf of $X_{(1)}$ is

$$f_{X_{(1)}}(x) = n[1 - F(x)]^{n-1}f(x).$$

One major application of the order statistics is to construct the *empirical cumulative distribution function* (ecdf) defined below.

$$F_n(x) = \begin{cases} 0, & \text{if } x < X_{(1)} \\ 1/n, & \text{if } x \in [X_{(1)}, X_{(2)}) \\ \vdots & \vdots \\ (n-1)/n, & \text{if } x \in [X_{(n-1)}, X_{(n)}) \\ 1, & \text{if } x \ge X_{(n)}. \end{cases} \tag{2.42}$$

Example 2.6 (continued) *For the data in Example 2.6, the ecdf is shown in Figure 2.2. From the plot, it can be seen that the ecdf is a step function with the jumps at the observed values in a sample.*

Clearly, the ecdf defined in (2.42) has the property that

$$F_n(x) = \frac{1}{n}\sum_{i=1}^{n} I(X_i \le x),$$

where $I(a)$ is the *indicator function* of a, and equals 1 when a is "true" and 0 otherwise. So, $F_n(x)$ is the proportion of observations in the sample that are smaller than or equal to x; it is the cdf of the data in the observed sample and is commonly used for estimating the population cdf F. As long as the sample $\{X_1, X_2, \ldots, X_n\}$ is a simple random sample, we have the following result:

$$P\left(\lim_{n\to\infty} \max_{x\in R} |F_n(x) - F(x)| = 0\right) = 1.$$

This result says that $F_n(x)$ converges to $F(x)$ almost surely (cf., Subsection 2.4.1) and uniformly over $x \in R$.

2.5.2 Goodness-of-Fit Tests

Some statistical methods are developed based on certain assumed distributions (cf., the maximum likelihood estimation method discussed in Subsection 2.4.2). To use these methods in practice, the assumed distributions should be verified in advance. Otherwise, the results could be unreliable. To this end, we consider testing the following hypotheses:

$$\begin{aligned} & H_0 : F(x) = F_0(x), && \text{for all } x \in R \\ \text{versus} \quad & H_1 : F(x) \ne F_0(x), && \text{for some } x \in R, \end{aligned} \tag{2.43}$$

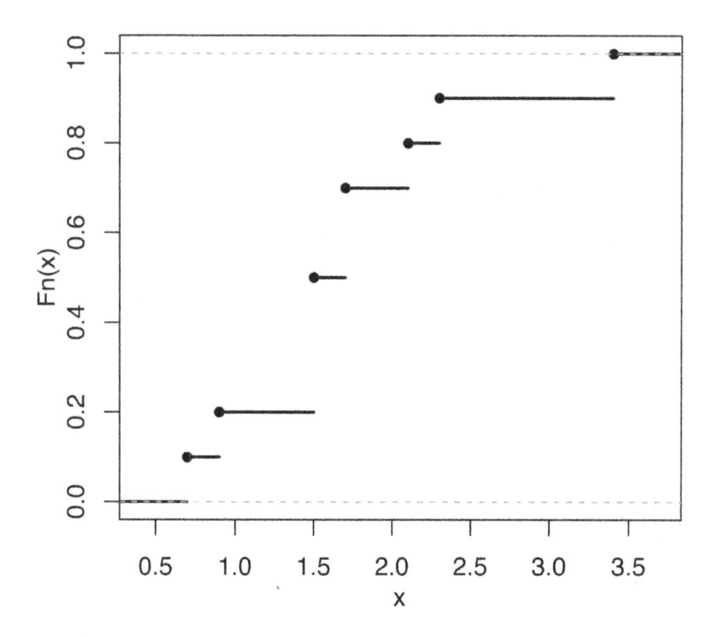

FIGURE 2.2
The ecdf constructed from the data in Example 2.6. The dark point at the beginning of each horizontal line segment denotes that the value of the ecdf at each jump position equals the height of the dark point.

where F denotes the true cdf of a population, and F_0 is a given cdf that is assumed completely specified. If F has a parametric form, then the testing problem of (2.43) can be addressed by the parametric methods discussed in Subsection 2.4.3. However, in many applications, such a parametric form is unavailable. Therefore, nonparametric testing procedures are needed. Because the hypotheses in (2.43) mainly concern about how well the actual population distribution F can be described by the assumed distribution F_0, tests for (2.43) are often called *goodness-of-fit tests.*

To test the hypotheses in (2.43), one approach is to divide the number line R into k intervals

$$(-\infty, a_1), [a_1, a_2), \ldots, [a_{k-1}, \infty),$$

where $a_1 < a_2 < \cdots < a_{k-1}$ are the given cut points. For a simple random sample $\{X_1, X_2, \ldots, X_n\}$, let O_j be the number of observations in the jth interval, for $j = 1, 2, \ldots, k$. If H_0 is true, then, on average, there should be

$$E_j = n\left[F_0(a_j) - F_0(a_{j-1})\right], \qquad \text{for } j = 1, 2, \ldots, k,$$

observations in the sample that fall into the jth interval, where $a_0 = -\infty$ and $a_k = \infty$. Therefore, to test the hypotheses in (2.43), we can compare the *observed counts* $\{O_j,\ j = 1, 2, \ldots, k\}$ with the *expected counts* $\{E_j,\ j = 1, 2, \ldots, k\}$. If H_0 is true, then their difference should be small. Otherwise, it is an indication that H_0 is false. Based on this intuition, we define the following test statistic:

$$X^2 = \sum_{j=1}^{k} \frac{(O_j - E_j)^2}{E_j}, \tag{2.44}$$

which provides a measure of the difference between $\{O_j,\ j = 1, 2, \ldots, k\}$ and $\{E_j,\ j = 1, 2, \ldots, k\}$. The test based on X^2 in (2.44) was first suggested by Pearson (1900) and is thus called the *Pearson's chi-square test* in the literature. Under H_0, the asymptotic null distribution of X^2 is proved to be χ^2_{k-1}. So, the Pearson's chi-square test can be implemented easily based on this null distribution, as discussed in Subsection 2.4.3.

After the number line R is divided into k intervals by the cut points $a_1 < a_2 < \cdots < a_{k-1}$, the LRT testing procedure (cf., (2.29) and (2.30)) can also be used for testing the hypotheses in (2.43). Let π_j be the probability that a randomly selected member from the population in question is included in the jth interval, for $j = 1, 2, \ldots, k$. Then, the observed counts $\{O_j,\ j = 1, 2, \ldots, k\}$ of the simple random sample $\{X_1, X_2, \ldots, X_n\}$ have a multinomial distribution (cf., Subsection 2.2.1), and the likelihood function of the sample is

$$L(\pi_1, \pi_2, \ldots, \pi_k; X_1, X_2, \ldots, X_n) = \frac{n!}{O_1!O_2!\cdots O_k!}\pi_1^{O_1}\pi_2^{O_2}\cdots\pi_k^{O_k}.$$

Let

$$\Lambda = \frac{\max_{H_0} L(\pi_1, \pi_2, \ldots, \pi_k; X_1, X_2, \ldots, X_n)}{\max_{H_0 \bigcup H_1} L(\pi_1, \pi_2, \ldots, \pi_k; X_1, X_2, \ldots, X_n)}$$

be the ratio of two maximized likelihoods, where $\max_{H_0}$ denotes "maximization under H_0" and $\max_{H_0 \bigcup H_1}$ denotes "maximization under $H_0 \bigcup H_1$". Then, it is easy to check that

$$\max_{H_0} L(\pi_1, \pi_2, \ldots, \pi_k; X_1, X_2, \ldots, X_n) = \frac{n!}{O_1!O_2!\cdots O_k!}\pi_{01}^{O_1}\pi_{02}^{O_2}\cdots\pi_{0k}^{O_k}$$

and

$$\max_{H_0 \bigcup H_1} L(\pi_1, \pi_2, \ldots, \pi_k; X_1, X_2, \ldots, X_n) = \frac{n!}{O_1!O_2!\cdots O_k!}\pi_{11}^{O_1}\pi_{12}^{O_2}\cdots\pi_{1k}^{O_k},$$

where

$$\begin{aligned} \pi_{0j} &= F_0(a_j) - F_0(a_{j-1}), \\ \pi_{1j} &= O_j/n, \qquad\qquad \text{for } j = 1, 2, \ldots, k. \end{aligned}$$

Therefore, the LRT test statistic becomes

$$G^2 = -2\log(\Lambda) = 2\sum_{j=1}^{k} O_j \log(O_j/E_j), \tag{2.45}$$

where $\{E_j,\ j = 1, 2, \ldots, k\}$ are the expected counts defined before. Similar to X^2, G^2 in (2.45) has an asymptotic null distribution of χ^2_{k-1}.

The X^2 and G^2 tests would give similar results when the sample size n is large. In the literature, the sample size is considered large if each expected count is at least 5 (i.e., $E_j \geq 5$, for each j). In cases when most E_j's are at least 5 and there are a small number of E_j's as small as 1, the X^2 test often gives a more reliable test, compared to the G^2 test. To best satisfy the large sample condition, in applications, the cut points $a_1 < a_2 < \cdots < a_{k-1}$ should be chosen such that the expected counts $\{E_j,\ j = 1, 2, \ldots, k\}$ are roughly the same, or equivalently, $\{\pi_{0j},\ j = 1, 2, \ldots, k\}$ are roughly the same. For detailed discussion on this topic, see Koehler (1986) and Koehler and Larntz (1980).

2.5.3 Rank Tests

The hypothesis testing procedures described in Subsection 2.4.3 are based on the assumption that the related population distribution has a parametric form (e.g., the normal distribution). In certain applications, however, the parametric form of the population distribution is unavailable, but we still want to test hypotheses about a population parameter. In such cases, an appropriate nonparametric testing procedure should be considered. This subsection introduces several commonly used nonparametric testing procedures.

Let us first focus on hypothesis testing of a population location parameter. In such cases, the population median, denoted as $\widetilde{\mu}$, is often more convenient to use, compared to the population mean μ, which can be seen from the description below. Assume that we have a simple random sample $\{X_1, X_2, \ldots, X_n\}$ from a population with the population median $\widetilde{\mu}$, and we are interested in testing

$$H_0 : \widetilde{\mu} = \widetilde{\mu}_0 \qquad \text{versus} \qquad H_1 : \widetilde{\mu} \neq \widetilde{\mu}_0 (> \widetilde{\mu}_0, < \widetilde{\mu}_0), \tag{2.46}$$

where $\widetilde{\mu}_0$ is a hypothesized value of $\widetilde{\mu}$. Define a test statistic Y by

$$Y = \text{the number of observations in the sample that exceeds } \widetilde{\mu}_0.$$

Then, under H_0, $Y \sim \mathit{Binomial}(n, 0.5)$. Therefore, the hypotheses in (2.46) can be tested using Y, with its critical value or the related p-value determined by the above binomial distribution. This testing procedure is called the *sign test*. When n is large in the sense that $n \geq 20$, the null distribution of Y is approximately normal, and consequently we can use the test statistic

$$Z = \frac{Y - n/2}{\sqrt{n}/2} \overset{H_0}{\sim} N(0, 1).$$

The sign test described above only uses the number of observations in the sample that exceeds $\widetilde{\mu}_0$ for testing the hypotheses in (2.46). It does not make use of the ordering information among all observations in the sample. In cases when the population distribution is symmetric, this ordering information can be used properly in the following two steps:

Step 1 Order all values of $\{|X_i - \widetilde{\mu}_0|,\ i = 1, 2, \ldots, n\}$ from the smallest to the largest, and then obtain the ranks of all observations from this ordered list.

Step 2 Define S_+ to be the summation of the ranks obtained in Step 1 that correspond to the nonnegative values of $\{X_i - \widetilde{\mu}_0,\ i = 1, 2, \ldots, n\}$, and S_- to be the summation of the ranks obtained in Step 1 that correspond to the negative values of $\{X_i - \widetilde{\mu}_0,\ i = 1, 2, \ldots, n\}$.

If H_0 is true (i.e., $\widetilde{\mu}_0$ is the true median of the population distribution), then the distributions of S_+ and S_- would be approximately the same. Since $S_+ + S_- = 1 + 2 + \cdots + n = n(n+1)/2$, the tests based on S_+, S_- or $S_+ - S_-$ are all asymptotically equivalent. For simplicity, we focus on the test using S_+ here. Obviously, if H_0 is true, then S_+ and S_- should be close to each other. If the value of S_+ is too large or too small, then it indicates that H_0 might be invalid. The null distribution of S_+ is given by Wilcoxon et al. (1972) in cases when $n \leq 50$. Table 2.4 gives some tail probabilities of this distribution when $5 \leq n \leq 20$. In cases when n is large (e.g., $n > 20$), the null distribution of S_+ can be regarded as a normal distribution with

$$\mu_{S_+} = n(n+1)/4, \qquad \sigma^2_{S_+} = n(n+1)(2n+1)/24.$$

The test described above, using either S_+, or S_-, or $S_+ - S_-$, is called the *Wilcoxon signed-rank test.*

Example 2.7 *Assume that we obtained the following 20 observations from a population with a symmetric distribution:*

$$8.7, 19.5, 12.7, 10.4, 12.6, 6.1, 11.1, 0.7, 2.2, 12.3,$$
$$11.5, 16.2, 16.0, 13.1, -0.8, 18.1, 8.1, 12.8, 11.6, 12.7.$$

We are interested in testing

$$H_0 : \widetilde{\mu} = 10 \qquad \textit{versus} \qquad H_1 : \widetilde{\mu} > 10.$$

To perform the Wilcoxon signed-rank test, we need to find the ranks of $\{|X_i - \widetilde{\mu}_0|,\ i = 1, 2, \ldots, n\}$, *which are listed in Table 2.5. From Table 2.5,*

$$S_+ = 19 + 9.5 + 1 + 8 + 2 + 7 + 4 + 15 + 14 + 12 + 17 + 11 + 5 + 9.5 = 134.$$

By Table 2.4, the p-value is $P_{H_0}(S_+ \geq 134) > P_{H_0}(S_+ \geq 140) = 0.101$. *Therefore, we fail to reject* H_0 *at the significance level of 0.05.*

To compare two population means μ_1 and μ_2, if we have two paired samples from the two populations, then the Wilcoxon signed-rank test can still be used, after the difference between the two paired samples is computed and the two-sample problem becomes the one-sample problem, as discussed at the end of Subsection 2.4.3, as long as it is reasonable to assume that the

TABLE 2.4
Some upper-tail probabilities $P_{H_0}(S_+ \geq s_+)$ of the null distribution of the Wilcoxon signed-rank test statistic S_+.

n	s_+	$P_{H_0}(S_+ \geq s_+)$	n	s_+	$P_{H_0}(S_+ \geq s_+)$	n	s_+	$P_{H_0}(S_+ \geq s_+)$
5	13	0.094	11	48	0.103	16	93	0.106
	14	0.062		52	0.051		94	0.096
	15	0.031		55	0.027		100	0.052
6	17	0.109		59	0.009		106	0.025
	20	0.031	12	56	0.102		112	0.011
	21	0.016		60	0.055		113	0.009
7	22	0.109		61	0.046		116	0.005
	24	0.055		64	0.026	17	104	0.103
	26	0.023		68	0.010		105	0.095
	28	0.008		71	0.005		112	0.049
8	28	0.098	13	64	0.108		118	0.025
	30	0.055		65	0.095		125	0.010
	32	0.027		69	0.055		129	0.005
	34	0.012		70	0.047	18	116	0.098
	35	0.008		74	0.024		124	0.049
	36	0.004		78	0.011		131	0.024
9	34	0.102		79	0.009		138	0.010
	37	0.049		81	0.005		143	0.005
	39	0.027	14	73	0.108	19	128	0.098
	42	0.010		74	0.097		136	0.052
	44	0.004		79	0.052		137	0.048
10	41	0.097		84	0.025		144	0.025
	44	0.053		89	0.010		152	0.010
	47	0.024		92	0.005		157	0.005
	50	0.010	15	83	0.104	20	140	0.101
	52	0.005		84	0.094		150	0.049
				89	0.053		158	0.024
				90	0.047		167	0.010
				95	0.024		172	0.005
				100	0.011			
				101	0.009			
				104	0.005			

"difference" population has a symmetric distribution. In cases when we have two independent samples from the two populations, there are two commonly used nonparametric tests in the literature, which are described below.

Assume that (i) $\{X_{11}, X_{12}, \ldots, X_{1n_1}\}$ and $\{X_{21}, X_{22}, \ldots, X_{2n_2}\}$ are two samples from the two populations, respectively, (ii) the two samples are independent of each other, and (iii) the two population distributions have exactly

TABLE 2.5
Ranks of $\{|X_i - \widetilde{\mu}_0|,\ i = 1, 2, \ldots, n\}$ for the observed data in Example 2.7.

X_i	$X_i - \widetilde{\mu}_0$	$\lvert X_i - \widetilde{\mu}_0\rvert$	Ranks
8.7	−1.3	1.3	3
19.5	9.5	9.5	19
12.7	2.7	2.7	9.5
10.4	0.4	0.4	1
12.6	2.6	2.6	8
6.1	−3.9	3.9	13
11.1	1.1	1.1	2
0.7	−9.3	9.3	18
2.2	−7.8	7.8	16
12.3	2.3	2.3	7
11.5	1.5	1.5	4
16.2	6.2	6.2	15
16.0	6.0	6.0	14
13.1	3.1	3.1	12
−0.8	−10.8	10.8	20
18.1	8.1	8.1	17
8.1	−1.9	1.9	6
12.8	2.8	2.8	11
11.6	1.6	1.6	5
12.7	2.7	2.7	9.5

the same shape and spread and their only difference is in their means. In such cases, we are interested in testing the hypotheses in (2.33). If H_0 is true, then the values of $\{X_{11} - \delta_0, X_{12} - \delta_0, \ldots, X_{1n_1} - \delta_0\}$ and the values of $\{X_{21}, X_{22}, \ldots, X_{2n_2}\}$ should be similar to each other, and they can be regarded as two independent samples from the same population. Otherwise, their values will be quite different. Based on this intuition, to test the hypotheses in (2.33), we can consider the combined sample

$$\{X_{11} - \delta_0, X_{12} - \delta_0, \ldots, X_{1n_1} - \delta_0, X_{21}, X_{22}, \ldots, X_{2n_2}\}.$$

Let W be the sum of the ranks of $\{X_{11} - \delta_0, X_{12} - \delta_0, \ldots, X_{1n_1} - \delta_0\}$ in the combined sample. Then, when the value of W is too large or too small, this implies that the values of $\{X_{11} - \delta_0, X_{12} - \delta_0, \ldots, X_{1n_1} - \delta_0\}$ are relatively large or small, compared to the values of $\{X_{21}, X_{22}, \ldots, X_{2n_2}\}$. Consequently, the observed data provide us evidence against H_0. Again, the null distribution of W has been tabulated by many authors, including Dixon and Massey (1969). Some of its tail probabilities are listed in Table 2.6 in cases when $4 \leq n_1 \leq n_2 \leq 8$. When both n_1 and n_2 are larger than 8, its null distribution can be well approximated by the normal distribution with

$$\mu_W = n_1(n_1 + n_2 + 1)/2, \qquad \sigma_W^2 = n_1 n_2 (n_1 + n_2 + 1)/12.$$

The test using W as its test statistic is called the *Wilcoxon rank-sum test.*

TABLE 2.6
Some upper-tail probabilities $P_{H_0}(W \geq w)$ of the null distribution of the Wilcoxon rank-sum test statistic W.

n_1	n_2	w	$P_{H_0}(W \geq w)$	n_1	n_2	w	$P_{H_0}(W \geq w)$
4	4	24	0.057	5	8	47	0.047
		25	0.029			49	0.023
		26	0.014			51	0.009
	5	27	0.056			52	0.005
		28	0.032	6	6	50	0.047
		29	0.016			52	0.021
		30	0.008			54	0.008
	6	30	0.057			55	0.004
		32	0.019		7	54	0.051
		33	0.010			56	0.026
		34	0.005			58	0.011
	7	33	0.055			60	0.004
		35	0.021		8	58	0.054
		36	0.012			61	0.021
		37	0.006			63	0.010
	8	36	0.055			65	0.004
		38	0.024	7	7	66	0.049
		40	0.008			68	0.027
		41	0.004			71	0.009
5	5	36	0.048			72	0.006
		37	0.028		8	71	0.047
		39	0.008			73	0.027
		40	0.004			76	0.010
	6	40	0.041			78	0.005
		41	0.026	8	8	84	0.052
		43	0.009			87	0.025
		44	0.004			90	0.010
	7	43	0.053			92	0.005
		45	0.024				
		47	0.009				
		48	0.005				

Under the conditions described above for the Wilcoxon rank-sum test, an alternative approach to test the hypotheses in (2.33) is to use the test statistic

$$U = \sum_{i=1}^{n_1} \sum_{j=1}^{n_2} I\left(X_{2j} < X_{1i} - \delta_0\right),$$

where $I(a)$ is the indicator function of a that equals 1 if $a =$ "True" and 0 otherwise. Similar to W, the statistic U makes use of the ordering information between the two samples. If the value of U is too large or too small, then it is an indication that H_0 might be invalid. This test is often called the *Mann-Whitney test.* As a matter of fact, it can be checked that

$$U = W - n_1(n_1 + 1)/2.$$

Therefore, the Wilcoxon rank-sum test and the Mann-Whitney test are actually equivalent to each other.

2.5.4 Nonparametric Density Estimation

Assume that a population distribution has a pdf f, and we are interested in estimating f from a simple random sample $\{X_1, X_2, \ldots, X_n\}$. If the pdf f has a parametric form, then it can be estimated by parametric methods, such as the maximum likelihood estimation method discussed in Subsection 2.4.2. In this subsection, we discuss estimation of f when its parametric form is unavailable, using *kernel density estimation* (cf. Parzen, 1962; Rosenblatt, 1956; Wand and Jones, 1995) described below.

For any $x \in R$, the *kernel density estimator* of $f(x)$ is defined by

$$\widehat{f}(x) = \frac{1}{nh_n} \sum_{i=1}^{n} K\left(\frac{x - X_i}{h_n}\right), \tag{2.47}$$

where $h_n > 0$ is a *bandwidth* and K is a *kernel function.* The kernel function K is often chosen to satisfy the following conditions:

(i) $K(x) \geq 0$, for any $x \in R$,

(ii) $\int_{-\infty}^{\infty} K(x)\, dx = 1$,

(iii) $K(x)$ is a decreasing function of x when $x > 0$, and

(iv) K is symmetric about 0 (i.e., $K(x) = K(-x)$, for any $x > 0$).

Therefore, such a kernel function K itself is a probability density function. From (2.47), it can be seen that the kernel density estimator $\widehat{f}(x)$ is an average of the kernel densities $K((x - X_i)/h_n)$ at the individual observations, and the values of the kernel densities are controlled by the kernel function K and the bandwidth h_n. Usually, the kernel function $K(x)$ is chosen to be a smooth density function that satisfies the conditions (i)–(iv) above. Commonly used kernel functions include the uniform kernel function $K(u) = I(-1/2 \leq u \leq 1/2)$, the Epanechnikov kernel function $K(u) = \frac{12}{11}(1 - u^2)I(-1/2 \leq u \leq 1/2)$, and the Gaussian kernel function $K(u) = \frac{1}{\sqrt{2\pi}}\exp(-u^2/2)$ or its truncated version $K(u) = 0.6171\exp(-u^2/2)I(-1/2 \leq u \leq 1/2)$, where $I(a)$ is an indicator function defined to be $I(a) = 1$ if a is "True" and 0 otherwise. By using the Epanechnikov kernel function or the Gaussian kernel function, observations closer to x would receive more weights in defining $\widehat{f}(x)$. Selection of the bandwidth h_n can be discussed in a similar way to that discussed in the next subsection.

2.5.5 Nonparametric Regression Analysis

In the regression model (2.20) discussed in Subsection 2.4.2, the regression function is assumed to be a linear function. In many applications, the true regression function may not have any parametric form. In such cases, *nonparametric regression analysis* would be more appropriate to use. Assume that bivariate observations $\{(x_i, Y_i),\ i = 1, 2, \ldots, n\}$ of the two variables (x, Y) have been collected and they follow the regression model

$$Y_i = f(x_i) + \varepsilon_i, \qquad \text{for } i = 1, 2, \ldots, n, \tag{2.48}$$

where $\{x_i,\ i = 1, 2, \ldots, n\}$ are the design points, $\{Y_i,\ i = 1, 2, \ldots, n\}$ are observations of the response variable Y, $\{\varepsilon_i,\ i = 1, 2, \ldots, n\}$ are i.i.d. random errors, and f is the true regression function. For simplicity of discussion, let us further assume that the design interval of Model (2.48) is $[0, 1]$ (i.e., all design points are in $[0, 1]$). Then, the major goal of nonparametric regression analysis is to estimate $f(x)$ in $[0, 1]$ from the observed data $\{(x_i, Y_i),\ i = 1, 2, \ldots, n\}$.

In cases when f is continuous in the entire design interval, intuitively, observations at the design points that are farther away from a given point x would provide less information about $f(x)$, compared to those whose design points are closer to x. Therefore, to estimate $f(x)$, one natural idea is to simply average observations whose design points are located in a neighborhood $[x - h_n/2, x + h_n/2]$ of x, and then use this average as an estimator of $f(x)$, where h_n is a bandwidth. The bandwidth is usually chosen relatively small, especially when the sample size n is large. Based on this idea, $f(x)$ can be estimated by the following simple average (SA):

$$\widehat{f}_{SA}(x) = \frac{1}{N_n(x)} \sum_{x_i \in [x - h_n/2, x + h_n/2]} Y_i,$$

where $N_n(x)$ denotes the number of design points in $[x - h_n/2, x + h_n/2]$. Based on (2.48), we have

$$\widehat{f}_{SA}(x) = \frac{1}{N_n(x)} \sum_{x_i \in [x - h_n/2, x + h_n/2]} f(x_i) + \frac{1}{N_n(x)} \sum_{x_i \in [x - h_n/2, x + h_n/2]} \varepsilon_i. \tag{2.49}$$

The estimator $\widehat{f}_{SA}(x)$ should estimate $f(x)$ well because of the following two facts:

- All values of $f(t)$ for $t \in [x - h_n/2, x + h_n/2]$ should be close to $f(x)$ since f is continuous in the design interval and h_n is small. Consequently, the first term on the right-hand side of (2.49) would be close to $f(x)$.

- The second term on the right-hand side of (2.49) would be close to zero as long as there are enough terms in the summation, which is guaranteed by the Central Limit Theorem discussed in Subsection 2.4.1. Intuitively, positive and negative errors would be canceled out in this term, and consequently the average of many i.i.d. error terms would be close to zero.

The above function estimation procedure that results in the estimator $\widehat{f}_{SA}(x)$ is a simple example of data smoothing. Almost all data smoothing procedures in the regression literature involve data averaging. For any given x in the design interval, procedures that use all observations in the design interval when estimating $f(x)$ are referred to as *global smoothing* procedures. The linear regression analysis discussed in Subsection 2.4.2 is an example of global smoothing. Other procedures only use observations in a neighborhood of x and are referred to as *local smoothing* procedures. So, $\widehat{f}_{SA}(x)$ is an example of local smoothing. The two facts mentioned above about the two terms on the right-hand side of (2.49) are commonly used when studying the properties of a local smoothing procedure.

By using $\widehat{f}_{SA}(x)$ to estimate $f(x)$, all observations outside the neighborhood $[x-h_n/2, x+h_n/2]$ are ignored completely, and all observations inside the neighborhood are treated equally. A natural generalization of $\widehat{f}_{SA}(x)$, which does not treat all observations in the neighborhood equally, is

$$\widehat{f}_{NW}(x) = \frac{\sum_{i=1}^{n} Y_i K\left(\frac{x_i - x}{h_n}\right)}{\sum_{i=1}^{n} K\left(\frac{x_i - x}{h_n}\right)}, \tag{2.50}$$

where K is a kernel function that has the support of $[-1/2, 1/2]$. The estimator $\widehat{f}_{NW}(x)$ is simply a weighted average of the observations in the neighborhood $[x - h_n/2, x + h_n/2]$, with the weights controlled by the kernel function. As in kernel density estimation, the kernel function K is often chosen to be a smooth density function that is symmetric about 0 and non-decreasing in $[-1/2, 0]$, such as those listed at the end of Subsection 2.5.4. Obviously, the estimator $\widehat{f}_{SA}(x)$ is a special case of $\widehat{f}_{NW}(x)$ when the uniform kernel function is used. The kernel estimator $\widehat{f}_{NW}(x)$ was first suggested by Nadaraya (1964) and Watson (1964). So it is often called a *Nadaraya-Watson (NW) kernel estimator* in the literature, as identified by the subscript of $\widehat{f}_{NW}(x)$.

It can be checked that the Nadaraya-Watson kernel estimator $\widehat{f}_{NW}(x)$ in (2.50) is the solution to a of the following minimization problem:

$$\min_{a \in R} \sum_{i=1}^{n} (Y_i - a)^2 K\left(\frac{x_i - x}{h_n}\right). \tag{2.51}$$

Therefore, $\widehat{f}_{NW}(x)$ has the property that, among all constants, its weighted distance to the observations in the neighborhood $[x - h_n/2, x + h_n/2]$ is the smallest. This is illustrated by Figure 2.3(a), in which the solid curve at the bottom denotes the weights $K((x_i - x)/h_n)$ and the dashed horizontal line denotes $\widehat{f}_{NW}(x)$.

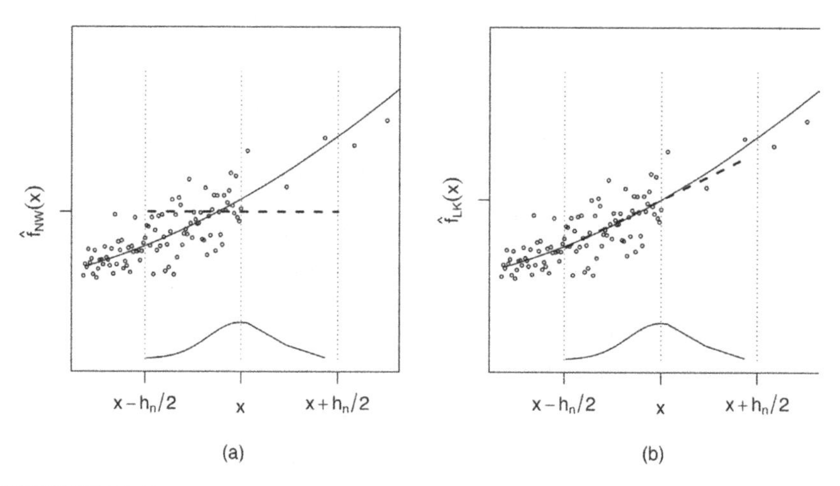

FIGURE 2.3
(a) The Nadaraya-Watson kernel estimator of $f(x)$ (dashed horizontal line) has the property that, among all constants, its weighted distance to observations in the neighborhood $[x - h_n/2, x + h_n/2]$ is the smallest. (b) The local linear kernel estimator equals the value of the dashed line at x. The dashed line has the property that its weighted distance to observations in the neighborhood $[x - h_n/2, x + h_n/2]$ is the smallest among all possible lines. The little circles in each plot denote the observations. The solid curve going through the data denotes the true regression function. The solid curve at the bottom denotes the weights that are controlled by a kernel function.

A natural generalization of (2.51) is the following minimization problem:

$$\min_{a, b_1, \ldots, b_m \in R} \sum_{i=1}^{n} \left[Y_i - (a + b_1(x_i - x) + \cdots + b_m(x_i - x)^m)\right]^2 K\left(\frac{x_i - x}{h_n}\right), \tag{2.52}$$

where m is a positive integer. Equation (2.52) is used to search for a polynomial function of order m whose weighted distance to the observed data in the neighborhood $[x - h_n/2, x + h_n/2]$ reaches the minimum. Then, the solution to a of (2.52) can be defined as an estimator of $f(x)$, which is called the *m-th order local polynomial kernel estimator*. As a by-product, the solution to b_j in (2.52) can be used as an estimator of $j!f^{(j)}(x)$, for $j = 1, 2, \ldots, m$, where $f^{(j)}(x)$ is the jth order derivative of f at x. Obviously, (2.51) is a special case of (2.52) when $m = 0$. That is, the Nadaraya-Watson kernel estimator is the zeroth order local polynomial kernel estimator, or the *local constant kernel estimator*.

In applications, the most commonly used local polynomial kernel estimator is the *local linear kernel (LK) estimator*, which is the solution to a in (2.52) when $m = 1$ and is denoted as $\widehat{f}_{LK}(x)$. This estimator is illustrated in Figure 2.3(b) by the dashed line. By some routine algebra, when $m = 1$, the solutions to a and b_1 of (2.52) have the following expressions:

$$\begin{aligned} \widehat{a}(x) &= \sum_{i=1}^{n} \frac{w_2 - w_1(x_i - x)}{w_0 w_2 - w_1^2} Y_i K\left(\frac{x_i - x}{h_n}\right), \\ \widehat{b}_1(x) &= \sum_{i=1}^{n} \frac{w_0(x_i - x) - w_1}{w_0 w_2 - w_1^2} Y_i K\left(\frac{x_i - x}{h_n}\right), \end{aligned} \tag{2.53}$$

where $w_j = \sum_{i=1}^{n}(x_i - x)^j K((x_i - x)/h_n)$, for $j = 0, 1$ and 2. Therefore, $\widehat{f}_{LK}(x) = \widehat{a}(x)$ and $\widehat{f'}(x) = \widehat{b}_1(x)$.

Compared to the local constant kernel estimator, the local linear kernel estimator defined in (2.53) has the benefit that the first-order derivative (i.e., the slope) of f would have little impact on its performance; by the definition, most of the slope effect has been accommodated in the estimation by fitting a local linear function. This benefit makes the local linear kernel estimator $\widehat{f}_{LK}(x)$ have the properties that (i) its bias would not be substantially larger when x is located in the boundary regions $[0, h_n/2)$ and $(1-h_n/2, 1]$, compared to its bias when x is in the interior region $[h_n/2, 1 - h_n/2]$, and (ii) its bias would not be substantially larger when the design points in $[x-h_n/2, x+h_n/2]$ are unequally distributed, compared to its bias when the design points in $[x-h_n/2, x+h_n/2]$ are equally distributed. As a comparison, the local constant kernel estimator $\widehat{f}_{NW}(x)$ does not have these properties.

Regarding the choice of the power m of a polynomial for the local polynomial kernel estimation, under some regularity conditions, it can be shown that: (i) the variance of a $(2k + 1)$-th order local polynomial kernel estimator is asymptotically the same as the variance of a $(2k)$-th order local polynomial kernel estimator, (ii) the variance of the $(2k + 1)$-th order local polynomial kernel estimator increases with k, and (iii) the bias of a higher order local polynomial kernel estimator is smaller than the bias of a lower order estimator. By these properties, the order of a local polynomial kernel estimator should be chosen to be an odd integer because a $(2k+1)$-th order estimator is generally better than a $(2k)$-th order estimator. In most cases, the local linear kernel estimator should be good enough among all $(2k+1)$-th order estimators because the bias reduction is limited by using a higher order estimator but the variability of a higher order estimator could be substantially larger.

The bandwidths used in the local polynomial kernel smoothing procedures control the size of the neighborhood around a given point used for data smoothing. If they are chosen larger, then the neighborhood is larger, implying that more observations are averaged for estimating the regression function at the given point, and vice versa. Therefore, the bandwidths control the amount of observations used in data smoothing. For this reason, they are often called *smoothing parameters.* If they are chosen too large, then the estimated regression function would become too smooth to capture local features of the true regression function, in which case we say that the estimator *oversmooths* the data. If the bandwidths are chosen too small, then the estimated regression function would capture too many details of the data, some of which are just noise, in which case the estimator *undersmooths* the data.

There are several existing procedures in the literature for choosing the bandwidths properly. We next introduce three of them: the cross-validation (CV) procedure, the Mallow's C_p criterion, and the plug-in algorithm. For simplicity, they are introduced only in the case of local linear kernel smoothing. Actually, these procedures are general and can be used for selecting bandwidths and other parameters used in most data smoothing procedures.

For bandwidth selection of the local linear kernel estimator $\widehat{f}_{LK}$, a natural criterion is the following residual mean squares (RMS):

$$\text{RMS}(h_n) = \frac{1}{n}\sum_{i=1}^{n}\left[Y_i - \widehat{f}_{LK}(x_i)\right]^2. \tag{2.54}$$

Since $\text{RMS}(h_n)$ measures the distance between the observed data and the estimator, the bandwidth h_n can be chosen by minimizing $\text{RMS}(h_n)$. However, it can be easily checked that the best bandwidth is $h_n = 0$ by this criterion, because the corresponding estimator connects all the data points in such a case and thus gets $\text{RMS}(h_n) = 0$. Obviously, this result is not what we want since no data smoothing is actually involved.

We can modify this criterion to allow for data smoothing as follows. Because $\widehat{f}_{LK}(x_i)$ is constructed by all observations in the neighborhood $[x_i - h_n/2, x_i + h_n/2]$, including Y_i, the residual $Y_i - \widehat{f}_{LK}(x_i)$ tends to be small for measuring the distance between the estimator and the data. This is a major reason why the criterion (2.54) is inappropriate for choosing h_n. As a remedy, let $\widehat{f}_{LK,-i}(x_i)$ be the local linear kernel estimator of $f(x_i)$ constructed from all observations in $[x_i - h_n/2, x_i + h_n/2]$ except Y_i, for $i = 1, 2, \cdots, n$. Then, a similar criterion to (2.54) is the following CV score:

$$CV(h_n) = \frac{1}{n}\sum_{i=1}^{n}\left(Y_i - \widehat{f}_{LK,-i}(x_i)\right)^2. \tag{2.55}$$

Consequently, the bandwidth h_n can be chosen to minimize the CV score in (2.55). This method for choosing the bandwidths or other procedure parameters is called the *CV procedure* in the literature (Allen, 1974).

We next discuss the Mallows' C_p criterion. Let $\mathbf{Y} = (Y_1, Y_2, \ldots, Y_n)'$ and write $(\widehat{f}_{LK}(x_1), \widehat{f}_{LK}(x_2), \ldots, \widehat{f}_{LK}(x_n))' = \mathbf{HY}$. Then, $\mathbf{H}$ is called a *hat matrix* in regression analysis. The Mallows' C_p criterion (Mallows, 1973) is defined to be

$$C_p(h_n) = \frac{1}{\sigma^2}\|(I_{n\times n} - \mathbf{H})\mathbf{Y}\|^2 - n + 2\,\mathrm{tr}(\mathbf{H}),$$

where $I_{n\times n}$ is the $n \times n$ identity matrix, $\|\cdot\|$ is the Euclidean norm, and $\mathrm{tr}(\mathbf{H})$ is the trace of the matrix $\mathbf{H}$ (i.e., the summation of all diagonal elements of $\mathbf{H}$). By this criterion, h_n is chosen to be the minimizer of $C_p(h_n)$.

The plug-in algorithm is based on the MSE criterion (cf., Subsection 2.4.1). It can be checked that the MSE of the local linear kernel estimator $\widehat{f}_{LK}(x)$ for estimating $f(x)$ is

$$\mathrm{MSE}\left(\widehat{f}_{LK}(x), f(x)\right) \sim \left[h_n^2 f''(x)\frac{K_{21}^2 - K_{11}K_{31}}{2(K_{01}K_{21} - K_{11}^2)}\right]^2 + (nh_n)^{-1}C(K)\sigma^2, \tag{2.56}$$

where $K_{j1} = \int_{-1/2}^{1/2} u^j K(u)du$, for $j = 0, 1, 2, 3$, $C(K) = \frac{1}{(K_{01}K_{21} - K_{11})^2}\int_{-1/2}^{1/2}(K_{21} - K_{11}u)^2 K^2(u)du$, and "$\sim$" denotes equality when certain high-order terms have been ignored on the right-hand side of (2.56). By the criterion (2.56), the optimal value of h_n that minimizes $\mathrm{MSE}\left(\widehat{f}_{LK}(x), f(x)\right)$ is asymptotically equal to the minimizer of the summation on the right-hand-side of (2.56) with respect to h_n, which has the expression

$$h_{n,opt} = \left(\frac{C_1(K)\sigma^2}{n[f''(x)]^2}\right)^{1/5}, \tag{2.57}$$

where $C_1(K) = C(K)(K_{01}K_{21} - K_{11}^2)^2/(K_{21}^2 - K_{11}K_{21})^2$. Because the quantity $f''(x)$ is unknown, the criterion (2.57) cannot be used directly for choosing h_n. One way to overcome this difficulty is to use the following iterative algorithm: (1) we assign an initial value for h_n and estimate $f''(x)$ by a local polynomial kernel estimator based on this initial bandwidth; (2) the value of h_n is updated by (2.57) after $f''(x)$ is replaced by its estimator; (3) we go back to step (1) using the updated bandwidth obtained from the previous step; and (4) steps (1)–(3) continue until some convergence criterion is satisfied. This *plug–in* bandwidth selection procedure has several different versions. For more discussions, read Härdle et al. (1992), Loader (1999), Ruppert et al. (1995), and the references cited therein.

2.6 Longitudinal Data Analysis

In medical studies, we often need to follow up individual patients multiple times to collect data on disease status, disease risk factors and so forth, in order to understand the temporal trajectory of the related variables and/or the numerical relationship among them. Such data with observations at multiple time points for individual subjects are often called *longitudinal data* in the literature. One major feature of longitudinal data is that their within-subject observations are often temporally correlated. Thus, an effective longitudinal modeling approach should accommodate the within-subject data correlation properly, which is often a major challenge in analyzing longitudinal data. In this section, some basic methods for analyzing longitudinal data that will be used by the methods discussed in later chapters are described. More comprehensive discussions on longitudinal data analysis can be found in books, such as Diggle et al. (2002) and Fitzmaurice et al. (2011).

2.6.1 Linear Mixed-Effects Modeling

Let Y_{ij} be the observed response of the ith subject at time $t_{ij} \in [0,1]$, for $j = 1, 2, \ldots, n_i$ and $i = 1, 2, \ldots, n$. For a given subject, let us assume that the response variable Y has a linear trend over time. But, different subjects are allowed to have different intercepts and slopes. Then, a natural model for describing such longitudinal data would be

$$\begin{aligned} Y_{ij} &= (\beta_0 + b_{i0}) + (\beta_1 + b_{i1})t_{ij} + \varepsilon_{ij} \\ &= (\beta_0 + \beta_1 t_{ij}) + (b_{i0} + b_{i1} t_{ij}) + \varepsilon_{ij}, \end{aligned} \tag{2.58}$$

where β_0 and β_1 are deterministic coefficients, b_{i0} and b_{i1} are zero-mean random coefficients, and $\{\varepsilon_{ij}, j = 1, 2, \ldots, n_i, i = 1, 2, \ldots, n\}$ are random errors. In Model (2.58), β_0 and β_1 denote the population (or mean) intercept and slope for describing the linear trend of the response variable Y over time, $\beta_0 + b_{i0}$ is the intercept of the ith subject, which has a random deviation of b_{i0} from the population intercept β_0, and $\beta_1 + b_{i1}$ is the slope of the ith subject that has a random deviation of b_{i1} from the population slope β_1. Model (2.58) is a specific *linear mixed-effects model*, in which β_0 and β_1 are the *fixed-effects* regression coefficients, and b_{i0} and b_{i1} are the *random-effects* regression coefficients. In this model, it is routinely assumed that (i) the random errors ε_{ij} are i.i.d., for all i and j, and (ii) $(b_{i0}, b_{i1})'$ are i.i.d., for all i. Thus, observations from different subjects are assumed to be independent; but, observations of a same subject at different observation times are allowed to be correlated, and the within-subject correlation is modeled using the random-effects coefficients.

In practice, usually there are covariates associated with the response variable Y. To accommodate such covariates, we can consider the following more general linear mixed-effects model:

$$Y_{ij} = \mathbf{X}_{ij}'\boldsymbol{\beta} + \mathbf{Z}_{ij}'\mathbf{b}_i + \varepsilon_{ij}, \quad \text{for } j = 1, 2, \ldots, n_i, i = 1, 2, \ldots, n, \tag{2.59}$$

where $\mathbf{X}$ is a p-dimensional fixed-effects covariate vector, $\mathbf{X}_{ij}$ is the value of $\mathbf{X}$ for the ith subject at time t_{ij}, $\boldsymbol{\beta}$ is the p-dimensional fixed-effects coefficient vector, $\mathbf{Z}$ is a q-dimensional random-effects covariate vector, $\mathbf{Z}_{ij}$ is the value of $\mathbf{Z}$ for the ith subject at time t_{ij}, and $\mathbf{b}_i$ is the q-dimensional random-effects coefficient vector for the ith subject. In Model (2.59), it is conventionally assumed that $\{\mathbf{b}_i, i = 1, 2, \ldots, n\}$ are i.i.d. with the common distribution $N_q(\mathbf{0}, \Sigma_b)$, and $\{\varepsilon_{ij}, j = 1, 2, \ldots, n_i, i = 1, 2, \ldots, n\}$ are i.i.d. with the common distribution $N(0, \sigma^2)$. Obviously, Model (2.58) is a special case of Model (2.59) when $p = q = 2$, $\mathbf{X}_{ij}' = (1, t_{ij})$ and $\mathbf{Z}_{ij}' = (1, t_{ij})$. Model (2.59) can be estimated by the maximum likelihood estimation procedure discussed in Subsection 2.4.2 under the conventional model assumptions given above, which can be accomplished by using the *R*-package **lme4** (Bates et al., 2020).

In the observed longitudinal data $\{(t_{ij}, \mathbf{X}_{ij}, \mathbf{Z}_{ij}, Y_{ij}), j = 1, 2, \ldots, n_i, i = 1, 2, \ldots, n\}$, some values might be missing for various reasons. This is the *missing value* problem in the literature. For instance, at t_{11}, the value of Y_{11} might be un-recorded for the first subject, although the values of $\mathbf{X}_{11}$ and $\mathbf{Z}_{11}$ are both available. In such cases, all observed data of the first subject at time t_{11} can be removed from data analysis; but, this simple method to handle missing values would result in loss of much useful information in the observed data. To avoid information loss, some *missing value imputation* methods have been developed in the literature (Carpenter and Kenward, 2013; Rubin, 1987) for replacing the missing values in the observed data by some sensible values so that all observed data can be used in data analysis. For Model (2.59), it should be noted that observation times $\{t_{ij}\}$ and their numbers $\{n_i\}$ are allowed to be different for different subjects. This flexibility greatly reduces the burden to handle missing values. For a given subject, if some variables used in the model are observed at a specific time point while the observations of some others are missing, then the missing values need to be properly imputed. In practice, the missing values in the related variables could be *missing completely at random* (e.g., due to negligence during data recording or data entry), *missing at random* (e.g., missingness in blood pressure could be random given a patient's age and gender), or *missing not at random* (e.g., status of a disease may be more likely to be missing for a patient without the disease). To accommodate these different kinds of missing values, many imputation methods are available (van Buuren, 2018; Rubin, 1987). One popular method is the *multiple imputation* approach that can be accomplished by using the *R*-package **mice** (van Buuren and Groothuis-Oudshoorn, 2011).

2.6.2 Nonparametric Mixed-Effects Modeling

In Model (2.59), the functional relationship between the response variable Y and the covariates $\mathbf{X}$ and $\mathbf{Z}$ is assumed to be linear, which could be too restrictive for certain applications. To overcome this limitation, several *non-parametric mixed-effects modeling* approaches have been developed in the literature (e.g., Lin and Carroll, 2000; Rice and Wu, 2001; Shi et al., 1996; Wu and Zhang, 2002). In this subsection, we briefly introduce the method discussed in Qiu et al. (2010).

To simplify the presentation, we choose to describe the method in cases with no covariates, and the described method can be generalized to cases with covariates. In the observed longitudinal data, assume that there are longitudinal observations of n subjects, the observed response variable of the ith subject at time $t_{ij} \in [0,1]$ is Y_{ij}, and it follows the model

$$Y_{ij} = f(t_{ij}) + g_i(t_{ij}) + \varepsilon_{ij}, \quad \text{for } j = 1, 2, \ldots, n_i, \; i = 1, 2, \ldots, n, \tag{2.60}$$

where $f(t)$ is the population mean function of the longitudinal response, $g_i(t)$ is a random function describing the deviation of the mean function of the ith subject from the population mean function, $f(t_{ij})$ and $g_i(t_{ij})$ are the values of $f(t)$ and $g_i(t)$ at t_{ij}, and $\{\varepsilon_{ij}, j = 1, 2, \ldots, n_i, i = 1, 2, \ldots, n\}$ are i.i.d. random errors with mean 0 and variance σ^2. In Model (2.60), $f(t_{ij})$ is considered as the fixed-effects term, $g_i(t_{ij})$ is the random-effects term, it is routinely assumed that the random-effects $\{g_i(t_{ij})\}$ and the random errors $\{\varepsilon_{ij}\}$ are independent of each other, and $\{g_i(t), t \in [0,1]\}$, for each i, is a realization of a mean 0 random process with the covariance function

$$\gamma(t', t'') = \mathrm{E}[g_i(t')g_i(t'')], \quad \text{for } t', t'' \in [0,1].$$

Model (2.60) does not require any parametric forms for describing the functions $f(t)$ and $g_i(t)$, although these functions are usually assumed to be continuous in $[0,1]$. It does not impose a parametric form on the random error distribution either. Therefore, it is fairly flexible.

Wu and Zhang (2002) suggested a method for estimating Model (2.60) by combining the linear mixed-effects modeling (cf., Subsection 2.6.1) and the local linear kernel smoothing (cf., Subsection 2.5.5). They demonstrated that their estimator of the population mean function $f(t)$ was often more efficient than some alternative estimators in terms of the mean squared errors. This model estimation method is briefly described below.

At a given time point $t \in [0,1]$, the functions $f(t)$ and $g_i(t)$ can be estimated by solving the following minimization problem:

$$\min_{\boldsymbol{\beta}, \boldsymbol{\alpha}_i, \mathbf{D}, \sigma^2} \sum_{i=1}^{n} \left\{ \frac{1}{\sigma^2} \sum_{j=1}^{n_i} \left[Y_{ij} - \boldsymbol{z}'_{ij}(\boldsymbol{\beta} + \boldsymbol{\alpha}_i) \right]^2 K_h(x_{ij} - s) \right. \tag{2.61}$$
$$\left. + \boldsymbol{\alpha}_i^T \mathbf{D}^{-1} \boldsymbol{\alpha}_i + \log |\mathbf{D}| + n_i \log(\sigma^2) \right\},$$

where $K_h(\cdot) = K(\cdot/h)/h$, $K(\cdot)$ is a symmetric density kernel function, h is a bandwidth, $\boldsymbol{z}'_{ij} = (1, t_{ij} - t)$, $\boldsymbol{\beta}$ is a deterministic two-dimensional coefficient vector, and $\boldsymbol{\alpha}_i \sim (\mathbf{0}, \mathbf{D})$ is a two-dimensional random coefficient vector. The minimization problem (2.61) can be solved by using the iterative algorithm described below.

Step 1. Set the initial values for $\mathbf{D}$ and σ^2, denoted as $\mathbf{D}_{(\mathbf{0})}$ and $\sigma^2_{(0)}$.

Step 2. At the kth iteration, for $k \geq 0$, compute the estimates of $\boldsymbol{\beta}$ and $\boldsymbol{\alpha}_i$ by solving the so-called mixed-model equation (Davidian and Giltinan, 1995; Wu and Zhang, 2002), and the resulting estimates are

$$\begin{aligned}
\widehat{\boldsymbol{\beta}}^{(k)} &= \left(\sum_{i=1}^{m} \boldsymbol{Z}_i'\boldsymbol{\Sigma}_i\boldsymbol{Z}_i\right)^{-1} \sum_{i=1}^{m} \boldsymbol{Z}_i'\boldsymbol{\Sigma}_i\boldsymbol{Y}_i, \\
\widehat{\boldsymbol{\alpha}}_i^{(k)} &= \left(\boldsymbol{Z}_i'\mathbf{K}_i\boldsymbol{Z}_i + \sigma^2_{(k)}[\mathbf{D}_{(k)}]^{-1}\right)^{-1} \boldsymbol{Z}_i'\mathbf{K}_i\left(\boldsymbol{y}_i - \boldsymbol{Z}_i\widehat{\boldsymbol{\beta}}^{(k)}\right),
\end{aligned}$$

where $\boldsymbol{Z}_i = (\boldsymbol{z}_{i1}', \boldsymbol{z}_{i2}', \ldots, \boldsymbol{z}_{in_i}')'$, $\boldsymbol{Y}_i = (Y_{i1}, Y_{i2}, \ldots, Y_{in_i})'$, $\boldsymbol{\Sigma}_i = (\boldsymbol{Z}_i\mathbf{D}_{(k)}\boldsymbol{Z}_i' + \sigma^2_{(k)}\mathbf{K}_i^{-1})^{-1}$ and $\mathbf{K}_i = \text{diag}\{K_h(t_{i1}-t), K_h(t_{i2}-t), \ldots, K_h(t_{in_i}-t)\}$.

Step 3. Based on $\widehat{\boldsymbol{\beta}}^{(k)}$ and $\widehat{\boldsymbol{\alpha}}_i^{(k)}$, update the estimates of $\mathbf{D}$ and σ^2 by

$$\begin{aligned}
\mathbf{D}_{(k+1)} &= \frac{1}{n}\sum_{i=1}^{n} \widehat{\boldsymbol{\alpha}}_i^{(k)}[\widehat{\boldsymbol{\alpha}}_i^{(k)}]' \\
\sigma^2_{(k+1)} &= \frac{1}{n}\sum_{i=1}^{n}\frac{1}{n_i}\left[\mathbf{Y}_i - \boldsymbol{Z}_i\left(\widehat{\boldsymbol{\beta}}^{(k)} + \widehat{\boldsymbol{\alpha}}_i^{(k)}\right)\right]'\mathbf{K}_i\left[\boldsymbol{y}_i - \boldsymbol{Z}_i\left(\widehat{\boldsymbol{\beta}}^{(k)} + \widehat{\boldsymbol{\alpha}}_i^{(k)}\right)\right].
\end{aligned}$$

Step 4. Repeat Steps 2–3 until the following stopping condition is satisfied:

$$\|\mathbf{D}_{(l)} - \mathbf{D}_{(l-1)})\|_1 / \|\mathbf{D}_{(l-1)}\|_1 \leq \epsilon,$$

where $\epsilon > 0$ is a pre-specified small positive number (e.g., $\epsilon = 10^{-4}$), and $\|\mathbf{A}\|_1$ denotes the summation of the absolute values of all elements of $\mathbf{A}$. If the above stopping condition is satisfied, then the algorithm stops at the lth iteration.

In Step 1 of the above iterative procedure, the initial values of $\mathbf{D}$ and σ^2 should be chosen properly. A simple but effective choice for these initial values is to set $\mathbf{D}_{(0)}$ to be the identity matrix and set

$$\sigma^2_{(0)} = \frac{1}{n}\sum_{i=1}^{n}\frac{1}{n_i}\sum_{j=1}^{n_i}\left[Y_{ij} - \widehat{f}_P(t_{ij})\right]^2,$$

where $\widehat{f}_P(t_{ij})$ is the standard local linear kernel estimator of $f(t_{ij})$ computed from the pooled observed data of all subjects, without considering the random-effects.

After obtaining estimates of $\boldsymbol{\beta}$ and $\boldsymbol{\alpha}_i$ using (2.61), we define

$$\widehat{f}(t) = \boldsymbol{e}_1'\widehat{\boldsymbol{\beta}}, \;\; \widehat{g}_i(t) = \boldsymbol{e}_1'\widehat{\boldsymbol{\alpha}}_i, \quad \text{for } t \in [0,1],$$

$$\widehat{\gamma}(t', t'') = \frac{1}{n}\sum_{i=1}^{n}\widehat{g}_i(t')\widehat{g}_i(t''), \quad \text{for any } t', t'' \in [0,1],$$

where $\boldsymbol{e}_1 = (1, 0)'$. Note that the variance estimator obtained from the above iterative algorithm depends on t. Since σ^2 is a parameter that does not depend on t, it can be estimated by

$$\widehat{\sigma}^2 = \frac{1}{n}\sum_{i=1}^{n}\frac{1}{n_i}\sum_{j=1}^{n_i}\left[Y_{ij} - \widehat{f}(t_{ij}) - \widehat{g}_i(t_{ij})\right]^2.$$

In the literature, there are some alternative methods for nonparametric modeling of univariate or multivariate longitudinal data. See, for instance, Hoover et al. (1998), Lin and Carroll (2000) and Xiang et al. (2013).

2.7 Parametric Spatio-Temporal Data Analysis

For disease surveillance, observations of the incidence of a disease in concern (e.g., COVID-19) are often collected daily, weekly, or in other time units at multiple spatial locations (e.g., major medical providers in US). Such data with observations collected at multiple times and multiple spatial locations are called *spatio-temporal data* in the literature. By analyzing an observed spatio-temporal dataset, we can study how the data distribution changes over both time and space. However, spatio-temporal data are often challenging to model properly, because of their complicated structure, including the complex spatial and/or temporal data variation, latent spatio-temporal data correlation, and unknown data distribution. In the literature, there has been much discussion on spatio-temporal data modeling. Some basic parametric methods on this topic that will be used in later chapters are introduced in this section. For more comprehensive discussions on spatio-temporal data modeling, see books, such as Cressie and Wikle (2011) and Diggle (2014).

In the literature, there are a number of parametric modeling and/or Bayesian modeling approaches for analyzing spatio-temporal data. Some of them are described in this section. Because the model setups of these methods are often complicated, our description is kept brief and the related references and *R* packages are introduced so that interested readers can further explore the related methods easily when it is needed.

One group of existing methods are based on linear regression modeling, by using temporal basis functions (Lindström et al., 2014; Sampson et al., 2011; Szpiro et al., 2010). Let $Y(t, \mathbf{s})$ be the spatio-temporal response variable with observations in the time interval $[0, T]$ and spatial region Ω. It can be decomposed into two components as follows:

$$Y(t, \mathbf{s}) = \mu(t, \mathbf{s}) + \varepsilon(t, \mathbf{s}), \qquad \text{for } (t, \mathbf{s}) \in [0, T] \times \Omega, \tag{2.62}$$

where $\mu(t, \mathbf{s})$ is the mean process, and $\varepsilon(t, \mathbf{s})$ is the zero-mean residual process. The residual process in (2.62) is often assumed to be a zero-mean Gaussian process whose observations at different time points are independent of each other and whose spatial covariance structure is stationary and has a parametric form.

The mean process in (2.62) can be expressed in the following linear form:

$$\mu(t, \mathbf{s}) = \sum_{k=1}^{p} a_k X_k(t, \mathbf{s}) + \sum_{l=1}^{q} b_l(\mathbf{s}) g_l(t), \qquad \text{for } (t, \mathbf{s}) \in [0, T] \times \Omega, \qquad (2.63)$$

where $\{X_k(t, \mathbf{s}), k = 1, 2, \ldots, p\}$ are p spatio-temporal covariates, $\{a_k, k = 1, 2, \ldots, p\}$ are regression coefficients, $\{g_l(t), l = 1, 2, \ldots, q\}$ are q pre-specified temporal basis functions with $g_1(t) \equiv 1$, and $\{b_l(\mathbf{s}), l = 1, 2, \ldots, q\}$ are spatially varying regression coefficients. In (2.63), the temporal basis functions $\{g_l(t)\}$ are used to capture the temporal data variation. They can be either pre-specified deterministic functions, or computed from the observed data using a numerical algorithm, such as the one by Fuentes et al. (2006). The cross-validation procedure (cf., its description in Subsection 2.5.5) can be used to determine their number q. The spatially varying regression coefficients $\{b_l(\mathbf{s})\}$ are often assumed to be mutually independent spatial Gaussian processes with pre-specified mean and covariance structures.

Estimation of Model (2.62) can be achieved by the maximum likelihood estimation (MLE) procedure (cf., Subsection 2.4.2). An R-package **SpatioTemporal** is available to implement this modeling approach (Lindström et al., 2015).

Another spatio-temporal modeling approach describes the observed spatio-temporal data as a log-Gaussian Cox process (LGCP) (Brix and Diggle, 2001; Diggle et al., 2005). Let $Y(t, \mathbf{s})$ be the number of cases of a specific event (e.g., occurrence of a given disease) in a unit time interval and within a unit spatial region around $(t, \mathbf{s}) \in [0, T] \times \Omega$. Then, the LGCP method assumes that

$$Y(t, \mathbf{s}) \sim Poisson(R(t, \mathbf{s})), \qquad (2.64)$$

where $R(t, \mathbf{s})$ is the rate parameter at $(t, \mathbf{s})$ and assumed to follow the model

$$R(t, \mathbf{s}) = \lambda(t)\gamma(\mathbf{s}) \exp[G(t, \mathbf{s})]. \qquad (2.65)$$

In (2.65), $\lambda(t)$ is a user-supplied temporal component, $\gamma(\mathbf{s})$ is a user-supplied spatial component and $G(t, \mathbf{s})$ is a stationary Gaussian process with a pre-specified parametric covariance function. Then, the models (2.64) and (2.65) can be estimated in the Bayesian framework, or by one of a number of estimation methods discussed in Brix and Diggle (2001) and Diggle et al. (2005). Implementation of this LGCP method can be achieved using the R-package **lgcp**, in which nonparametric estimates of $\lambda(t)$ and $\gamma(\mathbf{s})$ are also provided (Taylor et al., 2013).

Some existing methods for analyzing spatio-temporal data are based on the dynamic spatio-temporal modeling (DSTM) approach described below (Cressie and Wikle, 2011; Stroud et al., 2001; Wikle et al., 2019). Let $\mathbf{Y}_t$ be the vector of spatial observations at m_t spatial locations at time t. Then, a linear DSTM model assumes that

$$\mathbf{Y}_t = \mathbf{H}_t \boldsymbol{\mu}_t + \boldsymbol{\varepsilon}_t, \tag{2.66}$$

where $\boldsymbol{\mu}_t$ is an M-dimensional latent spatial process, $\mathbf{H}_t$ is an $m_t \times M$ mapping matrix, and $\boldsymbol{\varepsilon}_t$ is an m_t-dimensional error vector. In (2.66), $\boldsymbol{\mu}_t$ can be regarded as the vector of the values of a latent spatial process at M specific locations, and M is often chosen to be a large number so that the M spatial locations are dense in the spatial domain Ω. By (2.66), each observation in $\mathbf{Y}_t$ is a linear combination of the elements in $\boldsymbol{\mu}_t$ plus a random error. For specifying the mapping matrix $\mathbf{H}_t$, there are several possible ways. In cases when $m_t \leq M$ and the observation locations at time t are a subset of the M locations associated with $\boldsymbol{\mu}_t$, the elements of $\mathbf{H}_t$ are often chosen to be 0's and 1's, with the 0's corresponding to the spatial locations in the M locations of $\boldsymbol{\mu}_t$ but not in the m_t locations of $\boldsymbol{\mu}_t$.

In the DSTM model (2.66), the error vectors $\{\boldsymbol{\varepsilon}_t\}$ at different observation times are often assumed to be independent of each other, and $\boldsymbol{\varepsilon}_t \sim N_{m_t}(\mathbf{0}, \Sigma_{\boldsymbol{\varepsilon}_t})$, for each t. The latent spatial process $\boldsymbol{\mu}_t$ is often assumed to follow an evolution model, such as the following first-order vector autoregressive (AR) model:

$$\boldsymbol{\mu}_t = \Xi \boldsymbol{\mu}_{t-1} + \boldsymbol{\eta}_t, \quad \text{for } t \geq 2, \tag{2.67}$$

where Ξ is an $M \times M$ coefficient matrix, and $\boldsymbol{\eta}_t \sim N_M(\mathbf{0}, \Sigma_\eta)$ are the random error vectors that are assumed to be independent of each other at different observation times. The matrix Ξ in (2.67) has M^2 coefficients, where M^2 is often a large number. To simplify its estimation, we often need to impose a structure on Ξ. For instance, it is common to assume that Ξ is a diagonal or band matrix.

After some parametric forms are imposed on the covariance matrices $\Sigma_{\boldsymbol{\varepsilon}_t}$ and Σ_η, Models (2.66) and (2.67) can be estimated under the Bayesian framework or by a numerical algorithm based on the maximum likelihood estimation. To this end, some *R* packages, such as **MARSS, dse** and **KFAS** have been developed.

At the end of this section, we would like to point out that the spatio-temporal data in practice often have complicated structure, reflecting the complex impact of various confounding variables, such as weather, demographic variables, life styles, and other cultural and environmental factors in cases concerning infectious diseases. Therefore, the restrictive model assumptions required by the parametric spatio-temporal modeling approaches discussed in this section can rarely be valid in practice. To address this issue, some nonparametric spatio-temporal modeling approaches have been developed in the literature (e.g., Choi et al., 2013; Kafadar, 1996; Yang and Qiu, 2022). Several recent nonparametric spatio-temporal modeling approaches will be discussed in Section 8.2.

2.8 Exercises

2.1 Assume that a random variable X has the uniform distribution on $[a, b]$, i.e., $X \sim U[a, b]$.

(i)Find the cdf of X.

(ii)Using Formulas (2.6) and (2.7), verify the mean and variance of X given in Table 2.3.

(iii)If $X \sim U[5, 10]$, find $P(7 \leq X \leq 9)$.

2.2 Most statistical software packages can compute probabilities related to a standard normal distribution. For instance, in the software package *R*, the following commands compute $P(Z < 1)$ and $P(Z < 2)$, where Z denotes a random variable that has the standard normal distribution:

```
> pnorm(1)
[1] 0.8413447
```

```
> pnorm(2)
[1] 0.9772499
```

From the above R printouts, we know that $P(Z < 1) = 0.8413447$ and $P(Z < 2) = 0.9772499$. Assume that $X \sim N(1.5, 0.5^2)$. Find the following probabilities:

(i)$P(X < 2)$

(ii)$P(X < 2.5)$

(iii)$P(2 < X < 2.5)$

(iv)$P(-1 < X < 2.5)$

2.3 For the binomial distribution discussed in Subsection 2.2.1, derive the formulas in (2.12).

2.4 If $X \sim Binomial(n, \pi)$, then $\widehat{\pi} = X/n$ can be interpreted as the proportion of successes out of n Bernoulli trials, and $\widehat{\pi}$ should be a good estimator of π (cf., the related discussion in Subsection 2.4.1). Derive the mean and variance of $\widehat{\pi}$, and give some reasonable explanations why $\widehat{\pi}$ is a good estimator of π.

2.5 Assume that 10% of people in a given population would suffer a specific disease in their lifetimes. Let X denote the number of people among 20 randomly selected people from the population who will suffer that disease during their lifetimes.

(i)Find the mean and variance of X.

(ii)Find the probability $P(3 \leq X \leq 5)$.

2.6 Consider a dataset with the following 11 observations:

$$4, 6, 7, 6, 3, 5, 8, 2, 9, 9, 100.$$

(i) Compute the sample mean of the data.
(ii) Compute the sample standard deviation of the data.
(iii) Find the sample median.
(iv) Explain why the sample mean and the sample median are quite different in this case.

2.7 Consider a dataset with the following 20 observations:

$$\begin{array}{c} 10, 12, 15, 17, 20, 20, 23, 25, 28, 30, \\ 40, 43, 45, 48, 50, 50, 59, 61, 64, 70. \end{array}$$

(i) Find the first quartile, median, and the third quartile of the data.
(ii) Find the inter-quartile range.

2.8 A random sample will be selected from a population with mean $\mu = 50$ and standard deviation $\sigma = 10$. Determine the approximate probability that $\overline{X}$ will be larger than 51 when $n = 100$.

2.9 A survey designed to obtain information on π, which denotes the proportion of smokers in a related population, results in a sample of size $n = 400$. Of the 400 people sampled, 47 are smokers.

(i) Give a point estimate of π.
(ii) Calculate a 95% confidence interval for π.

2.10 A research project aims to estimate the mean height μ of all high school students in a state. Based on historical data, it is believed that the standard deviation of these students' heights is $\sigma = 4.5$ inches.

(i) Determine how large a sample is needed in order to have the 90% confidence interval for μ shorter than or equal to 2 inches.
(ii) If a sample of size $n - 100$ yields a sample average height of 65.4 inches, calculate a 90% confidence interval for μ.

2.11 The following summary statistics are obtained from a study for exploring the relationship between a predictor x and a response variable Y:

$$\begin{array}{ccc} n = 12, & \sum_{i=1}^{n} x_i = 241.1, & \sum_{i=1}^{n} x_i^2 = 4932.8, \\ \sum_{i=1}^{n} Y_i = 14.34, & \sum_{i=1}^{n} Y_i^2 = 17.288, & \sum_{i=1}^{n} x_i Y_i = 291.55. \end{array}$$

(i) Compute the estimated linear regression model using (2.21).

(ii) In the linear regression analysis, the *residual sum of squares (RSS)*, defined by

$$RSS = \sum_{i=1}^{n} \left[Y_i - \left(\widehat{\beta}_0 + \widehat{\beta}_1 x_i \right) \right]^2 = \sum_{i=1}^{n} \left(Y_i - \overline{Y} \right)^2 - \widehat{\beta}_1^2 \sum_{i=1}^{n} (x_i - \overline{x})^2 ,$$

can be used for measuring the variability in the observed data that is not explained by the estimated regression model. The *sum of squares of total (SST)*, defined by

$$SST = \sum_{i=1}^{n} \left(Y_i - \overline{Y} \right)^2 ,$$

can be used for measuring the total variability in the observed data. And, the *coefficient of determination* R^2, defined by

$$R^2 = 1 - \frac{RSS}{SST},$$

can be used for measuring the proportion of variability in the observed data that is explained by the estimated regression model. Using the summary statistics given above, compute the values of SST, RSS and R^2.

2.12 Let μ denote the mean cholesterol level of heart attack patients under the age of 50. Some research reports claim that a cholesterol level of 240 or higher would dramatically increase the risk of heart attacks. A random sample of cholesterol levels of 16 heart attack patients who are under the age of 50 yields $\overline{X} = 247$ and $s = 14$. Using $\alpha = 0.05$, test the hypotheses

$$H_0 : \mu = 240 \qquad \text{versus} \qquad H_1 : \mu > 240.$$

In the test, what assumptions have been made so that the test is valid?

2.13 In a paired treatment-control study to evaluate the effectiveness of a weight management intervention, 10 pairs of participants were randomly recruited to the project, who were paired by their initial weights, age and gender. People in the treatment group received the weight management intervention for 6 months, while people in the control group did not. The weights of all participants measured after the 6-month intervention period were presented in the table below. Assume that the population distributions of the treatment and control groups are both normal. Use $\alpha = 0.05$ to test whether there is a significant difference between the mean weights of the people in the two populations.

Pair ID	1	2	3	4	5	6	7	8	9	10
Treatment	154	138	183	212	121	138	172	220	146	178
Control	176	146	201	255	143	156	186	231	169	196

2.14 Assume that the following data are from a population with mean μ:

5.6, 2.5, 3.7, 7.9, 11.3, 6.4, 3.2, 2.7, 0.5, 5.7, 3.2, 2.4, 7.6, 3.8, 5.7, 5.8, 3.4, 5.1, 2.2, 4.0, 4.2, 4.2, 5.5, 1.5, 1.6, 6.3, 4.3, 5.0, 8.6, 6.3, 4.3, 6.4, 4.6, 2.0, 4.4.

(i) Using the delta method, construct a 95% confidence interval for $\theta=\mu(\mu+1)$.

(ii) Using the bootstrap method with the bootstrap sample size $B = 1000$, construct a 95% confidence interval for $\theta = \mu(\mu+1)$. Compare the result with that in part (i).

2.15 For the data in the previous problem, test whether they are from a population with the distribution $N(5, 3^2)$, using both the X^2 and G^2 tests (cf., Subsection 2.5.2) and the significance level $\alpha = 0.05$. In the tests, use five intervals to group the data.

2.16 For the data in Exercise 2.14, test $H_0 : \widetilde{\mu} = 5.5$ versus $H_1 : \widetilde{\mu} \neq 5.5$, using $\alpha = 0.05$ and

(i) the sign test,

(ii) the Wilcoxon signed-rank test.

2.17 Assume that two independent samples are obtained from two populations, respectively. Observations in the two samples are listed below.

Sample 1	1.2	8.0	0.9	2.1	2.7	7.3	7.6	
Sample 2	2.6	8.5	2.4	4.5	4.6	7.7	3.8	10.3

Assume that the two population distributions have the same shape and spread. Use the Wilcoxon rank-sum test and $\alpha = 0.05$ to test $H_0 : \mu_1 - \mu_2 = -1$ versus $H_1 : \mu_1 - \mu_2 < -1$, where μ_1 and μ_2 are the two population means.

2.18 For the data in Exercise 2.14, make a plot of the kernel density estimator of the population pdf, using the Epanechnikov kernel function and the bandwidth $h_n = 1.0$.

2.19 For the Nadaraya-Watson kernel estimator $\widehat{f}_{NW}(x)$ defined in (2.50), find its bias, variance and MSE for estimating the true regression function $f(x)$.

2.20 Provide an intuitive explanation regarding the fact that the bias of the local linear kernel estimator $\widehat{f}_{LK}(x)$ would not be substantially larger in the boundary regions $[0, h_n/2)$ and $(1-h_n/2, 1]$, compared to its bias in the interior region $[h_n/2, 1-h_n/2]$.

2.21 The folder "StrokeData" included in the book webpage contains the longitudinal data of 1055 patients from a medical study. Each patient was followed 7 times. At each follow-up time, four medical indices, including the systolic blood pressure (mmHg), diastolic blood pressure (mmHg), total cholesterol level (mg/100ml), and glucose level (mg/100ml), were recorded. In this example, the total cholesterol level is regarded as a response variable and the other three variables as predictors. Estimate model (2.59) using the *R*-package **lme4**. In the model, try two different setups with $\mathbf{Z} = 1$ and $\mathbf{Z} = (1, t)'$, respectively, and compare the two sets of results.

3

Basic Statistical Process Control Concepts and Methods

As discussed in Chapter 1, both disease screening and disease surveillance problems are related to sequential monitoring of longitudinal processes. In statistics, *statistical process control (SPC)* charts provide a major statistical tool for sequential process monitoring. In this chapter, we provide a brief introduction to some basic SPC concepts and methods that will be used in later chapters. More detailed discussions on SPC can be found in books, such as Hawkins and Olwell (1998), Montgomery (2012) and Qiu (2014).

3.1 Basic Concepts and Methods of Statistical Process Control

3.1.1 Some Basic SPC Concepts

SPC was pioneered by Walter A. Shewhart and some other people in 1920s as a tool for inspection and testing of manufactured or installed products and purchased materials of the AT&T Company (Wadsworth et al., 2002). A systematic description of the first control chart was given in the book Shewhart (1931), which is now known as the *Shewhart chart.* Since then, many other control charts have been developed. Noticeable progresses include the creation of the *cumulative sum (CUSUM) chart* (Page, 1954), the *exponentially weighted moving average (EWMA) chart* (Roberts, 1959), and the *changepoint detection (CPD) chart* (Hawkins et al., 2003). These charts and some other basic SPC concepts, terminologies and methods are described briefly in this section. Because they were developed mainly for monitoring production processes in the manufacturing industry, they are discussed here in that setup as well, although they will be used mainly for disease screening and disease surveillance in later chapters.

The main purpose to monitor a production process online by an SPC chart is to distinguish *special cause variation* from *common cause variation* in the observed data of the process. Common cause variation is mainly due to random noise and considered an inherent part of the process. In cases when only common cause variation is present in the observed data, the process under

DOI: 10.1201/9781003138150-3

monitoring is considered to be in statistical control, or simply *in-control* (IC). When some components of a production process become out of order (e.g., defective raw material, improper operation by workers), the distribution of the related quality variables of the process would have a systematic shift. This type of variation is called special cause variation. When a process has special cause variation present, the process is considered to be *out-of-control* (OC). So, SPC charts are mainly for detecting special cause variation. A signal is given by them once such variation is detected. After the signal is triggered, the production process needs to be stopped immediately for us to figure out the root causes of the detected special cause variation, and the production process should be adjusted accordingly before it is re-started.

When a production process is first installed, we do not know much about its performance. In such cases, we usually let the process to produce a small number of products and then analyze the observed quality variables of these products to check whether they meet the designed requirements. If the answer is "no", then the root causes should be figured out and the process should be adjusted accordingly. After the proper adjustments, the production process is allowed to produce another small batch of products, and their quality is evaluated again. This adjust-and-control step is repeated several times until the quality of the production process meets the designed requirements. This phase of SPC is often called *Phase I SPC*. After the Phase I SPC, the production process should be able to run stably and satisfactorily. Then, we let it keep produce products, and at the same time monitor its quality constantly, by sampling the products periodically, analyzing the observed quality variables of the sampled products properly, and making a decision about the process status (i.e., IC or OC) using a control chart immediately after the observed data at the current time point are collected and analyzed. This phase of SPC is often called *Phase II SPC*, and the related sequential decision-making process is called online process monitoring. In this chapter, if there is no further specification, we focus mainly on Phase II SPC to introduce the related control charts. For Phase I SPC methods, see Capizzi and Masarotto (2013), Jones-Farmer et al. (2014), and the references cited therein. In addition, only process mean shifts are concerned here for simplicity. For control charts designed for detecting shifts in variance or other process distribution characteristics, see the related discussions in Qiu (2014). Discussions about connections and differences between SPC and jump regression analysis (Qiu, 2005) can be found in Qiu (2018b).

3.1.2 Shewhart Charts

Assume that the observed data of a production process at the nth time point are

$$X_{n1}, X_{n2}, \ldots, X_{nm}, \qquad \text{for } n \geq 1,$$

where $m \geq 1$ is an integer. When $m > 1$, the data are often called *batch data* with the batch size of m, and they are often called *individual observation data* when $m = 1$. When the process is IC, its observations are routinely assumed to be independent and identically (i.i.d.) distributed with the common distribution $N(\mu_0, \sigma_0^2)$, where the IC parameters μ_0 and σ_0 are usually assumed known. Then, a Phase II Shewhart chart gives a signal of process mean shift if

$$\left|\overline{X}_n - \mu_0\right| > Z_{1-\alpha/2}\frac{\sigma_0}{\sqrt{m}}, \tag{3.1}$$

where $\overline{X}_n$ is the sample mean of $(X_{n1}, X_{n2}, \ldots, X_{nm})$, α is a significance level and $Z_{1-\alpha/2}$ is the $(1-\alpha/2)$-th quantile of the $N(0,1)$ distribution. In manufacturing applications, α is often chosen to be 0.0027. In such cases, $Z_{1-\alpha/2} = 3$. By the Shewhart chart (3.1), a signal will be given when the sample mean $\overline{X}_n$ at the current time point n is beyond an interval centered at μ_0 with the width $6\sigma_{\overline{X}_n} = 6\sigma_0/\sqrt{m}$. That is where the name of the popular quality management system *six-sigma* (e.g., Gygi et al., 2012) comes from.

For control charts such as the one in (3.1), their performance is usually measured by the *IC average run length (ARL)*, denoted as ARL_0, which is defined to be the average number of observation times from the beginning of Phase II monitoring to a signal from the control chart when the process is IC, and the *OC ARL*, denoted as ARL_1, which is defined to be the average number of observation times from the occurrence of a true shift to a signal from the control chart. Intuitively, ARL_0 should be as large as possible, and ARL_1 should be as small as possible for detecting a given shift. Similar to the probabilities of the two types of errors in hypothesis testing (cf., Subsection 2.4.3), ARL_1 will be larger if ARL_0 is set to be larger. To overcome this difficulty, ARL_0 is often pre-specified at a given level in the SPC literature. Then, a control chart performs better if its ARL_1 is smaller for detecting a given shift. For the Shewhart chart (3.1), it can be checked that its ARL_0 equals $1/\alpha$.

Example 3.1 *Assume that 10 samples of size 5 each are generated from the $N(0,1)$ distribution, and another 10 samples of size 5 each are generated from the $N(1,1)$ distribution. These samples are regarded as observed data collected at 20 consecutive time points from a production process, the IC distribution of the process is $N(0,1)$, and the process has a mean shift of size 1 at the 11th time point. Figure 3.1 shows the Shewhart chart (3.1) with $\alpha = 0.0027$ for monitoring the observed data. In the plot, the first 10 sample means are denoted by solid dots and connected by solid lines, and the second 10 sample means are denoted by little circles and connected by dotted lines. From the plot, it can be seen that the chart gives its first signal at the 12th time point. Thus, the production line needs to be stopped after the signal for people to figure out the root causes of the signal.*

The Shewhart chart (3.1) is for detecting both upward and downward shifts. In some applications, only one-sided shifts are of our concern. For

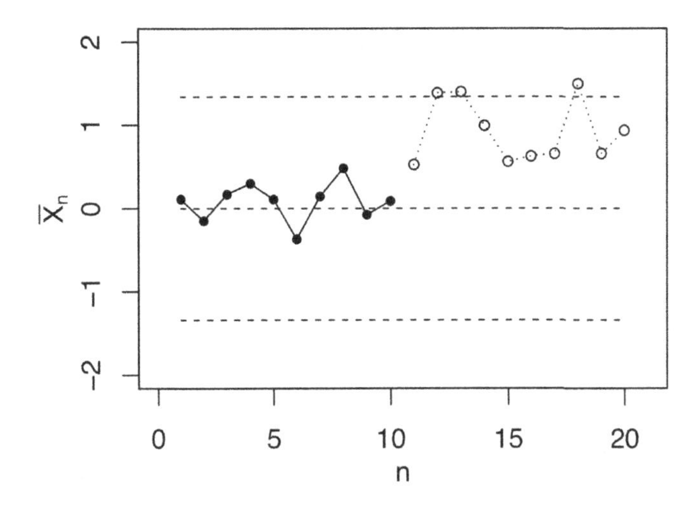

FIGURE 3.1
The Shewhart chart (3.1) with $\alpha = 0.0027$ for monitoring observed data of a process with the IC distribution of $N(0,1)$ and a true occurring at $n = 11$. In the plot, the first 10 sample means are IC and they are denoted by solid dots and connected by solid lines. The remaining 10 sample means are OC and they are denoted by little circles and connected by dotted lines. The dashed horizontal lines denote the upper control limit, the center line (i.e., $\mu_0 = 0$), and the lower control limit, respectively.

instance, for disease surveillance, we are usually concerned about upward shifts in the disease incidence rate. In such cases, one-sided Shewhart charts can be used. As an example, the Shewhart chart for detecting upward mean shifts with $ARL_0 = 1/\alpha$ would give a signal when

$$\overline{X}_n > \mu_0 + Z_{1-\alpha}\frac{\sigma_0}{\sqrt{m}}.$$

The Shewhart chart for detecting downward mean shifts can be defined in a similar way.

3.1.3 CUSUM Charts

One major limitation of the Shewhart chart (3.1) is that it uses the observed data at the current time point n only for making a decision about the process status (IC or OC) at n, and all historical data of the process have been completely ignored in its decision making process. To overcome this limitation, Page (1954) suggested the CUSUM chart, and its charting statistics are defined as: for $n \geq 1$,

$$\begin{aligned} C_n^+ &= \max\left(0, C_{n-1}^+ + \frac{\overline{X}_n - \mu_0}{\sigma_0/\sqrt{m}} - k_C\right), \\ C_n^- &= \min\left(0, C_{n-1}^- + \frac{\overline{X}_n - \mu_0}{\sigma_0/\sqrt{m}} + k_C\right), \end{aligned} \tag{3.2}$$

where $C_0^+ = C_0^- = 0$, and $k_C > 0$ is a constant that is often called the *reference value* or *allowance* in the literature (Qiu, 2014, Chapter 4). The chart gives a signal of process mean shift when

$$C_n^+ > \rho_C \qquad \text{or} \qquad C_n^- < -\rho_C, \tag{3.3}$$

where $\rho_C > 0$ is a control limit. To use the CUSUM chart (3.2)–(3.3), the constant k_C is often pre-specified, and the control limit ρ_C can then be determined to reach a given ARL_0 value. The value of k_C is usually chosen to be half of a target shift size. From expressions in (3.2), it is obvious that the CUSUM charting statistics C_n^+ and C_n^- have used all historical data in making its decision about the process status at the current time point n. For the statistic C_n^+ that is defined mainly for detecting upward mean shifts, its value is reset to 0 each time when

$$C_{n-1}^+ + (\overline{X}_n - \mu_0)/(\sigma_0/\sqrt{m}) \leq k_C,$$

i.e., when the observed data by the time n do not suggest an upward shift. Similarly, the statistic C_n^- is defined mainly for detecting downward mean shifts, and reset to 0 each time when

$$C_{n-1}^- + (\overline{X}_n - \mu_0)/(\sigma_0/\sqrt{m}) \leq -k_C,$$

i.e., when the observed data by the time n do not suggest a downward shift. This is the so-called *re-starting mechanism* of the CUSUM chart. Because of its re-starting mechanism, the CUSUM chart has been proved theoretically to be optimal under some regularity conditions, in the sense that its ARL_1 value would be the smallest, compared to the ARL_1 values of other control charts with the same ARL_0 value (Moustakides, 1986).

The CUSUM chart (3.2)–(3.3) is two-sided, and designed for detecting both upward and downward process mean shifts. If we are concerned about upward mean shifts only, then we can just use the upward CUSUM chart that gives a signal when $C_n^+ > \rho_C$. Similarly, the downward CUSUM chart gives a signal when $C_n^- < -\rho_C$. In these one-sided CUSUM charts, ρ_C needs to be chosen properly so that a pre-specified value of ARL_0 is reached. For some commonly used k_C and ARL_0 values, the corresponding values of ρ_C can be found from Table 4.1 in Qiu (2014). They can also be computed by using the *R*-package **spc**.

Example 3.2 *The dark dots in Figure 3.2(a) denote the individual observation data (i.e.,* $m = 1$*) of a process collected at the first 100 observation times. The first 50 observations are actually generated from the IC process distribution* $N(0,1)$*, and the remaining 50 observations are generated from the OC process distribution* $N(0.5,1)$*. So, the related process has an upward mean shift of size 0.5 at* $n = 51$*. To monitor the process observations, we use the upward CUSUM chart discussed above with* $k_C = 0.25$ *and* $ARL_0 = 200$*. From Table 4.1 in Qiu (2014), the corresponding value of* ρ_C *is 5.597. Then, the upward CUSUM charting statistic* C_n^+ *is computed by the related formula in (3.2), and its values are shown in Figure 3.2(b). From the plot, it can be seen that the chart gives its first signal at* $n = 56$*.*

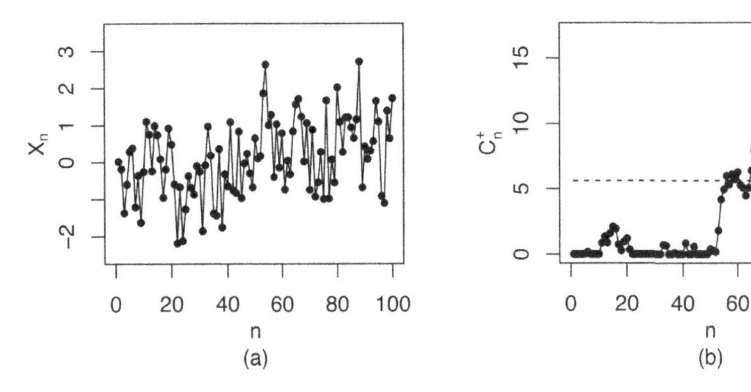

FIGURE 3.2
(a) Dark dots denote 100 process observations, where the first 50 observations are generated from the IC process distribution $N(0,1)$, and the remaining 50 observations are generated from the OC process distribution $N(0.5,1)$. (b) Dark dots denote the values of the upward CUSUM charting statistic C_n^+ defined in (3.2) with $k_C = 0.25$ and $ARL_0 = 200$, and the horizontal dashed line denotes the control limit $\rho_C = 5.597$.

3.1.4 EWMA Charts

Although the CUSUM chart (3.2)–(3.3) is effective, especially for detecting relatively small and persistent shifts (cf., Qiu, 2014, Chapter 4), it is quite complicated for us to study its statistical properties (e.g., the means and variances of its charting statistics C_n^+ and C_n^-), due mainly to the re-starting mechanism accomplished by using the "max" and "min" operations in the definition of its charting statistics (cf., (3.2)). As an alternative, Roberts (1959) suggested the EWMA chart described below. The EWMA charting statistic is defined to be

$$E_n = \lambda \frac{\overline{X}_n - \mu_0}{\sigma_0/\sqrt{m}} + (1-\lambda)E_{n-1} \qquad (3.4)$$
$$= \lambda \sum_{i=1}^{n} (1-\lambda)^{n-i} \frac{\overline{X}_i - \mu_0}{\sigma_0/\sqrt{m}}, \qquad \text{for } n \geq 1,$$

where $E_0 = 0$, and $\lambda \in (0, 1]$ is a weighting parameter. It is easy to check that $\mu_{E_n} = 0$ and $\sigma_{E_n} = \sqrt{\frac{\lambda}{2-\lambda}[1-(1-\lambda)^{2n}]}$. Then, the chart gives a signal of process mean shift if

$$|E_n| > \rho_E \sqrt{\frac{\lambda}{2-\lambda}[1-(1-\lambda)^{2n}]} \approx \rho_E \sqrt{\frac{\lambda}{2-\lambda}}, \qquad (3.5)$$

where $\rho_E > 0$ is a parameter. To use the EWMA chart (3.4)–(3.5), the weighting parameter λ is usually pre-specified, and ρ_E is determined to reach a pre-specified ARL_0 value. From (3.4), it can be seen that the EWMA charting statistic E_n is a weighted average of the current and all previous observations, and the weight of the observed data at the ith time point decays exponentially fast when i moves away from the current observation time n. In the literature, it has been shown that large values of λ are good for detecting relatively large shifts and small values are good for detecting relatively small shifts. Commonly used values for λ include 0.05, 0.1 and 0.2. For some commonly used λ and ARL_0 values, the corresponding values of ρ_E can be found from Table 5.1 in Qiu (2014). They can also be computed by using the *R*-package **spc**.

It has been verified in the literature that for the CUSUM chart (3.2)–(3.3) with a given value of k_C, we can always find an appropriate value of λ such that the ARL_1 value of the corresponding EWMA chart for detecting a given shift would be close to the ARL_1 value of the CUSUM chart. For this reason and the reason that it is relatively easy to study the statistical properties of the EWMA charting statistic E_n, the EWMA chart is popular in the SPC literature. Also, the EWMA chart (3.4)–(3.5) is designed for detecting both upward and downward mean shifts. One-sided EWMA charts can be defined easily by focusing on either positively large or negatively large values of E_n in their decision-making process, depending on whether upward or downward mean shifts are of our concern. For instance, the upward EWMA chart gives a signal when

$$E_n > \rho_E \sqrt{\frac{\lambda}{2-\lambda}[1-(1-\lambda)^{2n}]},$$

where $\rho_E > 0$ is a constant chosen to reach a pre-specified ARL_0 value. The downward EWMA chart can be defined in a similar way. See Chapter 5 of Qiu (2014) for a more detailed discussion about the issues discussed above.

Example 3.3 *For the data shown in Figure 3.2(a), the EWMA chart (3.4)-(3.5) with $\lambda = 0.5$ and $ARL_0 = 200$ is used for online process monitoring.*

From Table 5.1 in Qiu (2014), the corresponding value of ρ_E is 2.777. Then, the EWMA chart is shown in Figure 3.3, where the dotted horizontal line denotes the IC mean of 0 and the two dashed lines denote the control limits $\pm\rho_E\sqrt{\frac{\lambda}{2-\lambda}\left[1-(1-\lambda)^{2n}\right]}$. From the plot, it can be seen that the chart gives its first signal at $n = 54$.

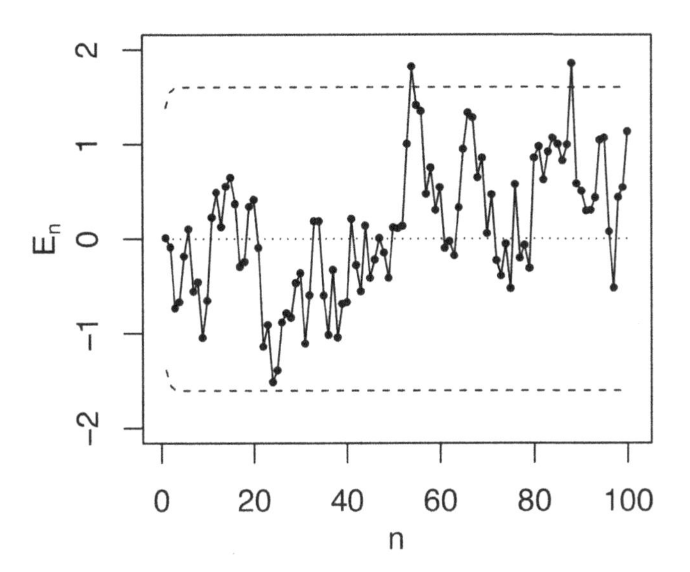

FIGURE 3.3
For the process observations shown in Figure 3.2(a), this plot shows the EWMA chart (3.4)–(3.5) with $\lambda = 0.5$ and $ARL_0 = 200$, where dark dots denote the values of E_n, the dotted horizontal line denotes the IC mean of 0, and the two dashed lines denote the control limits $\pm\rho_E\sqrt{\frac{\lambda}{2-\lambda}\left[1-(1-\lambda)^{2n}\right]}$.

3.1.5 CPD Charts

All the three charts discussed in Subsections 3.1.2–3.1.4 require that the IC parameters μ_0 and σ_0 are known, or can be estimated in advance from an IC dataset, which may cause inconvenience for their practical use. In addition, after a signal is given by these charts, the specific time at which the detected shift starts is still unknown and needs to be estimated afterwards. These limitations can be overcome by using the CPD chart suggested by Hawkins et al. (2003) described below. Assume that process observations by the current observation time n are $\{(X_{i1}, X_{i2}, \ldots, X_{im}), 1 \leq i \leq n\}$, and they follow the change-point model: for $1 \leq j \leq m$,

$$X_{ij} = \begin{cases} \mu_0 + \varepsilon_{ij}, & \text{if } i = 1, 2, \ldots, r, \\ \mu_1 + \varepsilon_{ij}, & \text{if } i = r+1, r+2, \ldots, n, \end{cases}$$

where $\{\varepsilon_{ij}, i = 1, 2, \ldots, n, j = 1, 2, \ldots, m\}$ are i.i.d. random errors with the common distribution $N(0, \sigma_0^2)$, and r is the *change-point* at which the process mean changes from μ_0 to μ_1. Then, the likelihood ratio test (LRT) statistic (cf., Subsection 2.4.3) for testing the existence of a possible change-point at r is

$$T_{max,n} = \max_{1 \leq \ell \leq n-1} \sqrt{\frac{\ell(n-\ell)}{n}} \left| \overline{\overline{X}}_\ell - \overline{\overline{X}}'_\ell \right| \Big/ \widehat{S}_\ell, \tag{3.6}$$

where $\overline{\overline{X}}_\ell$ and $\overline{\overline{X}}'_\ell$ are the sample means of the observed data before and after time ℓ, respectively,

$$\widehat{S}_\ell^2 = \sum_{i=1}^{\ell} (\overline{X}_i - \overline{\overline{X}}_\ell)^2 + \sum_{i=\ell+1}^{n} (\overline{X}_i - \overline{\overline{X}}'_\ell)^2,$$

and $\overline{X}_i = \frac{1}{m} \sum_{j=1}^{m} X_{ij}$, for each i. Then, the CPD chart gives a signal of process mean shift if

$$T_{max,n} > \rho_n, \tag{3.7}$$

where $\rho_n > 0$ is a control limit chosen to reach a given ARL_0 value. It should be pointed out that the control limit ρ_n generally depends on n. A table listing the values of ρ_n when n changes can be found in Section 6.3 of Qiu (2014). After the CPD chart (3.6)–(3.7) gives a signal, the change-point position r can be estimated by the maximizer of (3.6). Compared to the other three control charts described in Subsections 3.1.2–3.1.4, besides its two major strengths mentioned earlier in this subsection, the CPD chart (3.6)–(3.7) has a major limitation that a process mean shift could be left undetected if it is not detected early by the chart, especially when the shift size is small. In addition, computation involved in the maximization procedure described in (3.6) is quite intensive. So, recursive computation during online process monitoring by the CPD chart (3.6)–(3.7) is especially important. To implement the chart, the *R*-package **cpm** should be helpful. See Chapter 6 in Qiu (2014) for a more detailed discussion on the CPD chart (3.6)–(3.7) and some of its variants developed for handling other process monitoring problems.

As a summary, we have introduced four basic control charts for detecting process mean shifts when the process to monitor is univariate in this section. In the SPC literature, there are many modified versions of these control charts for solving various different SPC problems, including detection of scale shifts in univariate cases and detection of location and/or scale shifts in multivariate cases. In some SPC applications, quality variables of a process to monitor are binary or categorical, or they take count values. There are many control charts designed specifically for handling such process monitoring problems. Interested readers on these topics are referred to SPC books, such as Hawkins and Olwell (1998), Montgomery (2012) and Qiu (2005), for more comprehensive discussions.

3.2 Self-Starting and Adaptive Control Charts

3.2.1 Self-Starting Control Charts

The CUSUM and EWMA charts discussed in Section 3.1 assume that the IC mean μ_0 and variance σ_0^2 are both known. In practice, these IC parameters are rarely known. To overcome this difficulty, in the manufacturing industry, we usually let a production line produce a small amount of products after it is adjusted properly based on a Phase I SPC analysis (cf., Subsection 3.1.1). Then, observations of the quality variables to monitor can be collected from these products. Because the related products are produced immediately after a Phase I SPC analysis and their amount is quite small, they can be treated as IC products, and the related data are called *IC data* in the literature. Once an IC dataset is collected, the IC parameters μ_0 and σ_0^2 can be estimated from it, and they can be replaced by their estimates $\widehat{\mu}_0$ and $\widehat{\sigma}_0^2$ when the conventional control charts discussed in the previous section are used. However, Hawkins (1987) showed that the randomness in the estimates $\widehat{\mu}_0$ and $\widehat{\sigma}_0^2$ could have a substantial impact on the performance of the CUSUM chart (3.2)–(3.3). More specifically, when the size of the IC dataset is small, the estimates $\widehat{\mu}_0$ and $\widehat{\sigma}_0^2$ would have quite large variances and consequently the actual ARL_0 value of the CUSUM chart could be substantially different from the pre-specified value of ARL_0. Such impact of the IC dataset on the performance of the CUSUM chart would decrease when the IC data size gets larger. See Jensen et al. (2006), Jones et al. (2004) and Castagliola and Maravelakis (2011) for some related discussions.

In many applications, it is difficult to obtain a large IC dataset. To have a reliable process monitoring in such cases, Hawkins (1987) suggested the *self-starting CUSUM chart*. Its major idea is to constantly expand the IC dataset during online process monitoring, by combining the existing IC data at the previous time point $n-1$ with the observed data at the current time point n, in the case when the process is declared to be IC by the chart at time n. Then, the estimates of the IC parameters can be updated, using the expanded IC dataset for process monitoring at the next time point $n+1$.

Next, we briefly introduce the construction of the self-starting CUSUM chart for detecting mean shifts in cases when the process IC and OC distributions are $N(\mu_0, \sigma_0^2)$ and $N(\mu_1, \sigma_0^2)$, respectively, where all parameters μ_0, μ_1 and σ_0^2 are assumed unknown. For simplicity, assume that the batch size $m = 1$ in the observed data (i.e., cases with individual observation data), the related one-sided CUSUM chart designed for detecting upward mean shifts does not give a signal at the previous time point $n-1$, and a new observation X_n has been collected at the current time point n. So, we need to make a decision whether the process mean has an upward shift at time n. Because the process has been declared to be IC at time $n-1$, all observations collected by that time (i.e., observations $X_{n-1}, X_{n-2}, \ldots, X_1$) can be regarded as IC observations. Therefore, μ_0 and σ_0^2 can be estimated by their sample mean and sample variance, denoted as $\overline{X}_{n-1}$ and s_{n-1}^2, respectively, for $n \geq 3$. Then, it is natural to use

$$T_n = \frac{X_n - \overline{X}_{n-1}}{s_{n-1}}$$

to replace $(\overline{X}_n - \mu_0)/(\sigma_0/\sqrt{m})$ in (3.2) for constructing a CUSUM chart. In cases when $\{X_1, X_2, \ldots, X_n\}$ are i.i.d., it is easy to check that

$$\sqrt{\frac{n-1}{n}} T_n \sim t_{n-2},$$

since $X_n \sim N(\mu_0, \sigma_0^2)$, $\overline{X}_{n-1} \sim N(\mu_0, \sigma_0^2/(n-1))$, $(n-2)s_{n-1}^2/\sigma_0^2 \sim \chi_{n-2}^2$, and $(X_n, \overline{X}_{n-1}, s_{n-1}^2)$ are independent of each other (cf., the related discussions in Subsections 2.2.2 and 2.4.1). In addition, Hawkins (1969) showed that $\{T_n, n \geq 1\}$ were independent of each other. Therefore, by using some properties of the uniform distribution discussed in Subsection 2.2.2, it can be checked that the sequence of

$$Z_n = \Phi^{-1}\left[\Upsilon_{n-2}\left(\sqrt{\frac{n-1}{n}} T_n\right)\right], \qquad \text{for } n \geq 3, \tag{3.8}$$

would be i.i.d. with the common distribution $N(0,1)$, where Φ is the cdf of the $N(0,1)$ distribution, and Υ_{n-2} is the cdf of the t_{n-2} distribution. Because both Φ^{-1} and Υ_{n-2} used in (3.3) are increasing functions, any upward mean shift in the original observations $\{X_n\}$ will result in an upward mean shift in the transformed observations $\{Z_n\}$. Thus, detection of an upward mean shift in the original observations $\{X_n\}$ can be accomplished by detecting an upward mean shift in the transformed observations $\{Z_n\}$, and the latter sequence consists of i.i.d. observations with the common distribution $N(0,1)$ when the process under monitoring is IC. The resulting self-starting CUSUM chart for detecting a process mean shift can then be summarized in the box below.

Self-Starting CUSUM Chart for Detecting Mean Shifts

In cases when the IC process distribution is $N(\mu_0, \sigma_0^2)$ and the IC parameters μ_0 and σ_0^2 are unknown, the self-starting CUSUM chart for detecting process mean shifts is just the conventional CUSUM chart (cf., (3.2)–(3.3)) constructed from the transformed observations $\{Z_n, n \geq 3\}$ that are i.i.d. with the IC distribution of $N(0,1)$. This self-starting CUSUM chart requires at least 2 IC observations collected before online process monitoring.

Example 3.4 *For the data shown in Figure 3.2(a), the self-starting CUSUM chart constructed based on $\{Z_n, n \geq 3\}$ defined in (3.8) with $k_C = 0.25$ and*

ARL_0 = 200 is shown in Figure 3.4 by the dark dots. As a comparison, the conventional CUSUM chart (3.2)–(3.3) with the same values of k_C and ARL_0 is shown in the plot by the dotted line. In this example, the self-starting CUSUM chart gives its first signal at $n = 54$, and the conventional CUSUM chart gives its first signal at $n = 56$.

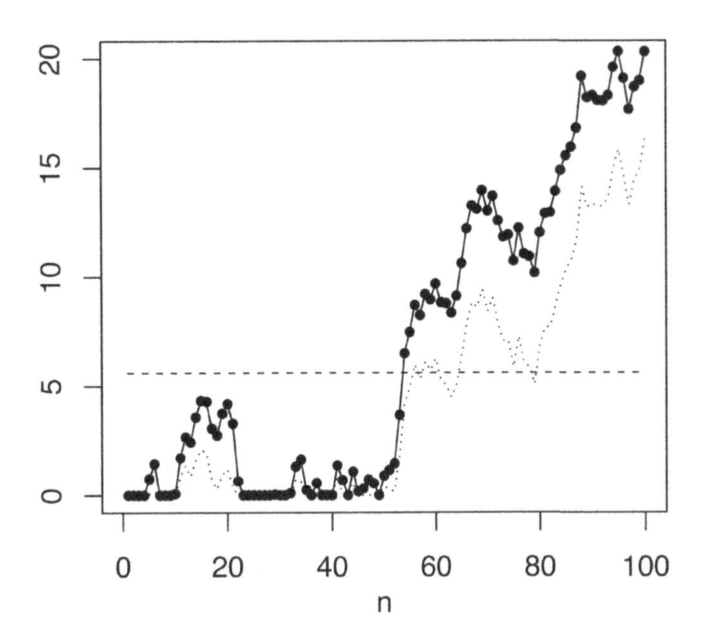

FIGURE 3.4
For the process observations shown in Figure 3.2(a), this plot shows the self-starting CUSUM chart constructed based on $\{Z_n, n \geq 3\}$ (cf., (3.8)) with $k_C = 0.25$ and $ARL_0 = 200$ (dark dots), and the conventional CUSUM chart (3.2)–(3.3) with the same values of k_C and ARL_0 (dotted line). The horizontal dashed line denotes the control limit of $\rho_C = 5.597$.

As pointed out in Section 4.5 of Qiu (2014), the self-starting CUSUM chart can indeed detect mean shifts in an effective way without knowing the IC parameter values. However, unlike the conventional CUSUM chart whose signal of mean shift is persistent over time, the signal of mean shifts from the self-starting CUSUM chart cannot last very long, which can be explained intuitively as follows. Assume that a mean shift occurs at the time point τ. Then, when $n \geq \tau$, the mean of $X_n - \overline{X}_{n-1}$ is

$$\mathrm{E}\left(X_n - \overline{X}_{n-1}\right) = \frac{\tau - 1}{n - 1}\left(\mu_1 - \mu_0\right). \tag{3.9}$$

From (3.8), it can be seen that the mean shift affects the performance of the self-starting CUSUM chart through $X_n - \overline{X}_{n-1}$. Therefore, from (3.9), it can be seen that such an effect becomes small when $(\tau - 1)/(n - 1)$ is small, or when n is large. As n increases, the mean of $X_n - \overline{X}_{n-1}$ tends to 0, making the mean shift more and more difficult to detect by the self-starting CUSUM chart. Thus, in practice, it is important to react to the signal from the self-starting CUSUM chart quickly. Otherwise, even a persistent mean shift can be missed by it. The expression (3.9) also implies that the impact of the mean shift on the self-starting CUSUM chart would be weak when τ is small. Therefore, it is a good idea to collect a dozen or more IC observations before the self-starting CUSUM chart is used.

Self-starting CUSUM control charts are popular in the SPC literature. Besides mean shifts, they can also be constructed for detecting shifts in process variance, or in both process mean and process variance. The idea of self-starting CUSUM charts discussed above is actually quite general. It can be applied to other types of control charts, including the Shewhart, EWMA and CPD charts, whose charting statistics depend on certain IC parameters. For related discussions, see Chatterjee and Qiu (2009), Hawkins and Maboudou-Tchao (2007), (Hawkins and Olwell, 1998, Section 7.3), (Qiu, 2014, Section 5.4) and Sullivan and Jones (2002).

3.2.2 Adaptive Control Charts

The conventional CUSUM chart (3.2)–(3.3) has the parameter k_C involved. In the literature, it has been demonstrated that the chart would have some good properties for detecting a target shift of size δ when k_C is chosen to be $\delta/2$ (Moustakides, 1986). In practice, however, δ is often unknown at the time when we design the CUSUM chart. In such cases, how can k_C be chosen properly? Sparks (2000) addressed this issue carefully, and proposed the *adaptive CUSUM chart* described below. For simplicity of presentation, our description here focuses on the specific case for detecting an upward mean shift of a process with a normal IC distribution by the CUSUM chart (3.2)–(3.3) (i.e., only the charting statistic C_n^+ is used in process monitoring). In addition, without loss of generality, it is assumed that the IC mean $\mu_0 = 0$ and the IC variance $\sigma_0^2 = 1$; otherwise, the standardized observations $\{(X_n - \mu_0)/\sigma_0, n \geq 1\}$ can be used for constructing the related CUSUM chart. It should also be pointed out that Sparks' adaptive CUSUM idea is quite general, and can be applied to other cases as well.

The major idea to construct the adaptive CUSUM chart is to estimate the shift size δ recursively at each observation time, and then choose the parameter k_C accordingly. To be more specific, let us first rewrite the charting statistic C_n^+ of the conventional CUSUM chart as

$$\widetilde{C}_n^+ = \max\left[0, \widetilde{C}_{n-1}^+ + (X_n - k_C)/\rho_C\right], \qquad \text{for } n \geq 1,$$

where $\widetilde{C}_n^+ = C_n^+/\rho_C$, and $\widetilde{C}_0^+ = 0$. Then, the chart gives a signal when $\widetilde{C}_n^+ > 1$. At the nth time point, if δ can be estimated by $\widehat{\delta}_n$, then it is natural to define the charting statistic of the upward CUSUM chart to be

$$C_{n,A}^+ = \max\left[0, C_{n-1,A}^+ + \left(X_n - \widehat{\delta}_n/2\right)/\xi(\widehat{\delta}_n)\right], \qquad \text{for } n \geq 1, \qquad (3.10)$$

where $C_{0,A}^+ = 0$ and $\xi(\widehat{\delta}_n)$ is the corresponding control limit chosen to achieve a given value of ARL_0. This chart gives a signal of process mean shift if

$$C_{n,A}^+ > 1. \qquad (3.11)$$

Then, Expressions (3.10)–(3.11) define the adaptive CUSUM chart for detecting upward mean shifts. In (3.10), k_C is chosen to be $\widehat{\delta}_n/2$, which can change its value at different time points, and the control limit $\xi(\widehat{\delta}_n)$ can change its value over time as well.

To compute the shift estimate $\widehat{\delta}_n$, Sparks suggested using the following recursive formula:

$$\widehat{\delta}_n = \max\left(\delta_{min}, \lambda X_n + (1-\lambda)\widehat{\delta}_{n-1}\right), \qquad \text{for } n \geq 1, \qquad (3.12)$$

where $\widehat{\delta}_0 = \delta_{min}$, $\delta_{min} \geq 0$ is the minimum shift size that we are interested in detecting, and $\lambda \in (0, 1]$ is a weighting parameter. In (3.12), we need to specify the minimum shift size δ_{min}, so that the resulting adaptive CUSUM chart (3.10)–(3.11) is effective in detecting upward mean shifts that are δ_{min} or larger. In practice, if shifts of all sizes should be detected, then we can simply set $\delta_{min} = 0$. From (3.12), it can be seen that process observations contribute to the estimate $\widehat{\delta}_n$ through the exponentially weighted moving average $\lambda X_n + (1-\lambda)\widehat{\delta}_{n-1}$. This weighted average guarantees that more recent observations receive more weights in the average. Based on the numerical study presented in Sparks (2000), the value of λ can be chosen between 0.1 and 0.2.

To use the adaptive CUSUM chart (3.10)–(3.11), we also need to determine the control limit $\xi(\widehat{\delta}_n)$. To this end, Sparks provided formulas to approximate $\xi(\widehat{\delta}_n)$ for different ARL_0 values, based on a large simulation study. For instance, when $ARL_0 = 200$, $\xi(\widehat{\delta}_n)$ can be approximated by

$$\begin{aligned} &-4.3883 + 25.4353 \Big/ \sqrt{1 + 8.895\widehat{\delta}_n - 0.8525\widehat{\delta}_n^2} + 0.7295\widehat{\delta}_n \\ &-1.5652\widehat{\delta}_n^2 + 1.5065\widehat{\delta}_n^3 - 0.7262\widehat{\delta}_n^4 + 0.1730\widehat{\delta}_n^5 - 0.0163\widehat{\delta}_n^6. \end{aligned}$$

By the Markov chain modeling approach, Shu and Jiang (2006) provided the following alternative formula for approximating $\xi(\widehat{\delta}_n)$:

$$\xi(\widehat{\delta}_n) \approx \frac{\log\left(1 + 2\widehat{\delta}_n^2 ARL_0 + 2.332\widehat{\delta}_n\right)}{2\widehat{\delta}_n} - 1.166. \qquad (3.13)$$

One advantage of the formula (3.13) is that it can be used for all values of ARL_0. As a matter of fact, Shu and Jiang (2006) pointed out that this formula could provide an accurate approximation to $\xi(\widehat{\delta}_n)$ when $\widehat{\delta}_n ARL_0 \gg \xi(\widehat{\delta}_n)$, which would be true in many applications.

The conventional EWMA chart (3.4)–(3.5) also has a parameter (i.e., λ) involved, which should be chosen in advance. As discussed in Section 3.1, it has been well demonstrated in the literature that large values of λ are good for detecting large shifts and small values are good for detecting small shifts. But, unlike the case with the CUSUM chart, the functional relationship between the optimal value of λ and the shift size δ is unavailable for the EWMA chart, although there are some existing numerical studies that try to explore such a relationship (e.g., Crowder, 1989; Lucas and Saccucci, 1990). To overcome this difficulty, Capizzi and Masarotto (2003) suggested an *adaptive EWMA chart* by choosing λ adaptively such that the resulting EWMA chart would perform reasonably well in a variety of different situations. Because the description of this method is quite intensive, it is omitted here. Interested readers can read Capizzi and Masarotto (2003) or (Qiu, 2014, Section 5.4).

3.3 Nonparametric Control Charts

The control charts discussed in Section 3.1 are constructed based on the assumption that the distribution of the process under monitoring is normal. As pointed out in Subsection 2.2.2, normal distributions play an important role in statistics because many continuous numerical variables in practice roughly follow normal distributions and many statistical methods and theory have been developed for normally distributed random variables. An intuitive explanation about the reason why many continuous numerical variables in our daily life roughly follow normal distributions can be given by using the Central Limit Theorem (CLT) discussed in Subsection 2.4.1. For instance, a person's height could be affected by the heights of that person's parents, diet, physical exercises during the person's teenage ages and many other factors. So, by the CLT, the distribution of the person's height should be roughly normal.

In practice, however, there are many variables whose distributions would be substantially different from normal distributions. For instance, disease incidence rates and other non-negative indices are often skewed to the right. In multivariate cases, the normality assumption is even more difficult to satisfy, because this assumption implies that all individual variables should follow normal distributions and all subsets of the related variables should follow joint normal distributions. In addition, a direct conclusion of the multivariate normal assumption is that the functional relationship between any two subsets of the individual variables must be linear, which is rarely valid in practice. When the normality assumption is invalid, it has been well demonstrated in the SPC literature that the conventional control charts constructed based on the normality assumption would be unreliable to use, in the sense that their actual ARL_0 values could be substantially different from the pre-specified ARL_0 values (cf., Capizzi and Masarotto, 2013; Chakraborti et al., 2001; Hackl and Ledolter, 1991; Qiu and Hawkins, 2001; Qiu and Li, 2011a,b). As an example, Figure 3.5 presents the actual ARL_0 values of the conventional upward CUSUM chart (3.2)–(3.3) when $k_C = 0.5$, its nominal ARL_0 value is 500 when the IC process distribution is assumed to be $N(0,1)$, but the true IC process distribution is actually the standardized version with mean 0 and standard deviation 1 of the χ^2_{df} or t_{df} distribution, where df denotes the degrees of freedom. From the plot, it can be seen that the actual ARL_0 values of the chart are indeed substantially different from the nominal ARL_0 value of 500, especially when df is small. To overcome the limitation of the conventional

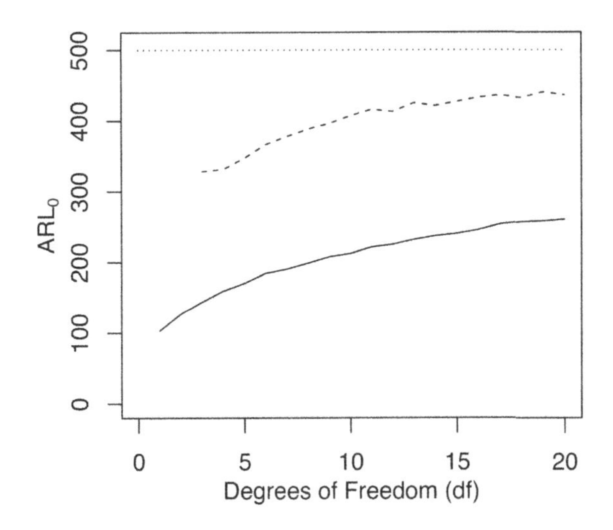

FIGURE 3.5
Actual ARL_0 values of the CUSUM chart (3.2)–(3.3) with $k_C = 0.5$ and its nominal $ARL_0 = 500$, in cases when the IC process distribution is assumed to be $N(0,1)$ but it is actually the standardized version with mean 0 and standard deviation 1 of the χ^2_{df} (solid curve) or t_{df} (dashed curve) distribution, where df is the degrees of freedom. The horizontal dotted line denotes the nominal ARL_0 value of 500.

SPC charts discussed above, many nonparametric control charts have been developed in the literature (Chakraborti and Graham, 2019; Qiu, 2014, 2018a). Some representative nonparametric control charts are introduced briefly in this section.

3.3.1 Univariate Nonparametric Control Charts

In the SPC literature, there have been many nonparametric control charts developed in recent years that do not require a parametric form to be imposed on the IC process distribution. Some of them are even distribution-free in the sense that distributions of their charting statistics do not depend on the true process distribution. In this subsection, we discuss some representative nonparametric control charts and their major properties when there is a single quality variable to monitor. For simplicity of presentation, our discussion focuses mainly on Phase II SPC, although Phase I SPC is also important which can be discussed similarly. For Phase I univariate nonparametric control charts, see papers such as Capizzi and Masarotto (2013), Jones-Farmer et al. (2009) and Ning et al. (2015).

Research on nonparametric SPC in univariate cases has a quite long history. For some early papers, see, e.g., Alloway and Raghavachari (1991); Bakir and Reynolds (1979) and Hackl and Ledolter (1991). Many methods in this area are based on the ranking/ordering information within different batches of the observed data of a process under monitoring. Let the batch of m independent and identically distributed process observations at the current time point n be

$$X_{n1}, X_{n2}, \ldots, X_{nm}, \qquad \text{for } n \geq 1.$$

Then, the sum of the Wilcoxon signed-ranks within the nth batch of observations is defined to be

$$\psi_n = \sum_{j=1}^{m} \text{sign}(X_{nj} - \eta_0) R_{nj}, \tag{3.14}$$

where η_0 is the median of the IC process distribution, $\text{sign}(u)$ is the indicator function that equals -1, 0 and 1, respectively, when $u < 0$, $= 0$ and > 0, and R_{nj} is the rank (cf., Subsection 2.5.1) of $|X_{nj} - \eta_0|$ in the sequence $\{|X_{n1} - \eta_0|, |X_{n2} - \eta_0|, \ldots, |X_{nm} - \eta_0|\}$. Obviously, the absolute value of ψ_n would be small if the process is IC, because the positive and negative values in the summation of (3.14) would be roughly the same and mostly canceled out. If there is an upward mean shift before or at time n, then the value of ψ_n will tend to be positively large. Its value will be negatively large if there is a downward mean shift. So, ψ_n in (3.14) carries useful information about potential mean shifts. Based on this statistic, Bakir (2004) and Chakraborti and Eryilmaz (2007) proposed their Shewhart charts for detecting process mean shifts, Bakir and Reynolds (1979) and Li et al. (2010) suggested two CUSUM charts and Graham et al. (2011) and Li et al. (2010) discussed the related EWMA charts. Because the IC distribution of ψ_n does not depend on the specific form of the IC process distribution as long as the IC process distribution is symmetric, most charts based on ψ_n are distribution-free in that sense.

To detect an upward mean shift in the process observations by a Shewhart chart based on ψ_n, the chart gives a signal when

$$\psi_n \geq U, \tag{3.15}$$

where $U > 0$ is an upper control limit. Similarly, the chart gives a signal of a downward process mean shift when $\psi_n \leq L$, and the two-sided chart gives a signal of an arbitrary process mean shift when $\psi_n \leq L$ or $\psi_n \geq U$, where $L < 0$ is a lower control limit. Since the distribution of ψ_n is symmetric about 0 when the process under monitoring is IC and the IC process distribution is symmetric about the IC median η_0, it is natural to choose $L = -U$. This control chart is called the *nonparametric signed-rank (NSR) chart* in the SPC literature.

The false alarm rate α^+ of the upward NSR chart (3.14)–(3.15) can be computed by

$$\alpha^+ = P(\psi_n \geq U),$$

where the probability is computed using the IC distribution of ψ_n, and the IC ARL value of the upward NSR chart, denoted as ARL_0^+, can be computed by

$$ARL_0^+ = 1/\alpha^+.$$

When $m = 5, 6, 8$ and 10, and U takes various integer values, the values of α^+ and ARL_0^+ have been computed in Bakir (2004), and they are presented in Table 3.1. From the table, it can be seen that, for a given batch size m, the upward NSR chart (3.14)–(3.15) can only reach a limited number of ARL_0 values. This phenomenon is common in cases when the charting statistic can only take a finite number of values. For the downward NSR chart, the results in Table 3.1 can also be used after the U values in the table are replaced by the $L = -U$ values. For the two-sided NSR chart, its false alarm rates, denoted as α, are 2 times the values of α^+ presented in the table, and consequently its ARL_0 values are halves of the ARL_0^+ values listed in the table.

Example 3.5 *The data shown in Figure 3.6(a) consist of 30 batches of observations with the batch size of $m = 10$. The first 20 batches of observations are generated from the t_4 distribution, and the remaining 10 batches of observations are generated from the $t_4 + 1.5$ distribution. So, these data can be regarded as observations from a production process with the IC process distribution of t_4, which is symmetric about the IC process median $\eta_0 = 0$, and the process has a mean shift of size 1.5 at the 21st time point. From the plot of Figure 3.6(a), it seems that the process distribution is indeed symmetric. Now, let us assume that η_0 is known to be 0, and we are interested in the online monitoring of the process mean. To this end, we would like to apply the upward NSR chart (3.14)–(3.15) to the observed data, and the values of the charting statistic ψ_n are then computed by the formula (3.14). The upward NSR chart (3.14)–(3.15) is shown in Figure 3.6(b) with the upper control limit of $U = 49$. By Table 3.1, this chart has the ARL_0 value of 204.0816. From*

TABLE 3.1
This table presents the values of α^+ and ARL_0^+ of the upward NSR chart (3.14)–(3.15) in various cases when $m = 5, 6, 8$ and 10.

$m=5$			$m=6$		
U	α^+	ARL_0^+	U	α^+	ARL_0^+
10	0.1563	6.3980	10	0.2188	4.5704
11	0.0938	10.6610	11	0.1563	6.3980
12	0.0938	10.6610	12	0.1563	6.3980
13	0.0625	16.0000	13	0.1094	9.1408
14	0.0625	16.0000	14	0.1094	9.1408
15	0.0313	32.0000	15	0.0781	12.8041
16	0.0000	∞	16	0.0781	12.8041
			17	0.0469	21.3220
			18	0.0469	21.3220
			19	0.0313	31.9489
			20	0.0313	31.9489
			21	0.0156	64.1026
			22	0.0000	∞

$m=8$			$m=10$		
U	α^+	ARL_0^+	U	α^+	ARL_0^+
18	0.1250	8.0000	25	0.1162	8.6059
20	0.0977	10.2354	27	0.0967	10.3413
22	0.0742	13.4771	29	0.0801	12.4844
24	0.0547	18.2815	31	0.0654	15.2905
26	0.0391	25.5755	33	0.0527	18.9753
28	0.0273	36.6300	35	0.0420	23.8095
30	0.0195	51.2821	37	0.0322	31.0559
32	0.0117	85.4701	39	0.0244	40.9836
34	0.0078	128.2051	41	0.0186	53.7634
36	0.0039	256.4103	43	0.0137	72.9927
> 36	0.0000	∞	45	0.0098	102.0408
			47	0.0068	147.0588
			49	0.0049	204.0816
			51	0.0029	344.8276
			53	0.0020	512.0328
			55	0.0010	1024.5900
			> 55	0.0000	∞

the plot, it can be seen that the first signal of the chart is given at the 22nd time point. So, the production process should be stopped at that time point for figuring out the possible root causes of the detected upward mean shift.

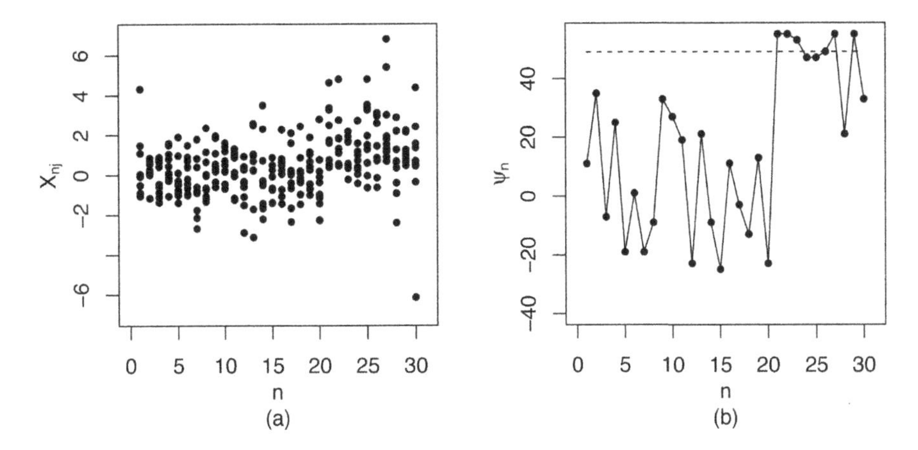

FIGURE 3.6
(a) Observed data from a production process with the IC process distribution of t_4. The data consist of 30 batches of observations with the batch size of $m = 10$. The process under monitoring has a mean shift of size 1.5 at the 21st time point. (b) The upward NSR chart (3.14)–(3.15) with the upper control limit of $U = 49$ (dashed horizontal line).

Besides ψ_n, some alternative nonparametric statistics would also be helpful for online process monitoring. For instance, Amin et al. (1995) and Lu (2015) considered using the sign test statistic (cf., Subsection 2.5.3) in their nonparametric control charts, and Liu et al. (2014) used sequential ranks. In cases when there is only one observation at each observation time (i.e., cases with individual observation data), several nonparametric control charts have been proposed using the ranking information among observations at different time points. For instance, Zou and Tsung (2010) proposed a nonparametric EWMA chart based on a nonparametric likelihood ratio test. Hawkins and Deng (2010) proposed a nonparametric CPD chart based on the nonparametric Mann-Whitney two-sample test.

All the nonparametric control charts mentioned above are based on the ranking information among different process observations. Another type of nonparametric control charts takes an alternative approach by first categorizing the original observations and then using the tool of categorical data analysis for constructing control charts (Qiu, 2008; Qiu and Li, 2011a). To be more specific, assume that the process observations at the current time point n are $\mathbf{X}_n = (X_{n1}, X_{n2}, \ldots, X_{nm})'$, where the batch size m can be 1 and the process observations are all numerical. First, we categorize the original observations into the following c intervals:

$$(-\infty, \xi_1], (\xi_1, \xi_2], \ldots, (\xi_{c-1}, \infty),$$

where $\xi_1 < \xi_2 < \cdots < \xi_{c-1}$ are $c - 1$ cut points. Let

$$Y_{njl} = I(X_{nj} \in (\xi_{l-1}, \xi_l]), \quad \text{for } j = 1, 2, \ldots, m,\ l = 1, 2, \ldots, c,$$

where $\xi_0 = -\infty$ and $\xi_c = \infty$. Then, $\mathbf{Y}_{nj} = (Y_{nj1}, Y_{nj2}, \ldots, Y_{njc})'$ has one component equal to 1, the remaining components are all 0, and the index of the component "1" is just the index of the interval that X_{nj} belongs to. The vector $\mathbf{Y}_{nj}$ can be regarded as the categorized version of X_{nj}, and its distribution can be described by $\mathbf{f} = (f_1, f_2, \ldots, f_c)'$, where f_l denotes the probability that X_{nj} belongs to the lth interval, for $l = 1, 2, \ldots, c$. When the process is IC, the distribution of $\mathbf{Y}_{nj}$ is denoted as $\mathbf{f}^{(0)} = (f_1^{(0)}, f_2^{(0)}, \ldots, f_c^{(0)})'$. Then, $g_{nl} = \sum_{j=1}^{m} Y_{njl}$ is the observed count of the original observations at the current time point that belong to the lth interval, and $mf_l^{(0)}$ is the corresponding expected count. The Pearson's chi-square test statistic (cf., (2.44) in Subsection 2.5.2) for measuring the discrepancy between the observed and expected counts is defined to be

$$\widetilde{X}_n^2 = \sum_{l=1}^{c} \left(g_{nl} - mf_l^{(0)}\right)^2 \Big/ \left(mf_l^{(0)}\right).$$

It has been verified in Qiu (2008) that a mean shift in the original process distribution would result in a shift in the distribution of $\mathbf{Y}_{nj}$ under some mild conditions. Then, based on $\widetilde{X}_n^2$, Qiu and Li (2011a) suggested a nonparametric CUSUM chart for detecting process mean shifts, as described below. Let $\mathbf{U}_0^{obs} = \mathbf{U}_0^{exp} = \mathbf{0}$ be two c-dimensional vectors, and

$$\begin{cases} \mathbf{U}_n^{obs} = \mathbf{0}, & \text{if } B_n \leq k_P, \\ \mathbf{U}_n^{exp} = \mathbf{0}, & \text{if } B_n \leq k_P, \\ \mathbf{U}_n^{obs} = \left(\mathbf{U}_{n-1}^{obs} + \mathbf{g}_n\right)(1 - k_P/B_n), & \text{if } B_n > k_P, \\ \mathbf{U}_n^{exp} = \left(\mathbf{U}_{n-1}^{exp} + m\mathbf{f}^{(0)}\right)(1 - k_P/B_n), & \text{if } B_n > k_P, \end{cases}$$

where

$$\begin{aligned} B_n &= \left\{\left(\mathbf{U}_{n-1}^{obs} - \mathbf{U}_{n-1}^{exp}\right) + \left(\mathbf{g}_n - m\mathbf{f}^{(0)}\right)\right\}' \left(\text{diag}\left(\mathbf{U}_{n-1}^{exp} + m\mathbf{f}^{(0)}\right)\right)^{-1} \\ & \quad \left\{\left(\mathbf{U}_{n-1}^{obs} - \mathbf{U}_{n-1}^{exp}\right) + \left(\mathbf{g}_n - m\mathbf{f}^{(0)}\right)\right\}, \end{aligned}$$

$\mathbf{g}_n = (g_{n1}, g_{n2}, \ldots, g_{nc})'$, $k_P \geq 0$ is an allowance constant, diag($\mathbf{a}$) denotes a diagonal matrix with its diagonal elements being the corresponding elements of the vector $\mathbf{a}$, and the superscripts "obs" and "exp" denote the observed and expected counts, respectively. Then, the nonparametric CUSUM charting statistic is defined to be

$$C_{n,P} = \left(\mathbf{U}_n^{obs} - \mathbf{U}_n^{exp}\right)' \left(\text{diag}(\mathbf{U}_n^{exp})\right)^{-1} \left(\mathbf{U}_n^{obs} - \mathbf{U}_n^{exp}\right), \tag{3.16}$$

and the chart gives a signal of process mean shift if

$$C_{n,P} > \rho_P, \tag{3.17}$$

where $\rho_P > 0$ is a control limit chosen to achieve a given ARL_0 value. The chart (3.16)–(3.17) is called the *nonparametric P-CUSUM chart* in this book, reflecting the fact that it is constructed based on the Pearson's chi-square test.

As a sidenote, it is obvious that (i) nonparametric Shewhart, EWMA and CPD charts can also be constructed based on $\widetilde{X}_n^2$, and (ii) these nonparametric charts can be used for detecting distributional shifts of processes with categorical observations as well, by simply skipping the data categorization step. From the above description about the construction of the chart (3.16)–(3.17), its IC properties depends on the $(c-1)$ IC parameters $f_1^{(0)}, f_2^{(0)}, \ldots, f_{c-1}^{(0)}$, after noting that $f_c^{(0)} = 1 - \sum_{l=1}^{c-1} f_l^{(0)}$. As well discussed in the categorical data analysis literature (Agresti, 2002), the Pearson's chi-square test statistic $\widetilde{X}_n^2$ would be most powerful for detecting distributional shifts in $\mathbf{Y}_{nj}$ when we choose $f_l^{(0)} = 1/c$, for all l. So, these parameter values are always recommended when using the chart (3.16)–(3.17). In that sense, the nonparametric charts based on the categorized data $\mathbf{Y}_{nj}$ are distribution-free. However, in practice, in order to categorize the observations, we need to determine the cut points $\{\xi_l, l = 1, 2, \ldots, c-1\}$, which are quantiles of the IC process distribution (e.g., ξ_1 is the $f_1^{(0)}$-th quantile). In some cases, these parameters can be determined easily. For example, if we know that the IC process distribution is symmetric and $c = 2$, then ξ_1 equals the IC process mean or median. But, in a general case, they depend on the IC process distribution and need to be estimated from an IC dataset, which is similar to the case with a conventional CUSUM chart where the IC mean and variance need to be estimated from an IC dataset. In that sense, the nonparametric charts based on $\mathbf{Y}_{nj}$ are not completely distribution-free, although only some IC parameters need to be determined in advance.

3.3.2 Multivariate Nonparametric Control Charts

Quality is a multifaceted concept. In most SPC applications, we are concerned about multiple quality characteristics. When process observations are multivariate, it is rare in practice that their distribution would be multivariate normal, as explained in the paragraph immediately before Subsection 3.3.1. In the statistical literature, existing methods for describing multivariate non-normal data or transforming multivariate non-normal data to multivariate normal data are limited. If a control chart based on the normality assumption is used in cases when the normality assumption is actually invalid, then its actual ARL_0 value could be substantially different from the pre-specified ARL_0 value, as demonstrated by Figure 3.5 in univariate cases. See the related discussion in Section 9.1 of Qiu (2014). Therefore, development of multivariate nonparametric control charts is important. In this subsection, we briefly introduce some existing multivariate nonparametric control charts and their major properties.

As in univariate cases, one natural idea to handle the multivariate nonparametric SPC (MNSPC) problem is to use the ranking/ordering information in the process observations. In multivariate cases, there are two types of ranking information. The *longitudinal ranking* refers to the one among observations at different time points, and the *cross-component ranking* refers to the one among different components of a multivariate observation at a given time point.

Boone and Chakraborti (2012) proposed a MNSPC Shewhart chart based on componentwise signs, described as follows. At the current time point n, assume that we have the following batch of m independent and identically distributed process observations:

$$\mathbf{X}_{n1}, \mathbf{X}_{n2}, \ldots, \mathbf{X}_{nm}, \qquad \text{for } n \geq 1,$$

where $\mathbf{X}_{nj} = (X_{nj1}, X_{nj2}, \ldots, X_{njp})'$, for $j = 1, 2, \ldots, m$. Then, for the lth component, the sign statistic is defined to be

$$\xi_{nl} = \sum_{j=1}^{m} \text{sign}(X_{njl} - \eta_{0l}), \qquad \text{for } l = 1, 2, \ldots, p,$$

where $\text{sign}(u) = -1, 0$ and 1, respectively, when $u < 0$, $= 0$ and > 0, and $\boldsymbol{\eta}_0 = (\eta_{01}, \eta_{02}, \ldots, \eta_{0p})'$ is the IC process median vector. Let $\boldsymbol{\xi}_n = (\xi_{n1}, \xi_{n2}, \ldots, \xi_{np})'$. Then, the Shewhart charting statistic is $\boldsymbol{\xi}_n' \widehat{\Sigma}_{\boldsymbol{\xi}_n}^{-1} \boldsymbol{\xi}_n$, where $\widehat{\Sigma}_{\boldsymbol{\xi}_n}$ is an estimate of the covariance matrix of $\boldsymbol{\xi}_n$. This chart is difficult to use in cases when $m = 1$ (i.e., a single observation is obtained at each observation time), due to the discreteness of its charting statistic. In addition, although Boone and Chakraborti (2012) provided a formula to compute the control limit of this Shewhart chart using the asymptotic χ_p^2 distribution of its charting statistic, this distribution is appropriate for describing the IC distribution of $\boldsymbol{\xi}_n' \widehat{\Sigma}_{\boldsymbol{\xi}_n}^{-1} \boldsymbol{\xi}_n$ only when m is large and $\widehat{\Sigma}_{\boldsymbol{\xi}_n}$ is close to $\Sigma_{\boldsymbol{\xi}_n}$. In practice, however, m is usually small (e.g., $m = 5$) and different components of $\boldsymbol{\xi}_n$ are correlated. In such cases, the IC distribution of $\boldsymbol{\xi}_n' \widehat{\Sigma}_{\boldsymbol{\xi}_n}^{-1} \boldsymbol{\xi}_n$ cannot be described well by its asymptotic distribution, and needs to be estimated properly from an IC dataset using a numerical approach (e.g., a bootstrap algorithm). (Qiu, 2014, Section 9.2) generalized the Shewhart chart discussed above to a multivariate EWMA chart as follows. First, we define the multivariate EWMA charting statistic to be

$$\mathbf{E}_n = \lambda \boldsymbol{\xi}_n + (1 - \lambda)\mathbf{E}_{n-1}, \qquad \text{for } n \geq 1, \tag{3.18}$$

where $\mathbf{E}_0 = \mathbf{0}$ and $\lambda \in (0, 1]$ is a weighting parameter. Then, the chart gives a signal of process mean shift when

$$\mathbf{E}_n' \Sigma_{\mathbf{E}_n}^{-1} \mathbf{E}_n > \rho, \tag{3.19}$$

where $\rho > 0$ is a control limit.

Boone and Chakraborti (2012) proposed another MNSPC Shewhart chart by generalizing the sum of the Wilcoxon signed-ranks (cf., (3.14)) into multivariate cases. In this chart, the sum of the Wilcoxon signed-ranks is computed for each component of the process observations, and the charting statistic is defined to be a quadratic form of the vector of these componentwise signed-rank sums. A similar MNSPC chart was discussed in Bush et al. (2010), and an

EWMA chart based on the Wilcoxon signed-rank sums is discussed recently in Chen et al. (2016).

The MNSPC charts discussed above use componentwise longitudinal ranking information in the observed data, and ignore the ordering among different components. To overcome this limitation, Zou and Tsung (2011) and Zou et al. (2012b) proposed two EWMA charts using the so-called *spatial sign* and *spatial rank*, respectively, discussed extensively in the nonparametric statistics literature (cf., Oja, 2010). Assume that a p-dimensional random vector $\mathbf{X}$ has the mean $\boldsymbol{\mu}_0$. Then, its spatial sign is defined to be

$$S(\mathbf{X}) = (\mathbf{X} - \boldsymbol{\mu}_0)/\|\mathbf{X} - \boldsymbol{\mu}_0\|$$

when $\mathbf{X} \neq \boldsymbol{\mu}_0$, and $\mathbf{0}$ otherwise, where $\|\cdot\|$ is the Euclidean norm. For a sample $(\mathbf{X}_1, \mathbf{X}_2, \ldots, \mathbf{X}_n)$ from the distribution of $\mathbf{X}$, the spatial rank of $\mathbf{X}_i$ is defined to be

$$\mathbf{r}_i = \frac{1}{n}\sum_{j=1}^{n} S(\mathbf{X}_i - \mathbf{X}_j), \qquad \text{for } i = 1, 2, \ldots, n.$$

Assume that the IC mean and the IC covariance matrix of $\mathbf{X}$ are $\boldsymbol{\mu}_0$ and Σ_0, respectively, and the "most robust" measure of scatter of the distribution of $\mathbf{X}$ defined by Tyler (1987) is A_0 which is an upper triangular $p \times p$ matrix with positive diagonal elements. Then, the EWMA charting statistic suggested by Zou and Tsung (2011) is defined to be $[(2-\lambda)p/\lambda]\mathbf{E}_n'\mathbf{E}_n$, where

$$\mathbf{E}_n = (1-\lambda)\mathbf{E}_{n-1} + \lambda S(A_0\mathbf{X}_n), \qquad \text{for } n \geq 1,$$

and $\mathbf{E}_0 = \mathbf{0}$. Zou and Tsung (2011) pointed out that this chart was distribution-free only in some special cases, and its control limit in a general case needed to be estimated from an IC dataset. The EWMA chart suggested by Zou et al. (2012b) replaced the spatial sign $S(A_0\mathbf{X}_n)$ in the above expression by a properly defined spatial rank of $\mathbf{X}_n$. For some alternative MNSPC charts constructed based on spatial signs or spatial ranks, see Li et al. (2013) and Holland and Hawkins (2014).

The control charts discussed above (e.g., the chart (3.18)–(3.19)) are all based on longitudinal ranking of the observed data. Qiu and Hawkins (2001) suggested an alternative strategy for nonparametric SPC based on cross-component ranking of the data. Let $\{\mathbf{X}_n = (X_{n1}, X_{n2}, \ldots, X_{np})', n \geq 1\}$ be the Phase II observations of a p-dimensional process with the IC mean vector $\boldsymbol{\mu}_0$ and the IC covariance matrix Σ_0, and $\boldsymbol{\mu} = (\mu_1, \mu_2, \ldots, \mu_p)'$ denotes the true mean of $\mathbf{X}_n$. Without loss of generality, assume that $\boldsymbol{\mu}_0 = \mathbf{0}$ and $\Sigma_0 = I_{p\times p}$ (otherwise, consider transformed observations $\widetilde{\mathbf{X}}_n = \Sigma_0^{-1/2}(\mathbf{X}_n - \boldsymbol{\mu}_0)$). It can be noticed that any mean shift in the observed data would violate either

$$H_0^{(1)} : \mu_1 = \mu_2 = \cdots = \mu_p$$

or

$$H_0^{(2)} : \sum_{j=1}^{p} \mu_j = 0,$$

where $H_0^{(1)}$ is related to the ranking among the p components of $\mathbf{X}_n$, and $H_0^{(2)}$ is related to their magnitudes. To detect mean shifts violating $H_0^{(1)}$, Qiu and Hawkins suggested using the antiranks (or called inverse ranks) of the p components of $\mathbf{X}_n$ (cf., Subsection 2.5.1). The first antirank A_{n1} is defined to be the index of the smallest component of $\mathbf{X}_n$ that takes its value in $(1, 2, \ldots, p)$, the last antirank A_{np} is the index of the largest component of $\mathbf{X}_n$ and so forth. While the p conventional ranks of $(X_{n1}, X_{n2}, \ldots, X_{np})$ are equally important in detecting a mean shift when no prior information is available about the shift, the antiranks would have the following properties: the first antirank is particularly sensitive to downward mean shifts in a small number of components of $\mathbf{X}_n$, and the last antirank is particularly sensitive to upward mean shifts in a small number of components of $\mathbf{X}_n$. If we do not know the direction of a shift, then the combination of the first and last antiranks should be sensitive to the shift. In other words, we can reduce the dimension of the SPC problem from p to 2 without losing much efficiency if the first and last antiranks are used for online process monitoring. Based on these properties of the antiranks, Qiu and Hawkins suggested a nonparametric CUSUM chart for detecting mean shifts violating $H_0^{(1)}$.

To detect mean shifts violating $H_0^{(2)}$, a regular CUSUM chart using $\sum_{j=1}^{p} X_{nj}$ should be effective. However, we usually do not know whether a future process mean shift would violate $H_0^{(1)}$ or $H_0^{(2)}$ in practice. So, in order to detect any process mean shift, we need to use two separate control charts designed for detecting mean shifts violating $H_0^{(1)}$ and $H_0^{(2)}$, respectively, making the entire process monitoring procedure inconvenient to use. To overcome this drawback, Qiu and Hawkins (2003) proposed a modification by using the antiranks of $(X_{n1}, X_{n2}, \ldots, X_{np}, 0)$. This modified CUSUM chart was shown to be effective for detecting arbitrary process mean shifts.

From the above description, it can be seen that the IC properties of the MNSPC charts based on the antiranks are determined completely by the IC distribution of the antiranks. In cases when the IC process distribution is exchangable in the sense that the distribution function is unchanged if the order of quality variables is changed, the IC distribution of the antiranks would be uniform in its domain. In such cases, the IC properties of the related control charts would be distribution-free (i.e., they do not depend on the IC process distribution). However, in a general case, parameters in the IC distribution of the antiranks should still be estimated from an IC dataset.

In cases when the joint distribution of $\mathbf{X}_n$ is not normal, its marginal distributions and the relationship between a pair of two subsets of the components of $\mathbf{X}_n$ could be complicated, which explains why multivariate nonnormal distributions are difficult to describe. However, if all components of $\mathbf{X}_n$ are categorical, this difficulty disappears because the log-linear modeling approach provides an effective tool for describing the relationship among categorical variables (e.g., Agresti, 2002). Based on this observation, Qiu (2008) proposed a general framework to construct MNSPC charts, by first categorizing the original process observations $\mathbf{X}_n$, and then describing the joint distribution of the categorized data using a log-linear model. If some quality variables are already categorical, then the first step can be skipped for these variables. Then, a control chart can be constructed accordingly by comparing the expected and observed counts of different categories, as discussed in Subsection 3.3.1 in univariate cases.

3.4 Control Charts for Monitoring Processes with Serially Correlated Data

It has been well demonstrated in the literature that traditional SPC charts designed for monitoring processes with independent observations at different observation times are unreliable to use in cases when serial correlation is present in the observed data (e.g., Harris and Ross, 1991; Johnson and Bagshaw, 1974). Therefore, it is important to develop control charts that can properly accommodate serial correlation in process observations. To this end, there have been some existing SPC methods developed for monitoring processes with serially correlated data. Most existing methods on this topic are based on parametric time series modeling and sequential monitoring of the resulting residuals. See, for instance, Apley and Shi (1999), Apley and Tsung (2002), Capizzi and Masarotto (2008), Montgomery and Mastrangelo (1991), Runger and Willemain (1995), Wardell et al. (1994) and more. One common limitation of these residual-based charts is that their performance is sensitive to the assumed parametric time series models. In practice, the assumed time series models could be invalid, resulting in unreliable process monitoring. In this section, we introduce a more flexible control chart suggested by Qiu et al. (2020a) for monitoring univariate processes with serially correlated data, which is labeled as QLL for simplicity. Some of its generalizations for monitoring multivariate processes with serially correlated data can be found in Li and Qiu (2020), Qiu and Xie (2022), Xie and Qiu (2023a), Xie and Qiu (2023b) and Xue and Qiu (2021).

The basic idea of the QLL method is to decorrelate process observations before a control chart is used, without imposing a parametric time series model and a parametric distribution on the observed data. To estimate the IC serial correlation structure and other IC properties (e.g., the IC mean and variance) of the process under monitoring, the QLL method assumes that an IC dataset

$$\boldsymbol{X}_{IC} = \{X_{-m_0+1}, X_{-m_0+2}, \ldots, X_0\}$$

is available before online process monitoring, which should be reasonable in many applications as discussed in Subsection 3.2.1. Then, the IC process mean μ_0 and variance σ_0^2 can be estimated by the sample mean and sample variance of the IC data, respectively, denoted as $\widehat{\mu}_0$ and $\widehat{\sigma}_0^2$. Let

$$\gamma(q) = Cov(X_i, X_{i+q})$$

be the covariance of two process observations X_i and X_{i+q} obtained at times i and $i+q$ when the process is IC, for any $i \geq -m_0+1$ and $q \geq 0$. Then, the QLL method further assumes that $\gamma(q)$ depends on q and does not depend on i when i changes (i.e., the serial correlation is stationary), and

$$\gamma(q) = 0, \qquad \text{when } q > T_{max},$$

i.e., the serial correlation is short-ranged, where $T_{max} > 0$ denotes the range of serial correlation. In practice, the correlation between X_i and X_{i+q} often decays when q increases. In such cases, $\gamma(q)$ is small when q is large. Thus, a proper value of T_{max} can be chosen such that $\gamma(q) \approx 0$ when $q > T_{max}$. Therefore, the assumption of short-range serial correlation should be reasonable for many applications, as long as T_{max} is not chosen too small. Then, $\gamma(q)$ can be estimated from the IC data by the following moment estimates:

$$\widehat{\gamma}_{m_0}(q) = \frac{1}{m_0 - q} \sum_{i=-m_0+1}^{-q} \left(X_i - \widehat{\mu}_0\right)\left(X_{i+q} - \widehat{\mu}_0\right), \qquad \text{for } 1 \leq q \leq T_{max}.$$

For convenience in notation, define $\widehat{\gamma}_{m_0}(0) = \widehat{\sigma}_0^2$. To use the above moment estimates, it is obvious that the IC sample size m_0 is required to be larger than T_{max}.

Let $\{X_n, n \geq 1\}$ be the Phase II process observations for online monitoring. They are allowed to be serially correlated as described above. Let us focus on detection of mean shifts in the Phase II process observations, although detection of a variance shift can be discussed similarly by using a proper variance monitoring chart (e.g., Yeh et al., 2010) to substitute the mean monitoring chart discussed below. As mentioned earlier, the basic idea of the QLL method is to decorrelate the Phase II process observations before a control chart is used for online process monitoring. Thus, the computational burden for data decorrelation could be heavy if a new process observation needs to be decorrelated with all of its previous T_{max} observations, especially when T_{max} is chosen relatively large. To partially overcome this difficulty, Qiu et al. (2020a) suggested using the concept of *spring length* that was originally discussed in Chatterjee and Qiu (2009). At the current time point n, let C_n be the conventional two-sided CUSUM charting statistic defined to be

$$C_n = \max\{C_n^+, -C_n^-\}, \tag{3.20}$$

where

$$\begin{aligned} C_n^+ &= \max\left[0, C_{n-1}^+ + (X_n - \widehat{\mu}_0)/\widehat{\sigma}_0 - k\right], \\ C_n^- &= \min\left[0, C_{n-1}^- + (X_n - \widehat{\mu}_0)/\widehat{\sigma}_0 + k\right], \text{ for } n \geq 1, \end{aligned}$$

$C_0^+ = C_0^- = 0$, and $k > 0$ is a constant. One important feature of the CUSUM charting statistic C_n is its re-starting mechanism discussed in Subsection 3.1.3. Namely, it will be reset to 0 each time when the cumulative information in all available process observations by the current time point n suggests that there is little evidence of a process mean shift in the sense that $C_{n-1}^+ + (X_n - \widehat{\mu}_0)/\widehat{\sigma}_0 \leq k$ and $C_{n-1}^- + (X_n - \widehat{\mu}_0)/\widehat{\sigma}_0 \geq -k$. Then, the spring length at time n is defined to be

$$T_n = \begin{cases} 0, & \text{if } C_n = 0, \\ b, & \text{if } C_n \neq 0, \ldots, C_{n-b+1} \neq 0, C_{n-b} = 0. \end{cases} \tag{3.21}$$

From the definition of T_n, it can be seen that process observations that are at least T_n time units before the current time point n would not be used for online process monitoring by the CUSUM chart (3.20) at time n. Thus, we only need to decorrelate the current observation X_n with its previous T_{n-1} observations. Here, T_{n-1} is used because T_n would be unavailable yet before data decorrelation and a decision is made about the process status at time n.

However, the CUSUM chart (3.20) and the spring length T_n are computed from the original process observations, instead of the decorrelated ones. In addition, data decorrelation at time n would depend on T_{n-1} which needs to be computed in advance. By taking all these considerations into account, Qiu et al. (2020a) suggested the following new SPC procedure for online monitoring of a sequential process with serially correlated data.

CUSUM Chart Proposed in Qiu et al. (2020a) for Online Monitoring of Processes with Serially Correlated Data

- For $n = 1$, define the standardized observation at time 1 to be $e_1 = (X_1 - \widehat{\mu}_0)/\sqrt{\widehat{\gamma}_{m_0}(0)}$. The CUSUM charting statistic at time 1 is defined to be
$$\widetilde{C}_1 = \max\left\{\widetilde{C}_1^+, -\widetilde{C}_1^-\right\}, \tag{3.22}$$
where $\widetilde{C}_1^+ = \max\{0, e_1 - \widetilde{k}\}$, $\widetilde{C}_1^- = \min\{0, e_1 + \widetilde{k}\}$, and $\widetilde{k} > 0$ is a constant. If $\widetilde{C}_1 = 0$, then define $\widetilde{T}_1 = 0$. Otherwise, define $\widetilde{T}_1 = 1$.

- For $n \geq 2$, consider the following two cases:

  (i) If $\widetilde{T}_{n-1} = 0$, then calculate e_n, $\widetilde{C}_n$ and $\widetilde{T}_n$ in the same way as that in the case when $n = 1$ discussed above.

  (ii) If $\widetilde{T}_{n-1} > 0$, define

$$\widehat{\boldsymbol{\Sigma}}_{n,n} = \begin{pmatrix} \widehat{\gamma}_{m_0}(0) & \cdots & \widehat{\gamma}_{m_0}(\widetilde{T}_{n-1}) \\ \vdots & \ddots & \vdots \\ \widehat{\gamma}_{m_0}(\widetilde{T}_{n-1}) & \cdots & \widehat{\gamma}_{m_0}(0) \end{pmatrix} =: \begin{pmatrix} \widehat{\boldsymbol{\Sigma}}_{n-1,n-1} & \widehat{\boldsymbol{\sigma}}_{n-1} \\ \widehat{\boldsymbol{\sigma}}_{n-1}' & \widehat{\gamma}_{m_0}(0) \end{pmatrix},$$

where $\widehat{\boldsymbol{\sigma}}_{n-1} = (\widehat{\gamma}_{m_0}(\widetilde{T}_{n-1}), \ldots, \widehat{\gamma}_{m_0}(1))'$. Then, the standardized and decorrelated observation at time n is defined to be

$$e_n = \left(X_n - \widehat{\mu}_0 - \widehat{\boldsymbol{\sigma}}'_{n-1}\widehat{\boldsymbol{\Sigma}}^{-1}_{n-1,n-1}\boldsymbol{e}^*_{n-1}\right) \Big/ d_n,$$

where $d_n^2 = \widehat{\gamma}_{m_0}(0) - \widehat{\boldsymbol{\sigma}}'_{n-1}\widehat{\boldsymbol{\Sigma}}^{-1}_{n-1,n-1}\widehat{\boldsymbol{\sigma}}_{n-1}$, and $\boldsymbol{e}^*_{n-1} = (X_{n-\widetilde{T}_{n-1}} - \widehat{\mu}_0, \ldots, X_{n-1} - \widehat{\mu}_0)$. According to Li and Qiu (2016), e_n is asymptotically uncorrelated with $e_{n-1}, e_{n-2}, \ldots, e_1$. This result is actually derived from the Cholesky decomposition of the estimated covariance matrix $\widehat{\boldsymbol{\Sigma}}_{n,n}$. Then, the CUSUM charting statistic is defined to be

$$\widetilde{C}_n = \max\left\{\widetilde{C}_n^+, -\widetilde{C}_n^-\right\}, \qquad \text{for } n \geq 2, \tag{3.23}$$

where

$$\widetilde{C}_n^+ = \max\{0, \widetilde{C}_{n-1}^+ + e_n - \widetilde{k}\}, \;\; \widetilde{C}_n^- = \min\{0, \widetilde{C}_{n-1}^- + e_n + \widetilde{k}\}.$$

If $\widetilde{C}_n = 0$, then define $\widetilde{T}_n = 0$. Otherwise, define $\widetilde{T}_n = \min(\widetilde{T}_{n-1} + 1, T_{max})$.

- The CUSUM chart gives a signal of process mean shift if

$$\widetilde{C}_n > \widetilde{\rho}, \qquad \text{for } n \geq 1, \tag{3.24}$$

where $\widetilde{\rho} > 0$ is a control limit.

In the CUSUM chart (3.22)–(3.24) discussed above, sequential data decorrelation and computation of the spring length are implemented simultaneously, and the charting statistic $\widetilde{C}_n$ is computed from the decorrelated data. Because each decorrelated observation e_n is a linear combination of the original process observations, its distribution would be closer to a normal distribution under some regularity conditions (cf., Wu, 2011), compared to the distribution of the original process observations. So, the CUSUM chart (3.22)–(3.24) should be more effective for monitoring the decorrelated data $\{e_n, n \geq 1\}$ than for monitoring the original data $\{X_n, n \geq 1\}$, since it has some optimal properties under the conventional assumptions that the IC process observations are independent and identically distributed with a normal distribution (cf., Qiu, 2014, Chapter 4).

In the CUSUM chart (3.22)–(3.24), the constant $\widetilde{k}$ is usually specified in advance, and the control limit $\widetilde{\rho}$ is determined such that a pre-specified ARL_0 value is reached. Because the distribution of the decorrelated data may not be exactly normal, Qiu et al. (2020a) suggested determining $\widetilde{\rho}$ from the IC data by a bootstrap procedure. Based on an intensive numerical study, it has been confirmed that the performance of the CUSUM chart (3.22)–(3.24) is stable in various cases when $m_0 \geq 2000$ and $T_{max} \geq 5$.

3.5 Exercises

3.1 Assume that we are interested in monitoring the daily operation of a hospital, and a single quality variable in concern is its daily number of patient visits. Use this example to discuss

- (i) the concepts of "common cause variation" and "special cause variation" in the observed data of the process, and
- (ii) the "in-control (IC)" and "out-of-control (OC)" process statuses.

3.2 Assume that we have collected the following 20 observations from a process whose IC distribution is $N(0, 1)$:

n	1	2	3	4	5	6	7	8
X_n	1.68	−0.15	−0.76	−1.31	−1.23	0.83	0.51	−0.26
n	9	10	11	12	13	14	15	16
X_n	−0.50	−0.62	1.20	2.19	1.77	1.40	2.61	−0.19
n	17	18	19	20				
X_n	1.88	2.45	1.55	1.29				

- (i) Use the Shewhart chart (3.1) with $m = 1$ and $\alpha = 0.005$ to detect a potential process mean shift. Does your Shewhart chart give any signal? What is the ARL_0 value of this chart?
- (ii) Use the CUSUM chart (3.2)–(3.3) with $k_C = 0.5$ and $\rho_C = 4.171$ to detect a potential process mean shift. This chart should have the same ARL_0 value as that of the Shewhart chart in part (i). Compare the results here with those in part (i).
- (iii) Use the EWMA chart (3.4)–(3.5) with $\lambda = 0.2$ and $\rho_E = 2.635$ to detect a potential process mean shift. This chart should have the same ARL_0 value as that of the chart in part (i). Compare the results here with those in parts (i) and (ii).

3.3 Use the property of the uniform distribution discussed in Subsection 2.2.2 to confirm Expression (3.8).

3.4 For the process monitoring problem discussed in Exercise 3.2, assume that we have the following 10 IC process observations collected before online process monitoring: −0.25, 0.93, −1.15, −0.77, 1.27, −1.28, 0.94, 0.73, 0.45, −0.76. Use the self-starting CUSUM chart discussed in Subsection 3.2.1 to monitor the 20 Phase II process observations given in Exercise 3.2, and compare the results here with those in part (ii) of Exercise 3.2.

3.5 For the process monitoring problem discussed in Exercise 3.2, use the adaptive CUSUM chart (3.10)–(3.11) with $ARL_0 = 200$ to monitor the 20 observations given in that exercise. In (3.10), you need to specify the function $\xi(\cdot)$. For that purpose, you can use the approximation in (3.13). Also, you need to specify δ_{min} and λ in (3.12). Try the following three sets of values for δ_{min} and λ, and summarize the major differences among the three sets of results:

(i) $\delta_{min} = 0$ and $\lambda = 0.1$,

(ii) $\delta_{min} = 0$ and $\lambda = 0.5$,

(iii) $\delta_{min} = 2.0$ and $\lambda = 0.1$.

3.6 The following $m = 10$ numbers constitute a batch of observations obtained from a process at time n for process monitoring:

$$3.718,\ 0.695,\ 1.094,\ 1.175,\ 2.888,\ -0.234,\ -0.231,\ 0.581,\ 0.307,\ -0.193$$

Assume that the IC process distribution is symmetric and the IC process median is $\eta_0 = 1$.

(i) Compute the value of ψ_n defined in (3.14).

(ii) Use the Shewhart chart (3.15) with $U = 49$ to detect a potential upward mean shift at time n. What is the conclusion from the Shewhart chart about the process status at time n?

(iii) Repeat part (ii) by using $U = 45$. Compare the result here with that in part (ii). If the two results are different, provide an explanation about the difference.

3.7 For a constant $\eta \in (0,1)$, the ηth *sample quantile* of an observed dataset is defined to be the number below which there are $\eta \times 100\%$ observations in the dataset. The ηth sample quantile of an IC dataset can be used to estimate the ηth quantile of the related IC process distribution. Assume that the (l/p)-th sample quantiles, for $p = 10$ and $l = 1, 2, \ldots, 9$, of an IC dataset of size $m_0 = 500$ obtained from a process under monitoring are listed below.

$$-1.172, -0.708, -0.454, -0.201, -0.040, 0.193, 0.397, 0.617, 1.088$$

Use this information and the nonparametric P-CUSUM chart (3.16)–(3.17) with $p = 10$, $k_P = 0.01$, and $\rho_P = 11.377$ to monitor the first 100 Phase II observations listed below for possible process mean shifts. Summarize your results.

−0.39, −0.05, 0.08, −0.37, −0.79, 0.36, −0.52, −0.30, 0.92, 0.50,
0.56, 0.95, −0.91, −0.86, −0.04, −0.12, 0.51, 0.24, 0.83, 1.60,
−0.44, −0.70, 0.02, −0.20, −0.91, −0.72, 0.00, 1.94, 0.48, −1.35,
0.62, 0.93, −0.11, 0.44, −0.22, −0.58, −1.85, 1.01, 0.85, −0.13,
−0.39, 0.36, 0.80, 2.49, 0.39, 0.82, −0.16, 0.07, 0.13, 0.20,
1.96, 1.20, 0.81, 0.89, 1.01, 1.09, 1.55, 1.17, 2.11, −0.29,
1.55, 0.18, 1.13, 2.34, 0.55, 0.44, 0.32, 1.13, 0.59, 0.28,
1.03, 1.03, 0.80, 1.69, 1.34, 1.01, 1.00, −0.23, 0.42, 0.46,
1.23, 0.57, 2.02, 1.33, 1.57, 0.37, 0.76, 1.51, 0.72, −2.86,
0.41, −0.25, 0.78, 0.78 , 1.67, 0.98, 1.77, 2.12, 0.40, 1.22

3.8 The following 10 vectors are observations from a 5-dimensional process:

$$
\begin{gathered}
(-0.502, -0.582, -0.202, -0.914, -0.814),\\
(0.132, 0.715, 0.740, 2.310, -0.438),\\
(-0.079, -0.825, 0.123, -0.438, -0.720),\\
(0.887, -0.360, -0.029, 0.764, 0.231),\\
(0.117, 0.090, -0.389, 0.262, -1.158),\\
(0.319, 0.096, 0.511, 0.773, 0.247),\\
(-2.091, -0.690, 1.065, -1.777, 0.637),\\
(-0.243, -0.222, 0.970, 0.623, 2.319),\\
(-2.138, 0.183, -0.102, -0.522, 1.044),\\
(-2.111, 0.417, 1.403, 1.322, -0.879).
\end{gathered}
$$

The first six vectors are actually generated from a distribution with mean $\mathbf{0}$ and covariance matrix $I_{5\times5}$, and the remaining four vectors are generated from the same distribution except that the mean changes to $(-2,0,0,0,1)'$. Therefore, there is a mean shift from $\boldsymbol{\mu}_0 = \mathbf{0}$ to $\boldsymbol{\mu}_1 = (-2,0,0,0,1)'$ at the 7th time point.

(i) Compute the five cross-component ranks for each observation vector.

(ii) Compute the five cross-component antiranks for each observation vector.

(iii) Comment on the useful information in the five ranks and the five antiranks about the mean shift.

3.9 For the CUSUM chart considered in the part (ii) of Exercise 3.2, compute the values of the spring length T_n (cf., (3.21)) at the 20 observation times.

4

Disease Screening by Dynamic Screening Systems

4.1 Introduction

As discussed in Chapter 1, medical disease screening methods aim to determine the chance of an individual person to have a particular disease, by applying a medical procedure or test to the person at a stage when no obvious disease symptoms can be observed. Many of these medical disease screening methods (e.g., mammography for detecting breast cancer) are invasive and can be potentially harmful for patients. In addition, they may not be effective in certain cases when disease symptoms are absent or weak. So, many alternative methods have been developed in predictive medicine (Ference et al., 2000; Warren, 2018) and preventive medicine (Shantharam et al., 2022; Soyiri and Reidpath, 2013), to predict the likelihood of a disease for individual patients based on the observed disease risk factors for disease early detection and prevention. This chapter introduces a recent analytic methodology, called *dynamic screening system (DySS)*, (DySS) for effective disease screening and/or early detection.

Disease screening is a sequential decision-making process, as described below. For a given patient, a set of disease risk factors can usually be observed sequentially over time, after regular or occasional clinical visits and/or medical tests. Each time after a new batch of data about the disease risk factors are collected, a decision about the disease status of the patient should be made based on the observed data. So, observations of the disease risk factors of each patient in such cases can be regarded as observations of a sequential process, and disease screening is mainly for monitoring this process online and detecting promptly any irregular longitudinal pattern of the process that may indicate the occurrence of the disease in concern. One important feature of such sequential processes is that their distributions usually change over time even for patients without the disease in concern. As an example, the distribution of cholesterol level readings of a patient would change when the patient gets older. Sequential processes with this feature are often called *dynamic processes* in the literature (Choi and Lee, 2004; Odiowei and Cao, 2010). So, disease screening is usually a dynamic process monitoring problem.

DOI: 10.1201/9781003138150-4

In the literature, there are three types of analytic methods that are relevant to disease screening. One is related to the longitudinal data analysis (LDA) (Li, 2011; Liang and Zeger, 1986; Lin and Carroll, 2001; Xiang et al., 2013), since the observed data of the disease risk factors are usually longitudinal. By an LDA method, we can first construct confidence intervals for the means of the disease risk factors at different time points based on an observed dataset of some people without the disease to detect. In this book, people without the disease to detect are called "non-diseased" people, and the ones with the disease to detect are called "diseased people", for simplicity of presentation. Then, a new patient can be claimed to have the disease if the patient's observed disease risk factors fall outside the respective confidence intervals. But, such LDA methods are retrospective; they make their decisions about a patient's disease status at a given time point by comparing the observed disease risk factors of the patient with those of some non-diseased people cross-sectionally at the given time point. These LDA methods have not made use of the historical data of the patient under monitoring in their decision-making process. For this reason, it has been well demonstrated in the literature that they are ineffective for prospective online monitoring of dynamic sequential processes like the observed disease risk factors in the disease screening problem (cf., Marshall et al., 2007).

The other relevant analytic tool is related to statistical process control (SPC) that was discussed in Chapter 3. By an SPC chart, the observed disease risk factors of a patient can be monitored sequentially, and a signal would be triggered once the chart detects a shift in the longitudinal pattern of the patient's observed disease risk factors from an in-control (IC) status to an out-of-control (OC) status (cf., Subsection 3.1.1). However, the conventional SPC charts cannot be applied to the disease screening problem directly for the following two main reasons. First, they are originally designed for monitoring production lines in the manufacturing industry and require the model assumptions that process observations at different time points are independent and identically distributed when the process under monitoring is IC. These assumptions are rarely valid in the disease screening problem. For instance, a patient's cholesterol level readings at different time points are usually serially correlated and the mean cholesterol level of the patient would change over time when the patient gets older. Although there are some recent SPC methods for handling cases when one or more of these model assumptions are violated, as discussed in Sections 3.3 and 3.4, they cannot be used for effectively monitoring the disease risk factors whose IC distributions can change over time in a complex way. Second, the conventional SPC charts are for monitoring a single process. They make their decisions about the process status by comparing the observed data at the current time point with all historical data of the process. In the disease screening problem, the disease risk factors of each patient can be regarded as a process, as discussed above. So, there are many processes involved in this problem since many individual patients need to be screened for disease early detection. To judge whether a patient has the specific disease to detect, besides the historical data of that patient, the observed data of some non-diseased people should also be used.

Another relevant analytic tool is related to machine learning methods (Aggarwal, 2018; Breiman, 2010; Carvalhoa et al., 2019; Cortes and Vapnik, 1995; Hastie et al., 2001; Mante et al., 2013) that have been used widely in different applications, including sequential process monitoring and disease prediction that are focused in this book. A conventional machine learning method tries to approximate a real-world problem by a computer algorithm after learning the data structure of the problem from a training dataset. Thus, its performance would depend heavily on how well the training dataset represents the population of interest. To partially overcome this limitation, much research effort has been made in several directions, including reinforcement learning (Francois-Lavet et al., 2018; Mnih et al., 2015), recurrent neural networks (Campolucci et al., 1999; Ostmeyer and Cowell, 2019), machine learning for analyzing sequential or longitudinal data (Chen and Bowman, 2011; Ngufor et al., 2019) and more. However, many of these methods are designed for monitoring a single non-dynamic process, instead of multiple dynamic processes as in the current disease screening problem. Some others cannot accommodate the complex data structure (e.g., time-varying process distribution and serial data correlation) in the current problem well, and thus would not be effective for monitoring dynamic sequential processes in disease screening.

The DySS method discussed in this chapter is developed specifically for disease screening and other applications that involve sequential monitoring of dynamic processes (Li and Qiu, 2016; Qiu and Xiang, 2014, 2015; Qiu et al., 2020b; Qiu and You, 2022; Qiu et al., 2018; You and Qiu, 2019, 2020a, 2021a). When sequentially monitoring the observed disease risk factors of a patient, it tries to use helpful information in all historical data of the patient. It can accommodate within-subject data correlation, time-varying process distribution, and other complex data structure. In the literature, several different versions of the DySS method have been developed to address different challenges of the disease screening problem. Several versions of this method that can detect the disease in concern by monitoring the observed disease risk factors of a patient directly are introduced in detail in this chapter. More specifically, in Section 4.2, the DySS method is introduced in the case when a single disease risk factor is monitored for disease screening. The case when multiple disease risk factors are monitored is discussed in Section 4.3. The DySS methods discussed in these two sections do not take into account possible serial data correlation and non-Gaussian process distribution explicitly in their method construction; thus, they would lose some efficiency in cases when serial data correlation is present in the observed data and/or the process distribution is substantially different from a normal distribution. A modified version of the DySS method to properly accommodate serial data correlation and nonparametric data distribution is introduced in Section 4.4. Another modified version to simplify the design of the DySS method is introduced in Section 4.5. Some concluding remarks are provided in Section 4.6.

4.2 Univariate Dynamic Screening System for Disease Screening

To detect a disease (e.g., stroke) by using the univariate DySS method, it is assumed that a major risk factor of the disease has been figured out and there is an *IC dataset* available in advance that contains the observed longitudinal data of the disease risk factor for some non-diseased people. The basic idea of the DySS method is that we first estimate the *regular longitudinal pattern* of the disease risk factor from the IC data, where the regular longitudinal pattern refers to the one for the non-diseased people. Then, to detect the disease for a specific patient, the patient's observed disease risk factor is first standardized using the estimated regular longitudinal pattern, and the standardized observations of the disease risk factor of the patient are then monitored by an SPC chart for disease early detection. By standardizing the observed disease risk factor of the patient under monitoring, the observed longitudinal pattern of the patient's disease risk factor is actually compared cross-sectionally with the estimated regular longitudinal pattern of the non-diseased people in the IC dataset. By using an SPC chart to sequentially monitor the standardized observations, the cumulative difference between the two longitudinal patterns up to the current observation time is actually used in determining the patient's disease status at the current observation time. So, all historical data of the patient under monitoring have been used in the decision-making process of the chart. See Figure 4.1 for a demonstration. The major steps of the univariate DySS method that was originally suggested in Qiu and Xiang (2014) are described in several parts below.

4.2.1 Estimation of the Regular Longitudinal Pattern

Assume that y is the disease risk factor of interest for detecting a given disease, and an IC dataset that contains observations of y for a group of m non-diseased people has been collected in advance. The observations of y in the IC data are assumed to follow the univariate nonparametric longitudinal model

$$y(t_{ij}) = \mu(t_{ij}) + \varepsilon(t_{ij}), \qquad \text{for } j = 1, 2, \ldots, J_i,\ i = 1, 2, \ldots, m, \tag{4.1}$$

where t_{ij} is the jth observation time of the ith person, $y(t_{ij})$ is the observed value of y at t_{ij}, $\mu(t_{ij})$ is the mean of $y(t_{ij})$, and $\varepsilon(t_{ij})$ is the error term. For simplicity of presentation, it is further assumed that all observation times are within the design interval $[0, 1]$. In Model (4.1), observations of different people are assumed to be independent, as in the LDA literature (e.g., Li, 2011). The error term $\varepsilon(t)$ is assumed to consist of two independent components, i.e., $\varepsilon(t) = \varepsilon_0(t) + \varepsilon_1(t)$, for any $t \in [0, 1]$, where $\varepsilon_0(t)$ is a random process with mean 0 and covariance function $V_0(s, t) = \text{Cov}(\varepsilon_0(s), \varepsilon_0(t))$, for any $s, t \in [0, 1]$, and $\varepsilon_1(t)$ is a zero-mean process satisfying the condition that $\varepsilon_1(s)$

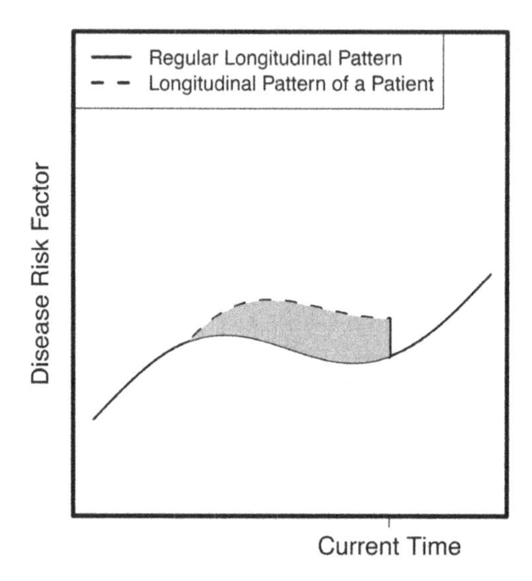

FIGURE 4.1
The DySS method makes its decision about a patient's disease status at the current time point based on the cumulative difference (shaded area) between the observed longitudinal pattern of the patient's disease risk factor and the estimated regular longitudinal pattern of the non-diseased people in the IC dataset.

and $\varepsilon_1(t)$ are independent of each other, for any $s \neq t \in [0,1]$. In this error decomposition, $\varepsilon_1(t)$ denotes the pure measurement error, and $\varepsilon_0(t)$ denotes all possible covariates that may affect y but are not included in Model (4.1). In such cases, the covariance function of $\varepsilon(t)$ is

$$V(s,t) = \text{Cov}\left(\varepsilon(s), \varepsilon(t)\right) = V_0(s,t) + \sigma_1^2(s) I(s=t), \quad \text{for } s,t \in [0,1], \qquad (4.2)$$

where $\sigma_1^2(s) = \text{Var}(\varepsilon_1(s))$, and $I(s=t)=1$ when $s=t$ and 0 otherwise.

For the nonparametric longitudinal model described by (4.1) and (4.2), Chen and Jin (2005) proposed a four-step model estimation procedure described below. In cases when $V(s,t)$ is assumed known, $\mu(t)$ can be estimated by the following local pth-order polynomial kernel estimator:

$$\widehat{\mu}(t;V) = \mathbf{e}_1' \left(\sum_{i=1}^{m} X_i' V_i^{-1} X_i \right)^{-1} \left(\sum_{i=1}^{m} X_i' V_i^{-1} \mathbf{y}_i \right), \qquad (4.3)$$

where $\mathbf{e}_1$ is a $(p+1)$-dimensional vector with 1 being the first element and 0 anywhere else,

$$X_i = \begin{pmatrix} 1 & (t_{i1}-t) & \dots & (t_{i1}-t)^p \\ \vdots & \vdots & \ddots & \vdots \\ 1 & (t_{iJ_i}-t) & \dots & (t_{iJ_i}-t)^p \end{pmatrix}_{J_i \times (p+1)},$$

$V_i^{-1} = K_{ih}^{1/2}(t)(I_i\Sigma_i I_i)^{-1}K_{ih}^{1/2}(t)$, $K_{ih}(t) = \text{diag}\{K((t_{i1}-t)/h),\ldots,K_h((t_{iJ_i}-t)/h)\}/h$, $K(\cdot)$ is a density kernel function, $h > 0$ is a bandwidth, $I_i = \text{diag}\{I(|t_{i1}-t| \leq 1),\ldots,I(|t_{iJ_i}-t| \leq 1)\}$, and Σ_i is the covariance matrix of $\mathbf{y}_i = (y(t_{i1}), y(t_{i2}),\ldots,y(t_{iJ_i}))'$ that can be computed from $V(s,t)$ in (4.2). In practice, we can simply choose $p = 1$. Throughout this section, the inverse of a matrix refers to the Moore-Penrose generalized inverse, which always exists.

The error covariance function $V(s,t)$ is usually unknown in practice. Thus, it should be estimated from the observed data in order to use the estimator $\widehat{\mu}(t;V)$ in (4.3). To this end, we can use the following four-step procedure. First, an initial estimator of $\mu(t)$, denoted as $\widetilde{\mu}(t)$, can be computed by (4.3) in which all Σ_i's are replaced by the identity matrix. In such cases, it is obvious that the resulting initial estimator $\widetilde{\mu}(t)$ is just the local pth-order polynomial kernel estimator based on the assumption that the error terms in Model (4.1) at different time points are i.i.d. for each individual person. Second, the residuals are defined to be

$$\widetilde{\varepsilon}(t_{ij}) = y(t_{ij}) - \widetilde{\mu}(t_{ij}), \qquad \text{for } j = 1,2,\ldots,J_i,\ i = 1,2,\ldots,m.$$

Third, when $s \neq t$, we can use the method originally proposed by Li (2011) to estimate $V_0(s,t)$ in (4.2) by

$$\begin{aligned}\widetilde{V}_0(s,t) &= [A_1(s,t)V_{00}(s,t) - A_2(s,t)V_{10}(s,t) - \\ &\quad A_3(s,t)V_{01}(s,t)]\, B^{-1}(s,t),\end{aligned} \tag{4.4}$$

where $A_1(s,t) = S_{20}(s,t)S_{02}(s,t) - S_{11}^2(s,t)$, $A_2(s,t) = S_{10}(s,t)S_{02}(s,t) - S_{01}(s,t)S_{11}(s,t)$, $A_3(s,t) = S_{01}(s,t)S_{20}(s,t) - S_{10}(s,t)S_{11}(s,t)$, $B(s,t) = A_1(s,t)S_{00}(s,t) - A_2(s,t)S_{10}(s,t) - A_3(s,t)S_{01}(s,t)$,

$$\begin{aligned}S_{l_1l_2}(s,t) &= \frac{1}{m}\sum_{i=1}^{m}\frac{1}{J_i(J_i-1)}\sum_{j=1}^{J_i}\sum_{j'\neq j}\left(\frac{t_{ij}-s}{h}\right)^{l_1}\left(\frac{t_{ij'}-t}{h}\right)^{l_2} \\ &\quad \times K_h(t_{ij}-s)\,K_h\left(t_{ij'}-t\right),\end{aligned}$$

$$\begin{aligned}V_{l_1l_2}(s,t) &= \frac{1}{m}\sum_{i=1}^{m}\frac{1}{J_i(J_i-1)}\sum_{j=1}^{J_i}\sum_{j'\neq j}\widetilde{\varepsilon}(t_{ij})\widetilde{\varepsilon}(t_{ij'})\left(\frac{t_{ij}-s}{h}\right)^{l_1}\left(\frac{t_{ij'}-t}{h}\right)^{l_2} \\ &\quad \times K_h(t_{ij}-s)\,K_h\left(t_{ij'}-t\right),\end{aligned}$$

$K_h(s) = K(s/h)/h$, and $l_1, l_2 = 0,1,2$. Note that the matrix $\widetilde{V}_0(s,t)$ in (4.4) may not be semipositive definite, and thus may not be a legitimate covariance matrix. To address this issue, the adjustment procedure in Li (2011) can effectively regularize it to be a well defined covariance matrix. When $s = t$, the variance of $y(t)$, denoted as $\sigma_y^2(t) = V_0(t,t) + \sigma_1^2(t)$, can be regarded as the mean function of $\varepsilon^2(t)$. It can be estimated from the data

$\{\widetilde{\varepsilon}^2(t_{ij}), j = 1, 2, \ldots, J_i, i = 1, 2, \ldots, m\}$ by (4.3), in which $\{\mathbf{y}_i\}$ are replaced by $\{(\widetilde{\varepsilon}^2(t_{i1}), \ldots, \widetilde{\varepsilon}^2(t_{iJ_i}))'\}$ and each Σ_i is replaced by the identity matrix. The resulting estimator is denoted as $\widetilde{\sigma}_y^2(t)$. Fourth, we can define the estimator of $V(s,t)$ by

$$\widetilde{V}(s,t) = \widetilde{V}_0(s,t)I(s \neq t) + \widetilde{\sigma}_y^2(t)I(s = t). \tag{4.5}$$

Consequently, the mean function $\mu(t)$ can be estimated by $\widehat{\mu}(t; \widetilde{V})$.

Note that, in the four-step model estimation procedure described above for computing $\widetilde{\mu}(t)$, $\widetilde{V}_0(s,t)$, $\widetilde{\sigma}_y^2(t)$, and $\widehat{\mu}(t; \widetilde{V})$, the kernel function $K(\cdot)$ could be chosen to be the Epanechnikov kernel function (cf., Subsection 2.5.4) and the bandwidth h could be chosen differently in each step by the conventional cross-validation procedure (cf., Subsection 2.5.5). We have not made it explicitly in the above description for simplicity.

By the estimation procedure described above, we can compute the local polynomial kernel estimator $\widehat{\mu}(t; \widetilde{V})$ of the mean function $\mu(t)$ in cases when the error covariance function $V(s,t)$ is unknown. After $\mu(t)$ is estimated, the variance function $\sigma_y^2(t)$ can be estimated in the same way as that described above for $\widetilde{\sigma}_y^2(t)$, except that $\{\widetilde{\varepsilon}^2(t_{ij}), j = 1, 2, \ldots, J_i, i = 1, 2, \ldots, m\}$ need to be replaced by

$$\widehat{\varepsilon}^2(t_{ij}) = \left[y(t_{ij}) - \widehat{\mu}\left(t_{ij}; \widetilde{V}\right)\right]^2, \qquad \text{for } j = 1, 2, \ldots, J_i, \ i = 1, 2, \ldots, m.$$

The resulting estimator of $\sigma_y^2(t)$ is denoted as $\widehat{\sigma}_y^2(t)$. Then, the *estimated regular longitudinal pattern* of the disease risk factor y is summarized in the box below.

Estimated Regular Longitudinal Pattern of the Disease Risk Factor y

The estimated regular longitudinal pattern of the disease risk factor y is described by its mean and variance function estimators $\widehat{\mu}(t; \widetilde{V})$ and $\widehat{\sigma}_y^2(t)$.

Example 4.1 *The Framingham Heart Study is a well-known, ongoing cardiovascular cohort study of residents of the city of Framingham in Massachusetts. The study started in 1948 and is currently on the fourth generation of the original participants. The main purpose of the study was to find key risk factors of heart disease (Cupples et al., 2007). In this example, we consider a dataset from the Framingham Heart Study. The dataset contains observations of 1055 participants. Each participant was followed up for 7 times (i.e., $J_i = 7$ for each i), and the follow-up times could be different for different participants. At each follow-up time, measurement of the total cholesterol level (in mg/100ml) was taken and the disease status of stroke was recorded as well. So, in this example, the disease in concern is stroke and there is a single disease risk factor (i.e.,* *the total cholesterol level) considered. Among the 1055 participants, 27 of them had strokes for at least once and the remaining people did not have any strokes during the study period. So, the observed data of the 1028 non-stroke participants can be used as the IC data, from which we can estimate the IC mean function* $\mu(t)$ *and the IC variance function* $\sigma_y^2(t)$*. To this end, the covariance function* $V(s,t)$ *is first estimated by* $\widetilde{V}(s,t)$ *in (4.5), and then* $\mu(t)$ *and* $\sigma_y^2(t)$ *are estimated by* $\widehat{\mu}(t;\widetilde{V})$ *and* $\widehat{\sigma}_y^2(t)$*, respectively, as described above. The 95% pointwise confidence band of* $\mu(t)$*, defined to be* $\widehat{\mu}(t;\widetilde{V}) \pm 1.96\widehat{\sigma}_y(t)$*, and the mean function estimator* $\widehat{\mu}(t;\widetilde{V})$ *are presented in Figure 4.2, together with the observed total cholesterol levels of the 27 stroke patients. So, the three bold lines in the figure describe the regular longitudinal pattern of the total cholesterol level for non-stroke participants of the study. From the figure, it can be seen that observations of some stroke participants exceed the upper confidence levels, and there are no stroke participants whose observed total cholesterol levels exceed the lower confidence levels, which implies that the total cholesterol level is indeed an effective risk factor of stroke.*

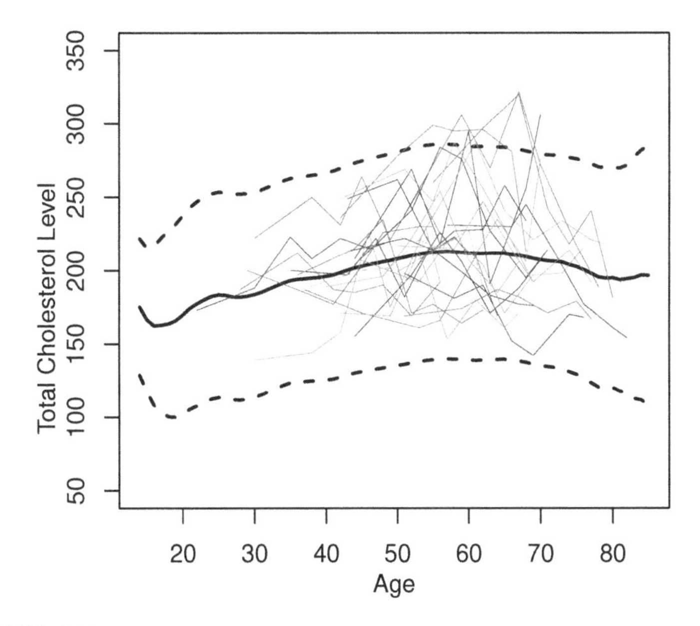

FIGURE 4.2
Pointwise 95% confidence intervals of the mean total cholesterol level $\mu(t)$ (dark dashed lines), the point estimator $\widehat{\mu}(t;\widetilde{V})$ of $\mu(t)$ (dark solid line), and the observed total cholesterol levels of the 27 stroke participants (thin lines).

4.2.2 Data Standardization for Disease Early Detection

To detect the disease in concern for a new patient, we need to standardize the patient's observed disease risk factor using the estimated regular longitudinal pattern. To this end, let the observed disease risk factor of the new patient be $\{y(t_j^*), j \geq 1\}$, where $t_j^* \in [0,1]$, for all j, are the observation times. The superscript "*" is used here to imply that observation times of the new patient could be different from those in the IC data. In cases when the new patient's longitudinal pattern of the disease risk factor is IC, or when the new patient is non-diseased, the patient's observed data of the disease risk factor should follow Model (4.1). For convenience of discussion, that model is re-written as

$$y(t_j^*) = \mu(t_j^*) + \sigma_y(t_j^*)\epsilon(t_j^*), \qquad \text{for } j \geq 1, \tag{4.6}$$

where $\sigma_y(t)\epsilon(t)$ here equals $\varepsilon(t)$ in Model (4.1). Thus, $\epsilon(t)$ in Model (4.6) has mean 0 and variance 1 at each t. Then, the standardized observations of the new patient are defined in the box below.

Standardized Observations of the New Patient

The standardized observations of the new patient under monitoring are defined to be

$$\widehat{\epsilon}(t_j^*) = \frac{y(t_j^*) - \widehat{\mu}(t_j^*; \widetilde{V})}{\widehat{\sigma}_y(t_j^*)}, \qquad \text{for } j \geq 1, \tag{4.7}$$

where $\widehat{\mu}(t; \widetilde{V})$ and $\widehat{\sigma}_y(t)$ are defined in Subsection 4.2.1.

As described in Subsection 4.2.1, both $\widehat{\mu}(t; \widetilde{V})$ and $\widehat{\sigma}_y(t)$ are estimated from the IC data for describing the regular longitudinal pattern of the disease risk factor y for non-diseased people. Thus, the standardized observations of the new patient defined in (4.7) actually compare the observed longitudinal pattern of the new patient with the estimated regular longitudinal pattern of the non-diseased people cross-sectionally at individual observation times $\{t_j^*, j \geq 1\}$. Intuitively, if the new patient does not have the disease to detect, then the absolute values of the standardized observations should be small. Otherwise, their absolute values would be relatively large. Therefore, the standardized observations can be used for disease early detection, which is discussed in the next subsection.

4.2.3 Sequential Monitoring of the Observed Disease Risk Factor for Disease Early Detection

Cases with independent observations. For simplicity, let us first consider cases when the observations of the disease risk factor, $\{y(t_j^*), j \geq 1\}$, are assumed to be independent of each other at different time points and each of them has a normal distribution. In such cases, the standardized observations $\{\widehat{\epsilon}(t_j^*), j \geq 1\}$ would be a sequence of asymptotically i.i.d. random variables with the common asymptotic distribution of $N(0, 1)$. If we further assume that $\{t_j^*, j \geq 1\}$ are equally spaced, then $\{\widehat{\epsilon}(t_j^*), j \geq 1\}$ can be monitored by a conventional control chart, such as the conventional CUSUM, EWMA or CPD chart discussed in Section 3.1. For instance, the conventional CUSUM chart for detecting upward mean shifts in $\{\widehat{\epsilon}(t_j^*), j \geq 1\}$ is presented in the box below.

A CUSUM Chart for Disease Early Detection

If an upward mean shift in the disease risk factor y would indicate an increased chance of the disease in concern, then the charting statistic of the upward CUSUM chart for disease early detection can be defined to be

$$C_j^+ = \max\left(0, C_{j-1}^+ + \widehat{\epsilon}(t_j^*) - k\right), \qquad \text{for } j \geq 1, \tag{4.8}$$

where $C_0^+ = 0$, and $k > 0$ is an allowance constant. The chart gives a signal of an upward mean shift if

$$C_j^+ > \rho, \tag{4.9}$$

where $\rho > 0$ is a control limit.

To evaluate the performance of the CUSUM chart (4.8)–(4.9), we can use the IC average run length ARL_0 and the OC average run length ARL_1, as discussed in Subsection 3.1.2, when the observation times are equally spaced. In practice, however, the observation times $\{t_j^*, j \geq 1\}$ are often unequally spaced. In such cases, ARL_0 and ARL_1 are obviously inappropriate for measuring the performance of the CUSUM chart (4.8)–(4.9), since they only count the observation times which cannot well reflect how fast the chart can detect a shift when the observation times are unequally spaced. Thus, new performance measures are needed. To this end, let $\omega > 0$ be a *basic time unit* in a given application, which is the largest time unit that all observation times are its integer multiples. Define

$$n_j^* = t_j^*/\omega, \qquad \text{for } j \geq 1.$$

Then, $t_j^* = n_j^*\omega$, for all j, and n_j^* is the jth observation time in the basic time unit ω. In cases when the new patient is IC but the CUSUM chart (4.8)–(4.9) gives a signal at the sth observation time, then n_s^* is a random variable measuring the time to a false signal. Its mean $\mathrm{E}(n_s^*)$ measures the IC average time to signal (ATS), denoted as ATS_0. If the new patient has an upward mean shift starting at the τth observation time and the CUSUM chart (4.8)–(4.9) gives a signal at the sth time point with $s \geq \tau$, then the OC

ATS, denoted as ATS_1, is defined to be the mean $E(n_s^* - n_\tau^*)$. To measure the performance the chart (4.8)–(4.9), its ATS_0 value can be pre-specified at a given level, and the chart performs better if its ATS_1 value is smaller when detecting a shift of a given size. It is obvious that the values of ATS_0 and ATS_1 are constant multiples of the corresponding values of ARL_0 and ARL_1 in cases when the observation times are equally spaced. In such cases, the two sets of measures are thus equivalent.

In cases when the IC mean function $\mu(t)$ and the IC variance function $\sigma_y^2(t)$ are known, the standardized observations $\{\widehat{\epsilon}(t_j^*), j \geq 1\}$ can be regarded as a sequence of i.i.d. standard normal random variables when the new patient under monitoring is IC. In such cases, as long as the distribution of the observation times $\{t_j^*, j = 1, 2, \ldots\}$ is specified properly, for a given k value in (4.8) and a given ATS_0 value, we can compute the corresponding value of the control limit ρ in (4.9) easily by Monte Carlo simulations such that the pre-specified ATS_0 value is reached. For instance, when the distribution of the observation times is specified by the sampling rate d, which is defined to be the average number of observation times within every 10 basic time units, the computed ρ values in cases when $ATS_0 = 20, 50, 100, 150, 200$, $k = 0.1, 0.2, 0.5, 0.75, 1.0$, and $d = 2, 5, 10$ are presented in Table 4.1. From the table, it can be seen that ρ increases with ATS_0 and d, and decreases with k. In cases when $\mu(t)$ and $\sigma_y^2(t)$ are unknown, they need to be estimated from the IC dataset by $\widehat{\mu}(t; \widetilde{V})$ and $\widehat{\sigma}_y^2(t)$, as discussed in Subsection 4.2.1. In such cases, the standardized observations $\{\widehat{\epsilon}(t_j^*), j \geq 1\}$ would have the asymptotic $N(0, 1)$ distribution when the new patient under monitoring is IC. When the IC sample size is moderate to large, we can still use the control limit values presented in Table 4.1, which has been justified by the numerical studies presented in Qiu and Xiang (2014).

Next, we make several remarks about the DySS method discussed above. First, the above description about the CUSUM chart (4.8)–(4.9) focuses only on cases to detect upward shifts in the process mean function $\mu(t)$. Control charts for detecting downward mean shifts or arbitrary mean shifts can be developed in the same way, except that the upward charting statistic in (4.8) and the decision rule in (4.9) need to be changed to the downward or two-sided version of the chart (cf., Subsection 3.1.3). Second, control charts for detecting shifts in the process variance function $\sigma_y^2(t)$, or shifts in both $\mu(t)$ and $\sigma_y^2(t)$, can be developed in a similar way, after (4.8) and (4.9) are replaced by the appropriate charting statistics and the related decision rules. See, for instance, Gan (1995) and Yeh et al. (2004) for the related discussions about such control charts. Third, although a CUSUM chart is used above, charts of other types (e.g., the Shewhart, EWMA and CPD charts) can also be used in the DySS method. Fourth, to use the proposed DySS method, the observation times $\{t_j^*, j \geq 1\}$ of the new patient to monitor cannot be larger than the largest value of the observation times $\{t_{ij}, j = 1, 2, \ldots, J_i, i = 1, 2, \ldots, m\}$ in the IC data, to avoid extrapolation in the data standardization in (4.7). In other words, it is inappropriate to use the DySS method to monitor the new

TABLE 4.1
Values of the control limit ρ of the CUSUM chart (4.8)–(4.9) for various combinations of ATS_0, k, and d in cases when the IC mean and variance functions are assumed known and the IC process distribution is assumed to be normal.

d	k	$ATS_0 = 20$	50	100	150	200
	0.1	0.929	1.844	2.820	3.552	4.171
	0.2	0.774	1.571	2.351	2.928	3.396
2	0.5	0.382	0.986	1.493	1.822	2.088
	0.75	0.118	0.654	1.064	1.312	1.507
	1.0	0.001	0.355	0.718	0.936	1.101
	0.1	1.844	3.215	4.612	5.631	6.445
	0.2	1.571	2.664	3.713	4.381	5.005
5	0.5	0.986	1.685	2.234	2.586	2.898
	0.75	0.654	1.200	1.612	1.869	2.072
	1.0	0.355	0.837	1.189	1.404	1.562
	0.1	2.820	4.612	6.407	7.649	8.612
	0.2	2.351	3.713	4.937	5.744	6.408
10	0.5	1.493	2.235	2.852	3.245	3.542
	0.75	1.061	1.610	2.039	2.310	2.509
	1.0	0.718	1.192	1.538	1.738	1.894

patient outside the following time range of the IC data:

$$\left[\min_{i,j} t_{ij},\ \max_{i,j} t_{ij}\right].$$

From the above description about the DySS method, it can be seen that this methodology actually combines cross-sectional comparison between the new patient to monitor and the m non-diseased people in the IC data with sequential process monitoring in a dynamic way. Therefore, to use the DySS method to monitor the longitudinal pattern of the new patient at time t, there should be some existing observations around t in the IC data to make the cross-sectional comparison possible.

It should be pointed out that construction of the CUSUM chart (4.8)–(4.9) has not taken into account the possibility that observation times could be unequally spaced, although its performance metrics ATS_0 and ATS_1 can accommodate unequally spaced observation times. As explained in Subsection 3.1.3, the CUSUM charting statistic C_j^+ defined in (4.8) tries to make use of all historical data of the process under monitoring by using the cumulative sum $C_{j-1}^+ + \widehat{\epsilon}(t_j^*)$. However, the cumulative sum does not use any information about the distribution of observation times. Or, it assumes the observation times are equally spaced. In cases when the observation times are unequally spaced, intuitively process observations collected at times that are farther away from the current observation time should receive less weights in C_j^+ or an alternative charting statistic. Based on this intuitive idea, Qiu et al. (2018) developed an EWMA chart for the univariate DySS method, which can well accommodate unequally spaced observation times in its construction.

Cases when observations are serially correlated and follow an AR(1) time series model. The CUSUM chart (4.8)–(4.9) is appropriate to use when the observations $\{y(t_j^*), j \geq 1\}$ are independent of each other at different time points. In practice, however, this assumption is rarely valid. Next, we discuss how to use the DySS method in cases when the longitudinal observations $\{y(t_j^*), j \geq 1\}$ follow an AR(1) time series model. In a conventional time series model, observation times are usually assumed to be equally spaced. In the current disease screening problem, however, they can be unequally spaced. In such cases, proper time series modeling is challenging (cf., Maller et al., 2008; Vityazev, 1996). This is the main reason why the DySS method is developed for the case when the observed disease risk factor is assumed to follow the simple AR(1) time series model only in this part.

Let us first discuss estimation of the regular longitudinal pattern from the IC dataset when the observed longitudinal data are serially correlated and follow an AR(1) model. In such cases, for the error term in Model (4.1), let $\varepsilon(t_{ij}) = \sigma_y(t_{ij})\epsilon(t_{ij})$, for each i and j, where $\epsilon(t_{ij})$ has mean 0 and variance 1 for each $t_{ij} \in [0,1]$. Then, it is assumed that $\epsilon(t_{ij})$ follows the AR(1) model

$$\epsilon(t_{ij}) = \phi\epsilon(t_{ij} - \omega) + e(t_{ij}), \qquad \text{for } j = 1, 2, ..., J_i, \; i = 1, 2, ..., m, \tag{4.10}$$

where ϕ is a coefficient, ω is the basic time unit defined earlier, and $e(t)$ is a zero-mean white noise process in $[0,1]$ (i.e., $e(t)$ and $e(t')$ are independent for any $t, t' \in [0,1]$). Model (4.10) is the conventional AR(1) model for the equally spaced observation times in the basic time unit ω. It does not have a constant term on the right-hand-side because the mean of $\epsilon(t_{ij})$ is 0. In the current disease screening problem, it is inconvenient to work with Model (4.10) directly because there may not be observation at the time $t_{ij} - \omega$ that is used in (4.10). To overcome this difficulty, we can transform the AR(1) model (4.10) to the following time series model that uses the actual observation times $\{t_{ij}\}$:

$$\epsilon(t_{ij}) = \phi^{\Delta_{i,j-1}}\epsilon(t_{i,j-1}) + \widetilde{\Theta}_{ij}(z)e(t_{ij}), \tag{4.11}$$

where $\Delta_{i,j-1} = (t_{ij} - t_{i,j-1})/\omega$, z is the lag operator used in time series modeling (e.g., $z\epsilon(t) = \epsilon(t - \omega)$), and

$$\widetilde{\Theta}_{ij}(z) = 1 + \phi z + \cdots + \phi^{\Delta_{i,j-1}-1} z^{\Delta_{i,j-1}-1}$$

is a lag polynomial. As discussed in Subsections 4.2.1 and 4.2.2, let $\widehat{\mu}(t;\widetilde{V})$ and $\widehat{\sigma}_y^2(t)$ be the local pth-order polynomial kernel estimators of $\mu(t)$ and $\sigma_y^2(t)$, and

$$\widehat{\epsilon}(t_{ij}) = \frac{y(t_{ij}) - \widehat{\mu}(t_{ij};\widetilde{V})}{\widehat{\sigma}_y(t_{ij})}, \qquad \text{for } j = 1, 2, \ldots, J_i, \; i = 1, 2, \ldots, m$$

be the standardized values of the observations in the IC dataset. Then, the least squares (LS) estimator of ϕ, denoted as $\widehat{\phi}$, is the solution of the following minimization problem:

$$\min_{\phi} \sum_{i=1}^{m} \sum_{j=2}^{J_i} \left[\widehat{\epsilon}(t_{ij}) - \phi^{\Delta_{i,j-1}} \widehat{\epsilon}(t_{i,j-1})\right]^2.$$

Next, we use the estimated regular longitudinal pattern described by $\widehat{\mu}(t;\widetilde{V})$, $\widehat{\sigma}_y^2(t)$ and $\widehat{\phi}$ to monitor a new patient's observed longitudinal pattern of y. Assume that the new patient's y observations follow Model (4.6), in which the error term $\epsilon(t_j^*)$ follows the AR(1) model

$$\epsilon(t_j^*) = \phi\epsilon(t_j^* - \omega) + e(t_j^*), \qquad \text{for } j \geq 1,$$

where ϕ is the same coefficient as the one in (4.10). Then, similar to the relationship between Models (4.10) and (4.11), the above AR(1) model implies that

$$\epsilon(t_j^*) = \phi^{\Delta_{j-1}^*} \epsilon(t_{j-1}^*) + e_j^*, \tag{4.12}$$

where $\Delta_{j-1}^* = (t_j^* - t_{j-1}^*)/\omega$, $e_j^* = \widetilde{\Theta}_j^*(z) e(t_j^*)$, and

$$\widetilde{\Theta}_j^*(z) = 1 + \phi z + \cdots + \phi^{\Delta_{j-1}^* - 1} z^{\Delta_{j-1}^* - 1}.$$

It can be checked that, when the new patient is IC, the error terms in $\{e_j^*, j = 1, 2, \ldots\}$ are independent of each other, and e_j^* has mean 0 and variance $\sigma_{e^*}^2 = 1 - \phi^{2\Delta_{j-1}^*}$, for each j. In the SPC literature, it has been well demonstrated that, when $\epsilon(t_j^*)$ follows the time series model (4.12), to detect an upward mean shift in $\epsilon(t_j^*)$, we can just monitor $\{e_j^*, j = 1, 2, \ldots\}$ (e.g., Lu and Reynolds, 2001). Based on these results, to detect an upward mean shift in the original observations of the disease risk factor y, the charting statistic of the upward CUSUM chart can be defined to be: for $j \geq 2$,

$$C_j^+ = \max\left\{0, C_{j-1}^+ + \left[\widehat{\epsilon}(t_j^*) - \widehat{\phi}^{\Delta_{j-1}^*} \widehat{\epsilon}(t_{j-1}^*)\right] \Big/ \sqrt{1 - \widehat{\phi}^{2\Delta_{j-1}^*}} - k\right\}, \tag{4.13}$$

where $C_1^+ = 0$, $k > 0$ is an allowance constant, and $\widehat{\epsilon}(t_j^*) = (y(t_j^*) - \widehat{\mu}(t_j^*;\widetilde{V}))/\widehat{\sigma}_y(t_j^*)$. The chart gives a signal when

$$C_j^+ > \rho, \tag{4.14}$$

where $\rho > 0$ is a control limit chosen to achieve a pre-specified ATS_0 value.

Example 4.2 *For the stroke data considered in Example 4.1, after $\mu(t)$ and $\sigma_y^2(t)$ are estimated, we can compute the standardized observations by*

$$\widehat{\epsilon}(t_{ij}) = \frac{y(t_{ij}) - \widehat{\mu}(t_{ij};\widetilde{V})}{\widehat{\sigma}_y(t_{ij})}, \qquad \textit{for } j = 1, ..., J_i,\ i = 1, ..., m.$$

To address the possible autocorrelation among $\{\widehat{\epsilon}(t_{ij})\}$, we consider the AR(1) model (4.10), and the coefficient ϕ in the model is estimated by the LS procedure described above to be $\widehat{\phi} = 0.9217$. The goodness-of-fit of the AR(1) model is studied as follows. First, the predicted values of the model (cf., (4.11)) are computed by

$$\widetilde{\epsilon}(t_{ij}) = \widehat{\phi}^{\Delta_{i,j-1}} \widehat{\epsilon}(t_{i,j-1}).$$

They are first ordered from the smallest to the largest, and then divided into g groups of the same size. Namely, the kth group includes all predicted values in the interval $I_k = [q_{k-1}, q_k)$, for $k = 1, 2, \ldots, g$, where q_k is the (k/g)-th quantile of all predicted values $\{\widetilde{\epsilon}(t_{ij})\}$, for $k = 1, 2, \ldots, g-1$, $q_0 = -\infty$, and $q_g = \infty$. Let O_k be the number of standardized residuals $\{\widehat{\epsilon}(t_{ij})\}$ in the interval I_k, and $E_k = \sum_{i=1}^{m} J_i/g$ be the expected number of the standardized residuals in I_k if the AR(1) model is valid, for $k = 1, 2, \ldots, g$. Then, the following Pearson's chi-square test statistic (cf., Subsection 2.5.2):

$$X^2 = \sum_{k=1}^{g} \frac{(O_k - E_k)^2}{E_k}$$

measures the discrepancy between the distribution of the standardized residuals and the distribution of their predicted values by the AR(1) model. If the AR(1) model fits the data well, then the null distribution of X^2 should be approximately χ^2_{g-2}, where the degrees of freedom is $g-2$ because there is one parameter (i.e., ϕ) in the AR(1) model that needs to be estimated beforehand. If we choose $g = 12$, then the observed value of X^2 is 0.2265, giving a p-value of about 1.0. We also tried other g values in the interval $[5, 50]$, and similarly large p-values were obtained. Therefore, the AR(1) model seems to fit the standardized observations well.

After $\mu(t)$, $\sigma_y^2(t)$ and ϕ are all estimated, next we design a CUSUM chart to detect any irregular longitudinal patterns of the total cholesterol level for the 27 stroke participants. In this example, because we are concerned about the upward shifts in the total cholesterol levels, only the upward CUSUM chart (4.13)–(4.14) is considered here. Since each stroke participant has an average of 2.3 observations every 10 years, we choose $d = 2$. In the CUSUM chart, we choose $k = 0.1$ and $ATS_0 = 25$. In such cases, the control limit ρ is computed to be 0.927. The CUSUM charts for monitoring the 27 stroke patients are presented in Figure 4.3, from which we can see that 22 out of the 27 stroke participants are detected to have upward mean shifts. The 22 signal times, computed from the starting point of each process monitoring, are listed in Table 4.2. The average signal time is 13.818 years.

Calculation of the control limit using a block bootstrap procedure. In the previous two parts, we assume that the original observations $\{y(t_j^*), j \geq 1\}$ of a new patient are either independent or serially correlated with the autocorrelation described by the AR(1) model (4.10). In addition, the process distribution is assumed to be normal. In practice, however, these

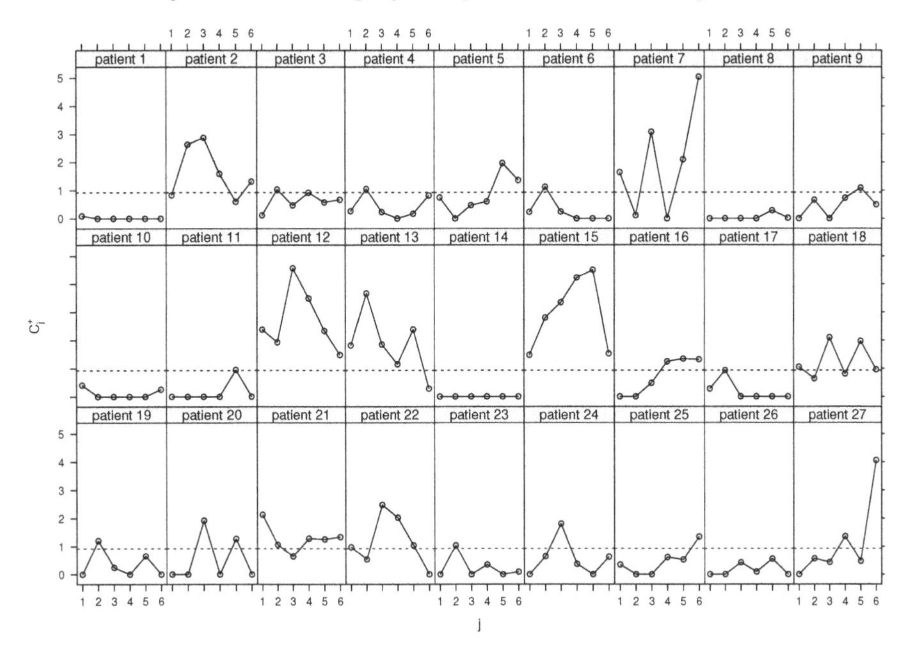

FIGURE 4.3
The CUSUM chart (4.13)–(4.14) with $(k, \rho, ATS_0) = (0.1, 0.927, 25)$ for monitoring the 27 stroke participants. The dashed horizontal lines in the plots denote the control limit ρ.

assumptions could be violated. If one or more such model assumptions are violated, then the related control charts (4.8)–(4.9) and (4.13)–(4.14) would not be reliable to use because their actual ATS_0 values could be substantially different from the pre-specified ATS_0 values. See the related discussions in Sections 3.3 and 3.4. Next, we introduce a numerical approach to compute the control limit ρ of the chart (4.8)–(4.9) from an IC data such that the chart is still reliable to use even in cases when the observed data are serially correlated with an arbitrary autocorrelation and a parametric form is unavailable to describe the process distribution.

As discussed in Subsection 4.2.1, assume that there is an IC dataset consisting of a group of m non-diseased people whose observations of y follow Model (4.1). The data of the first m_1 people are then used for obtaining estimators $\widehat{\mu}(t; \widetilde{V})$ and $\widehat{\sigma}_y^2(t)$, as discussed in Subsection 4.2.1. The control limit ρ of the chart (4.8)–(4.9) can be computed from the observed data of the remaining $m_2 = m - m_1$ people using a block bootstrap procedure (e.g., Lahiri, 2003) described below, where all observations of a single person are re-sampled together as a block.

TABLE 4.2
Signal times (years) of the 22 stroke participants who receive signals from the CUSUM chart (4.13)–(4.14).

Patient ID	Signal Time	Patient ID	Signal Time
2	12	16	19
3	13	17	12
4	12	18	8
5	22	19	12
6	11	20	16
7	8	21	8
9	23	22	9
11	24	23	11
12	8	24	16
13	7	25	26
15	8	27	19

Step 1 Compute the standardized observations of the m_2 non-diseased people by

$$\widehat{\epsilon}(t_{ij}) = \frac{y(t_{ij}) - \widehat{\mu}(t_{ij}; \widetilde{V})}{\widehat{\sigma}_y(t_{ij})}, \quad \text{for } j = 1, 2, \ldots, J_i, \ i = m_1 + 1, m_1 + 2, \ldots, m.$$

Step 2 Randomly select B people with replacement from the m_2 non-diseased people, apply the chart (4.8)–(4.9) to their standardized observations, and use a numerical searching algorithm (e.g., the bisection searching algorithm) to compute the value of ρ so that a pre-specified ATS_0 level is reached. Such a searching algorithm has been well discussed in Qiu (2008) and Section 4.2 of Qiu (2014). Basically, we first give an initial value to ρ, and compute the actual ATS_0 value of the chart (4.8)–(4.9) from the standardized observations of the B re-sampled people. If the actual ATS_0 value is smaller than the pre-specified ATS_0 value, then the previous value of ρ is increased; otherwise, the value of ρ is decreased. Then, the actual ATS_0 value of the chart is computed again, using the updated value of ρ. This process is repeated until the pre-specified ATS_0 level is reached.

Based on our numerical experience, the performance of the above block bootstrap procedure should be reasonably good if we choose $m_1 = m/2$ and $B = 1000$.

4.3 Multivariate Dynamic Screening System for Disease Screening

The DySS method discussed in Section 4.2 considers only one disease risk factor for disease early detection. In practice, there are often multiple disease risk factors that are associated with the occurrence of a given disease, and thus should be monitored jointly for detecting the given disease. As an example, for early detection of strokes considered in Examples 4.1 and 4.2, besides the total cholesterol level, the systolic blood pressure, the diastolic blood pressure, and the glucose level should all be important disease risk factors. Thus, it should be helpful for effective early detection of strokes in such cases by monitoring all these disease risk factors jointly. To this end, Qiu and Xiang (2015) suggested a multivariate DySS method, which is described in several parts below.

4.3.1 Estimation of the Regular Longitudinal Pattern

Let $\boldsymbol{y}$ be the vector of q risk factors of a disease in concern. Assume that an IC dataset has been collected in advance, which contains the observed longitudinal data of m non-diseased people. The observations of $\boldsymbol{y}$ in the IC dataset are assumed to follow the multivariate nonparametric longitudinal model

$$\boldsymbol{y}(t_{ij}) = \boldsymbol{\mu}(t_{ij}) + \boldsymbol{\varepsilon}(t_{ij}), \qquad \text{for } j = 1, 2, \ldots, J_i,\ i = 1, 2, \ldots, m, \tag{4.15}$$

where t_{ij} is the jth observation time of the ith person, $\boldsymbol{y}(t_{ij}) = (y_1(t_{ij}), y_2(t_{ij}), \ldots, y_q(t_{ij}))'$ is the observed vector of $\boldsymbol{y}$ at t_{ij}, $\boldsymbol{\mu}(t_{ij}) = (\mu_1(t_{ij}), \mu_2(t_{ij}), \ldots, \mu_q(t_{ij}))'$ is its mean vector, and $\boldsymbol{\varepsilon}(t_{ij}) = (\varepsilon_1(t_{ij}), \varepsilon_2(t_{ij}), \ldots, \varepsilon_q(t_{ij}))'$ is the q-dimensional error term. In Model (4.15), it is assumed that observations of different people are independent of each other. For simplicity, it is further assumed that all observation times are in the unit time interval $[0, 1]$.

The regular longitudinal pattern of $\boldsymbol{y}$ can be described jointly by the mean function $\boldsymbol{\mu}(t)$ and the covariance matrix function $\Sigma(s,t) = \text{Cov}(\boldsymbol{y}(s), \boldsymbol{y}(t))$, for any $s, t \in [0, 1]$. In univariate cases (i.e., $q = 1$), nonparametric estimation of the mean and variance functions of $\boldsymbol{y}$ has been discussed extensively in the literature (cf., Subsection 2.6.2). In multivariate cases (i.e., $q > 1$), there is not much existing discussion on estimating a multivariate nonparametric longitudinal model. Next, we briefly describe the method proposed by Xiang et al. (2013) for estimating Model (4.15).

For $i = 1, 2, \ldots, m$, let

$$K_i = \text{diag}\left\{K_{h_l}(t_{ij} - t), j = 1, 2, \ldots, J_i, l = 1, 2, \ldots, q\right\}$$

be a diagonal matrix, and

$$W_i = \left(K_i^{-\frac{1}{2}} V_i K_i^{-\frac{1}{2}}\right)^{-1},$$

where $K_{h_l}(u) = K(u/h_l)/h_l$, for $l = 1, 2, \ldots, q$, $K(\cdot)$ is a kernel function, $\{h_l, l = 1, 2, \ldots, q\}$ are q bandwidths, $V_i = \text{Cov}(\boldsymbol{Y}_i)$, $\boldsymbol{Y}_i = (y_1(t_{i1}), \ldots, y_1(t_{iJ_i}), \ldots, y_q(t_{i1}), \ldots, y_q(t_{iJ_i}))'$ is a long vector of all observations of the ith person, and the inverse of a matrix is the Moore-Penrose generalized inverse that always exists. Then, for any $t \in [0,1]$, $\boldsymbol{\mu}(t)$ can be estimated by the following pth order local polynomial kernel smoothing procedure:

$$\min_{\boldsymbol{\beta} \in R^{q(p+1)}} \sum_{i=1}^{m} \left[\boldsymbol{Y}_i - (I_{q\times q} \otimes X_i)\boldsymbol{\beta}\right]' W_i \left[\boldsymbol{Y}_i - (I_{q\times q} \otimes X_i)\boldsymbol{\beta}\right], \tag{4.16}$$

where $\otimes$ denotes the Kronecker product, $I_{q\times q}$ is the $q \times q$ identity matrix,

$$\boldsymbol{\beta} = \left(\left(\beta_0^{(1)}, \ldots, \beta_p^{(1)}\right), \ldots, \left(\beta_0^{(q)}, \ldots, \beta_p^{(q)}\right)\right)',$$

and

$$X_i = \begin{pmatrix} 1 & (t_{i1} - t) & \ldots & (t_{i1} - t)^p \\ \vdots & \vdots & \ddots & \vdots \\ 1 & (t_{iJ_i} - t) & \ldots & (t_{iJ_i} - t)^p \end{pmatrix}_{J_i \times (p+1)}.$$

The solution of (4.16) to $\boldsymbol{\beta}$ has the expression

$$\widehat{\boldsymbol{\beta}} = \left[\sum_{i=1}^{m} (I_{q\times q} \otimes X_i)' W_i (I_{q\times q} \otimes X_i)\right]^{-1} \left[\sum_{i=1}^{m} (I_{q\times q} \otimes X_i)' W_i \boldsymbol{Y}_i\right].$$

Then, the pth order local polynomial kernel estimator of $\boldsymbol{\mu}(t)$ is

$$\widehat{\boldsymbol{\mu}}(t) = (I_{q\times q} \otimes \boldsymbol{e}_1')\,\widehat{\boldsymbol{\beta}}, \tag{4.17}$$

where $\boldsymbol{e}_1$ is the $(p+1)$-dimensional vector with its 1st element being 1 and all other elements being 0. In the above estimation procedure, $K(\cdot)$ can be chosen to be the Epanechnikov kernel function or some alternative kernel functions discussed in Subsection 2.5.4, and the bandwidths $\{h_l, l = 1, 2, \ldots, q\}$ can be determined by the conventional cross-validation (CV) procedure discussed in Subsection 2.5.5. In the kernel smoothing literature (cf. Qiu, 2005, Chapter 2), it has been well discussed that p can be chosen to be 1 in the model estimation procedure (4.16) without sacrificing much effectiveness of the kernel estimator $\widehat{\boldsymbol{\mu}}(t)$.

In practice, the matrix V_i contained in W_i is usually unknown and needs to be estimated. To this end, Xiang et al. (2013) suggested the following estimation method. First, the local linear kernel smoothing procedure (i.e., $p = 1$ in (4.16)) is used to obtain an initial estimator of $\boldsymbol{\mu}(t)$, denoted as $\widetilde{\boldsymbol{\mu}}(t) = (\widetilde{\mu}_1(t), \widetilde{\mu}_2(t), \ldots, \widetilde{\mu}_q(t))$. Then, its residuals are defined to be

$$\widetilde{\varepsilon}_{ijl} = y_{ijl} - \widetilde{\mu}_l(t_{ij}), \;\; j = 1, 2, \ldots, J_i, \; l = 1, 2, \ldots, q, \; i = 1, 2, \ldots, m.$$

Finally, the (l_1, l_2)-th element of $\Sigma(s,t) = (\sigma_{l_1,l_2}(s,t))$, for $l_1, l_2 = 1, 2, \ldots, q$, can be estimated by the following kernel estimator:

$$\widetilde{\sigma}_{l_1,l_2}(s,t) = \frac{\sum_{i=1}^{m} \sum_{j=1}^{J_i} \sum_{k=1}^{J_i} \widetilde{\varepsilon}_{ijl_1} \widetilde{\varepsilon}_{ikl_2} K\left(\frac{t_{ij}-s}{g_{l_1}}\right) K\left(\frac{t_{ik}-t}{g_{l_2}}\right)}{\sum_{i=1}^{m} \sum_{j=1}^{J_i} \sum_{k=1}^{J_i} K\left(\frac{t_{ij}-s}{g_{l_1}}\right) K\left(\frac{t_{ik}-t}{g_{l_2}}\right)}, \tag{4.18}$$

where $K(\cdot)$ is a kernel function, and $\{g_l, l = 1, 2, \ldots, q\}$ are bandwidths. In (4.18), $K(\cdot)$ can still be chosen to be the Epanechnikov kernel function, and the bandwidth g_l can still be chosen by the CV procedure for estimating the variance of $y_l(t)$ from the quantities $\{\widetilde{\varepsilon}^2_{ijl}, j = 1, 2, \ldots, J_i, i = 1, 2, \ldots, m\}$, for $l = 1, 2, \ldots, q$, using the local linear kernel smoothing procedure. From $\widetilde{\Sigma}(s,t) = (\widetilde{\sigma}_{l_1,l_2}(s,t))$, the corresponding estimator of V_i can be computed. The resulting estimator of $\boldsymbol{\mu}(t)$ computed by (4.17) is denoted as

$$\widehat{\boldsymbol{\mu}}(t, \widetilde{\Sigma}) = \left(\widehat{\mu}_1(t, \widetilde{\Sigma}), \widehat{\mu}_2(t, \widetilde{\Sigma}), \ldots, \widehat{\mu}_q(t, \widetilde{\Sigma})\right)'.$$

Then, the estimator of $\Sigma(s,t)$ can be updated by (4.18), after $\{\widetilde{\varepsilon}_{ijl}, j = 1, 2, \ldots, J_i, l = 1, 2, \ldots, q, i = 1, 2, \ldots, m\}$ are replaced by

$$\widehat{\varepsilon}_{ijl} = y_{ijl} - \widehat{\mu}_l(t_{ij}, \widetilde{\Sigma}), \;\; j = 1, 2, \ldots, J_i, \;\; l = 1, 2, \ldots, q, \;\; i = 1, 2, \ldots, m.$$

The resulting estimator of $\Sigma(s,t)$ is denoted as $\widehat{\Sigma}(s,t)$.

Model (4.15) and its estimation procedure described above are quite general. It does not impose any structure on the random error term $\boldsymbol{\varepsilon}(t)$, and allows the error covariance matrix $\Sigma(s,t)$ to change with both s and t in $[0,1]$. As a comparison, the alternative mixed-effects modeling approach discussed in Subsection 2.6.3 assumes that $\boldsymbol{\varepsilon}(t)$ consists of two independent parts: one is the random-effects and the other is the pure measurement error, and the variance/covariance of the pure measurement error is time-independent. So, model (4.15) is more general than most existing mixed-effects models in the literature. In some applications, it might be reasonable to specify the correlation structure among observations of $\boldsymbol{y}(t)$ by a parametric model (e.g., a parametric time series model). In such cases, the specified correlation structure can be accommodated when estimating the covariance matrix V_i. For instance, in the SPC literature, it is often assumed that observations of $\boldsymbol{y}(t)$ within a given person are independent of each other at different time points. If that assumption is valid, then the covariance matrix V_i is uniquely determined by the covariance matrix function $\Sigma(t,t)$, for $t \in [0,1]$. Its (l_1, l_2)-th element $\sigma_{l_1,l_2}(t,t)$, for $l_1, l_2 = 1, 2, \ldots, q$, can be estimated by

$$\widetilde{\sigma}_{l_1,l_2}(t,t) = \frac{\sum_{i=1}^{m}\sum_{j=1}^{J_i} \widetilde{\varepsilon}_{ijl_1}\widetilde{\varepsilon}_{ijl_2} K\left(\frac{t_{ij}-t}{g_{l_1}}\right) K\left(\frac{t_{ij}-t}{g_{l_2}}\right)}{\sum_{i=1}^{m}\sum_{j=1}^{J_i} K\left(\frac{t_{ij}-t}{g_{l_1}}\right) K\left(\frac{t_{ij}-t}{g_{l_2}}\right)},$$

where the kernel function $K(\cdot)$ and the bandwidths $\{g_l, l = 1, 2, \ldots, q\}$ can be chosen in the same way as that for those in (4.18).

4.3.2 Data Standardization for Disease Early Detection

The estimated regular longitudinal pattern of the q disease risk factors in $\boldsymbol{y}$ can be described by the estimated mean function $\widehat{\boldsymbol{\mu}}(t; \widetilde{\Sigma})$ and the estimated covariance matrix function $\widehat{\Sigma}(s,t)$, for $s,t \in [0,1]$, as discussed in the previous subsection. Next, we discuss how to detect the disease in concern effectively for a new patient by using the estimated regular longitudinal pattern. To this end, the new patient's observed disease risk factors need to be standardized first, which is discussed below.

Assume that observations of $\boldsymbol{y}$ of a new patient under monitoring are obtained at times $\{t_j^*, j \geq 1\}$ in the design interval $[0,1]$. If the new patient does not have the disease in concern, then the longitudinal pattern of the observed disease risk factors is reasonable to be considered as IC. In such cases, the observed longitudinal data should follow Model (4.15), which can be re-written as

$$\boldsymbol{y}(t_j^*) = \boldsymbol{\mu}(t_j^*) + \Sigma^{\frac{1}{2}}(t_j^*, t_j^*)\boldsymbol{\epsilon}(t_j^*), \qquad \text{for } j = 1, 2, \ldots, \tag{4.19}$$

where $\Sigma^{\frac{1}{2}}(t,t)\boldsymbol{\epsilon}(t)$ equals $\boldsymbol{\varepsilon}(t)$ in Model (4.15). Thus, $\boldsymbol{\epsilon}(t)$ in Model (4.19) has mean $\mathbf{0}$ and the identity covariance matrix $I_{q\times q}$ at each t. For the $\boldsymbol{y}$ observations of the new patient, their *standardized values* are then defined to be

$$\widehat{\boldsymbol{\epsilon}}(t_j^*) = \widehat{\Sigma}^{-\frac{1}{2}}(t_j^*, t_j^*)\left[\boldsymbol{y}(t_j^*) - \widehat{\boldsymbol{\mu}}\left(t_j^*; \widetilde{\Sigma}\right)\right], \qquad \text{for } j = 1, 2, \ldots. \tag{4.20}$$

As discussed in Subsection 4.2.2, by using these standardized observations of the new patient, we have actually compared its observed longitudinal pattern cross-sectionally with the estimated regular longitudinal pattern at the observation times $\{t_j^*, j \geq 1\}$. In cases when the observed longitudinal pattern of the new patient is IC, the mean and covariance matrix of each q-dimensional standardized observation in $\{\widehat{\boldsymbol{\epsilon}}(t_j^*), j \geq 1\}$ would be asymptotically $\mathbf{0}$ and $I_{q\times q}$, respectively.

4.3.3 Online Monitoring of Multiple Disease Risk Factors for Disease Early Detection

To detect the disease in concern for a new patient, we need to sequentially monitor the patient's observed disease risk factors to see whether the observed longitudinal pattern of the new patient is substantially different from the estimated regular longitudinal pattern. For simplicity, our discussion focuses on mean shifts only when comparing the two longitudinal patterns. Scale shifts can be discussed in a similar way. To this end, we consider monitoring the standardized observations $\{\boldsymbol{\epsilon}(t_j^*), j \geq 1\}$ since any shift in the mean function of the original observations of the new patient from the mean function of the regular longitudinal pattern would result in a shift in the mean function of the standardized observations, and vice versa. To detect a mean shift in the standardized observations $\{\boldsymbol{\epsilon}(t_j^*), j \geq 1\}$ of the new patient, there are some existing multivariate control charts in the SPC literature (cf., Qiu, 2014, Chapter 7). The conventional multivariate SPC charts are constructed based on the model assumptions that process observations at different time points are independent and identically distributed when the process under monitoring is IC, the IC process distribution is normal, and the observation times are equally spaced. In order to use these conventional charts, let us first discuss cases when the original process observations $\{\boldsymbol{y}(t_j^*), j \geq 1\}$ meet these assumptions. In such cases, the standardized observations $\{\widehat{\boldsymbol{\epsilon}}(t_j^*), j \geq 1\}$ would be asymptotically i.i.d. with the normal distribution $N(\mathbf{0}, I_{q\times q})$ when the longitudinal pattern of the new patient is IC. To use the multivariate exponentially weighted moving average (MEWMA) chart by Lowry et al. (1992), let us define its charting statistic to be

$$\boldsymbol{E}_j = \lambda\widehat{\boldsymbol{\epsilon}}(t_j^*) + (1-\lambda)\boldsymbol{E}_{j-1}, \qquad \text{for } j \geq 1, \tag{4.21}$$

where $\boldsymbol{E}_0 = \mathbf{0}$, and $\lambda \in (0,1]$ is a weighting parameter. The chart gives a signal when

$$\boldsymbol{E}_j'\Sigma_{0,\boldsymbol{E}_j}^{-1}\boldsymbol{E}_j > \rho_E, \tag{4.22}$$

where $\rho_E > 0$ is a control limit, and $\Sigma_{0,\boldsymbol{E}_j}$ is the IC covariance matrix of $\boldsymbol{E}_j$. It can be checked that

$$\Sigma_{0,\boldsymbol{E}_j} = \frac{\lambda}{2-\lambda}[1-(1-\lambda)^{2j}]\Sigma_{0,\widehat{\boldsymbol{\epsilon}}(t_j^*)},$$

where $\Sigma_{0,\widehat{\boldsymbol{\epsilon}}(t_j^*)} \approx I_{q\times q}$ is the IC covariance matrix of $\widehat{\boldsymbol{\epsilon}}(t_j^*)$. When j is large, $[1-(1-\lambda)^{2j}] \approx 1$. So, in such cases, (4.22) can be replaced by

$$\frac{2-\lambda}{\lambda}\boldsymbol{E}_j'\boldsymbol{E}_j > \rho_E. \tag{4.23}$$

By using the MEWMA chart (4.21) and (4.23), the observed disease risk factors of the new patient are monitored sequentially and all historical data of the patient up to the current time point t_j^* have been used in the decision-making process of the chart, after the patient's observed longitudinal pattern is compared cross-sectionally with the estimated regular longitudinal pattern.

For the MEWMA chart (4.21) and (4.23), its control limit ρ_E can be determined by Monte Carlo simulations in cases when the original process observations $\{\boldsymbol{y}(t_j^*), j \geq 1\}$ are assumed to be independent and normally distributed and when the sampling rate d (cf., its definition in Subsection 4.2.3) is pre-specified. In cases when the original process observations are serially correlated, this chart can still be used, but its control limit ρ_E should be determined properly from the IC data using a numerical algorithm such as the block bootstrap procedure discussed at the end of Subsection 4.2.3. Besides the MEWMA chart (4.21) and (4.23), other multivariate SPC charts can also be considered. In Qiu and Xiang (2015), the one by combining q univariate EWMA charts designed for monitoring the q individual disease risk factors and the LASSO-based MEWMA chart originally discussed in Zou and Qiu (2009) were also discussed. Based on an extensive numerical study, it was found that the MEWMA chart (4.21) and (4.23) and the LASSO-based MEWMA chart had similar numerical performance and the one by combining the q univariate EWMA charts had the worst performance in most cases considered.

4.4 Cases with Serially Correlated and Nonparametrically Distributed Data

The univariate and multivariate DySS methods discussed in the previous two sections are constructed based on the assumption that observations of the disease risk factors are either serially independent or serially correlated but the serial correlation can be described by an AR(1) model. They also require the data distribution to be normal. In reality, these assumptions are rarely valid. In cases when one or more such assumptions are violated, the related DySS methods would be unreliable to use if they are designed based on the invalid assumptions, because their actual ATS_0 values could be substantially different from the pre-specified ATS_0 values. See some related discussions in Section 3.3. If the control limit values of the related control charts in the DySS methods are determined numerically from an IC dataset using a numerical algorithm, as discussed at the end of Subsection 4.2.3, then the DySS methods would be reliable when the IC data are reasonably large, but their effectiveness could be compromised since their construction does not take into account the structure of the observed data properly. To overcome this limitation, Li and Qiu (2016) suggested a modified version of the univariate DySS method for disease early detection in cases when the observed data of the related disease risk factor are serially correlated and there are no parametric forms available for describing the data autocorrelation and data distribution. This method is introduced below, and its multivariate version was discussed in Li and Qiu (2017).

Let us assume that the regular longitudinal pattern of the disease risk factor y has been estimated from the IC data $\{y(t_{ij}), j = 1, 2, \ldots, J_i, i = 1, 2, \ldots, m\}$, and the estimated mean and variance functions are $\widehat{\mu}(t; \widetilde{V})$ and $\widehat{\sigma}_y^2(t)$, respectively, as discussed in Subsection 4.2.1. To detect the disease in concern for a new patient whose observed data are $\{y(t_j^*), j \geq 1\}$, the DySS method discussed in Section 4.2 used the standardized observations $\{\widehat{\epsilon}(t_j^*), j \geq 1\}$ computed by (4.7). These standardized observations could be serially correlated in a complex way and their IC distribution could be non-normal. So, instead of sequentially monitoring the standardized observations $\{\widehat{\epsilon}(t_j^*), j \geq 1\}$ directly, Li and Qiu (2016) suggested a sequential data decorrelation and standardization procedure to obtain decorrelated and standardized observations from the original observed data $\{y(t_j^*), j \geq 1\}$. This procedure is described below, which is similar to the one discussed in Section 3.4, although the former is for the disease screening problem while the latter is for the conventional SPC problem.

- When $j = 1$, the standardized value of $y(t_1^*)$ is defined to be

$$e^*(t_1^*) = \frac{y(t_1^*) - \widehat{\mu}(t_1^*; \widetilde{V})}{\widehat{\sigma}_y(t_1^*)}.$$

- When $j > 1$, let $\boldsymbol{y}_j = (\boldsymbol{y}'_{j-1}, y(t_j^*))'$, where $\boldsymbol{y}_1 = y(t_1^*)$. Then, the covariance matrix of $\boldsymbol{y}_j$ has the expression

$$\Sigma_{jj} = \begin{pmatrix} \Sigma_{j-1,j-1} & \boldsymbol{\sigma}_{j-1,j} \\ \boldsymbol{\sigma}'_{j-1,j} & \sigma_{jj} \end{pmatrix},$$

where $\Sigma_{j-1,j-1} = \text{Cov}(\boldsymbol{y}_{j-1})$, $\boldsymbol{\sigma}_{j-1,j} = \text{Cov}(\boldsymbol{y}_{j-1}, y(t_j^*)) = (V(t_1^*, t_j^*), V(t_2^*, t_j^*), \cdots, V(t_{j-1}^*, t_j^*))'$, and $\sigma_{jj} = \text{Var}(y(t_j^*)) = V(t_j^*, t_j^*)$. The estimator of Σ_{jj}, denoted as $\widehat{\Sigma}_{jj}$, can be obtained by replacing $V(s,t)$ in the above expression of Σ_{jj} by its estimator $\widetilde{V}(s,t)$ defined in (4.5). Then, the Cholesky decomposition of $\widehat{\Sigma}_{jj}$ can be written as

$$\Phi_j \widehat{\Sigma}_{jj} \Phi'_j = D_j,$$

where

$$\begin{aligned} \Phi_j &= \begin{pmatrix} \Phi_{j-1} & \boldsymbol{0} \\ -\widehat{\boldsymbol{\sigma}}'_{j-1,j}\widehat{\Sigma}^{-1}_{j-1,j-1} & 1 \end{pmatrix}, \\ D_j &= \text{diag}\left(d_1^2, d_2^2, \ldots, d_j^2\right), \\ d_j^2 &= \widehat{\sigma}_{jj} - \widehat{\boldsymbol{\sigma}}'_{j-1,j}\widehat{\Sigma}^{-1}_{j-1,j-1}\widehat{\boldsymbol{\sigma}}_{j-1,j}, \end{aligned}$$

and Φ_{j-1} and $\text{diag}(d_1^2, d_2^2, \ldots, d_{j-1}^2)$ are from the Cholesky decomposition of $\widehat{\Sigma}_{j-1,j-1}$. Therefore, if we define

$$e(t_j^*) = -\widehat{\boldsymbol{\sigma}}'_{j-1,j}\widehat{\Sigma}^{-1}_{j-1,j-1}(\boldsymbol{y}_{j-1} - \widehat{\boldsymbol{\mu}}_{j-1}) + \left(\boldsymbol{y}_j - \widehat{\mu}(t_j^*; \widetilde{V})\right),$$

where

$$\widehat{\boldsymbol{\mu}}_{j-1} = (\widehat{\mu}(t_1^*; \widetilde{V}), \widehat{\mu}(t_2^*; \widetilde{V}), \ldots, \widehat{\mu}(t_{j-1}^*; \widetilde{V}))',$$

then

$$\begin{aligned} \boldsymbol{e}_j &= (e(t_1^*), e(t_2^*), \ldots, e(t_j^*))' \\ &= (\boldsymbol{e}'_{j-1}, e(t_j^*))' \\ &= \begin{pmatrix} \Phi_{j-1} & \boldsymbol{0} \\ -\widehat{\boldsymbol{\sigma}}'_{j-1,j}\widehat{\Sigma}^{-1}_{j-1,j-1} & 1 \end{pmatrix} \begin{pmatrix} \boldsymbol{y}_{j-1} - \widehat{\boldsymbol{\mu}}_{j-1} \\ \boldsymbol{y}_j - \widehat{\mu}(t_j^*; \widetilde{V}) \end{pmatrix} \\ &= \Phi_j(\boldsymbol{y}_j - \widehat{\boldsymbol{\mu}}_j), \end{aligned}$$

and $\text{Cov}(\boldsymbol{e}_j) = D_j$. (Note that the last equation is only asymptotically true in the sense that it is true when $\widehat{\Sigma}_{jj}$ and Σ_{jj} are the same.) Thus, we define the standardized and decorrelated observation at time t_j^* to be

$$e^*(t_j^*) = \frac{e(t_j^*)}{d_j} = \frac{-\widehat{\boldsymbol{\sigma}}'_{j-1,j}\widehat{\Sigma}^{-1}_{j-1,j-1}(\boldsymbol{y}_{j-1} - \widehat{\boldsymbol{\mu}}_{j-1}) + \left(\boldsymbol{y}_j - \widehat{\mu}(t_j^*; \widetilde{V})\right)}{d_j}.$$

Then, $e^*(t_j^*)$ has the properties that (i) it is asymptotically uncorrelated with $\{e^*(t_1^*), e^*(t_2^*), \ldots, e^*(t_{j-1}^*)\}$, and (ii) it has the asymptotic mean 0 and the asymptotic variance 1.

By the above sequential data decorrelation and standardization procedure, the original process observations $\{y(t_j^*), j \geq 1\}$ are decorrelated into $\{e^*(t_j^*), j \geq 1\}$. For each j, because $e^*(t_j^*)$ is a linear combination of the original observations $y(t_1^*), y(t_2^*), \ldots, y(t_j^*)$, its distribution would be asymptotically normal under some regularity conditions. Therefore, the sequence $\{e^*(t_j^*), j \geq 1\}$ would be asymptotically i.i.d. with the common asymptotic distribution of $N(0,1)$ when the related process under monitoring is IC. In such cases, the conventional CUSUM chart (cf., Subsection 3.1.3) is reasonable to use. For example, to detect upward mean shifts in $\{y(t_j^*), j \geq 1\}$, the CUSUM charting statistic can be defined to be

$$C_j^+ = \max\left(0, C_{j-1}^+ + e^*(t_j^*) - k\right), \qquad \text{for } j \geq 1, \tag{4.24}$$

where $C_0^+ = 0$ and $k > 0$ is an allowance constant. The CUSUM chart gives a signal if

$$C_j^+ > \rho_C, \tag{4.25}$$

where $\rho_C > 0$ is a control limit chosen to achieve a pre-specified ATS_0 value. The control charts for detecting downward and/or arbitrary mean shifts in the original process observations $\{y(t_j^*), j \geq 1\}$ can be constructed in similar ways. See the related discussion in Subsection 3.1.3.

In the data standardization and decorrelation procedure discussed above, we need to compute $\widehat{\Sigma}_{j-1,j-1}^{-1}$ at time t_j^*. To reduce computational burden in computing this matrix, the following recursive formula can be used: for $j > 2$,

$$\widehat{\Sigma}_{j-1,j-1}^{-1} =$$
$$\begin{pmatrix} \widehat{\Sigma}_{j-2,j-2}^{-1} + \widehat{\Sigma}_{j-2,j-2}^{-1}\widehat{\boldsymbol{\sigma}}_{j-2,j-1}D_{j-1}^{-1}\widehat{\boldsymbol{\sigma}}_{j-2,j-1}'\widehat{\Sigma}_{j-2,j-2}^{-1}, & -\widehat{\Sigma}_{j-2,j-2}^{-1}\widehat{\boldsymbol{\sigma}}_{j-2,j-1}D_{j-1}^{-1} \\ -D_{j-1}^{-1}\widehat{\boldsymbol{\sigma}}_{j-2,j-1}'\widehat{\Sigma}_{j-2,j-2}^{-1}, & D_{j-1}^{-1} \end{pmatrix},$$

where

$$D_{j-1} = \widehat{\sigma}_{j-1,j-1} - \widehat{\boldsymbol{\sigma}}_{j-2,j-1}'\widehat{\Sigma}_{j-2,j-2}^{-1}\widehat{\boldsymbol{\sigma}}_{j-2,j-1} = d_{j-1}^2,$$

and

$$\widehat{\boldsymbol{\sigma}}_{j-2,j-1} = \widehat{\text{Cov}}\left(\boldsymbol{y}_{j-2}, y(t_{j-1}^*)\right) = \left(\widetilde{V}(t_1^*, t_{j-1}^*), \widetilde{V}(t_2^*, t_{j-1}^*), \ldots, \widetilde{V}(t_{j-2}^*, t_{j-1}^*)\right)'.$$

From its construction, it can be seen that the CUSUM chart (4.24)–(4.25) can accommodate arbitrary covariance structure in the observed data. Li and Qiu (2016) showed that this chart was actually equivalent to the chart (4.13)–(4.14) when the serial correlation in the observed data followed an AR(1) model.

Next, we discuss how to determine the control limit ρ_C used in (4.25). From the construction of the chart, it can be seen that the decorrelated and standardized observations $\{e^*(t_j^*), j \geq 1\}$ used in (4.24) are serially uncorrelated. If it is reasonable to assume that the original process observations $\{y(t_j^*), j \geq 1\}$ have a normal IC distribution, then $\{e^*(t_j^*), j \geq 1\}$ would be asymptotically i.i.d. with the standard normal IC distribution, as pointed out earlier. So, in such cases, the control limit ρ_C can be determined by

Monte Carlo simulations, as discussed in Subsection 4.2.3. If the IC distribution of the original process observations is unknown but the number of observations of each patient is large, then we can still use the above Monte Carlo method to determine the control limit ρ_C, since each decorrelated and standardized observation (e.g., $e^*(t_j^*)$) is a linear combination of the original process observations at the current and all previous observation times and thus its IC distribution would be asymptotically normal. However, if the IC process distribution is unknown and the number of observations of each patient is small, the distribution of $e^*(t_j^*)$ could be substantially different from normal. In such cases, we can use a bootstrap procedure to determine the control limit ρ_C from an IC dataset, which is briefly described below. The IC dataset with m non-diseased people is first divided into two parts. The first part with m_1 non-diseased people is used for obtaining the estimates of the mean and covariance functions, as discussed in Subsection 4.2.1. Based on these estimates, we can obtain the decorrelated and standardized observations $\{e^*(t_{ij}), j = 1, 2, \ldots, J_i, i = m_1+1, m_1+2, \ldots, m\}$ of the second part of the IC data. These decorrelated and standardized observations are asymptotically uncorrelated, and can be used to approximate the IC distribution of $e^*(t_j^*)$ used in (4.24). Therefore, to determine the control limit ρ_C such that a pre-specified ATS_0 value is achieved, we can use the following numerical algorithm. (i) Obtain a bootstrap sample by randomly selecting a sequence of observations with replacement from $\{e^*(t_{ij}), j = 1, 2, \ldots, J_i, i = m_1+1, m_1+2, \ldots, m\}$. (ii) Apply the CUSUM chart (4.24)–(4.25) with a given value of ρ_C to the bootstrap sample and record the time to signal (TS) value. (iii) Repeat steps (i) and (ii) B times and compute the actual ATS_0 value by averaging the B TS values. (iv) Search the value of ρ_C by a numerical algorithm (e.g., the bisection search algorithm) such that the pre-specified ATS_0 value is reached.

Example 4.3 *For the stroke data considered in Example 4.1, the observed total cholesterol levels (in mg/100ml) of the* $m = 1028$ *non-stroke patients are considered as the IC data. Then, the observed data of the first* $m_1 = 800$ *non-stroke patients are used for estimating Model (4.1) by the model estimation procedure described in Subsection 4.2.1. When computing the estimated IC mean function* $\widehat{\mu}(t; \widetilde{V})$ *and the estimated IC covariance function* $\widetilde{V}(s,t)$*, the bandwidth is set to be* $h = 0.15$ *in both cases. Based on the estimated regular longitudinal pattern described by* $\widehat{\mu}(t; \widetilde{V})$ *and* $\widetilde{V}(s,t)$*, the data decorrelation and standardization procedure discussed above is applied to the observed data of the remaining* $m_2 = 228$ *non-stroke patients in the IC dataset to obtain the decorrelated and standardized IC observations* $\{e^*(t_{ij}), j = 1, 2, \ldots, J_i, i = m_1 + 1, m_1 + 2, \ldots, m\}$*. The control limit* ρ_C *of the CUSUM chart (4.24)–(4.25) is then determined to be 0.763 from these decorrelated and standardized IC observations by the bootstrap procedure described above when we choose* $k = 0.1$, $ATS_0 = 25$ *and* $d = 2$*, as in Example 4.2. The CUSUM chart (4.24)–(4.25) is then applied to the observed data of the 27 stroke patients for disease early detection. The resulting CUSUM charts for monitoring the 27 stroke patients are presented in Figure 4.4. From the figure, it can be seen* *that 23 out of the 27 stroke patients are detected to have upward mean shifts in the total cholesterol level. The signal times of these 23 stroke patients are reported in Table 4.3, and their average is 9.96 years. Compared to the results in Example 4.2, it can be seen that more stroke patients receive signals from the CUSUM chart (4.24)–(4.25) after the observed data are decorrelated by the data decorrelation and standardization procedure discussed above. In addition, the average signal time is also shorter here than that in Example 4.2.*

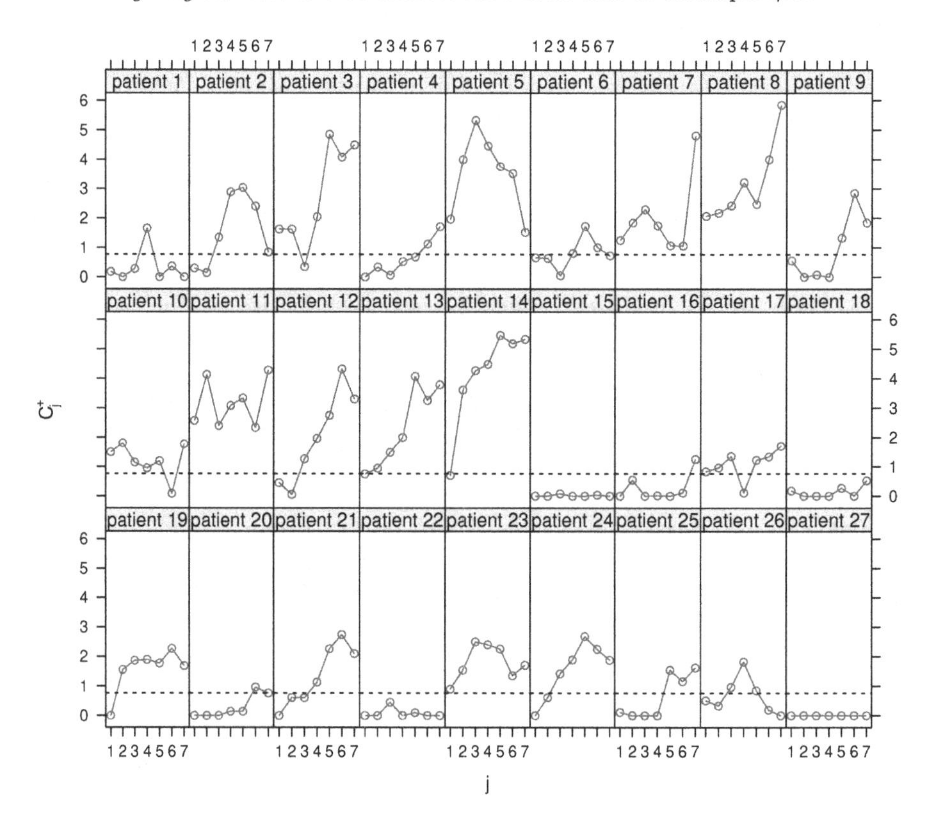

FIGURE 4.4
CUSUM chart (4.24)–(4.25) with $(k, \rho_C, ATS_0) = (0.1, 0.763, 25)$ for monitoring the 27 stroke patients. The dashed horizontal lines in the plots denote the control limit ρ_C.

4.5 Robust Disease Screening by Estimation of Longitudinal Data Distribution

In all the DySS methods discussed in the previous sections, the regular longitudinal pattern of the dynamic process of the disease risk factor(s) is

TABLE 4.3
Signal times (years) of the 23 stroke patients who receive signals from the CUSUM chart (4.24)–(4.25).

Patient ID	Signal Time	Patient ID	Signal Time
1	16	13	7
2	12	14	8
3	0	16	26
4	23	17	0
5	0	19	8
6	15	20	24
7	0	21	16
8	0	23	0
9	19	24	12
10	0	25	19
11	0	26	12
12	12		

described by the mean and covariance functions. This is appropriate when the time-varying distribution of the dynamic process is normal, since a normal distribution is uniquely determined by its mean and variance (cf., Subsection 2.2.2). But, in cases when the distribution of a dynamic process is non-normal, which is often the case in practice, the mean and covariance functions could be ineffective in describing the regular longitudinal pattern of the dynamic process. To overcome this limitation, a natural idea is to describe the regular longitudinal pattern by the entire time-varying IC process distribution, and then apply a control chart to the process observations after they have been decorrelated and standardized properly by the estimated IC process distribution. Based on this idea, You and Qiu (2021a) developed a robust DySS method in cases with a single disease risk factor, which is introduced below in several parts.

4.5.1 Description and Estimation of the Regular Longitudinal Pattern

Let y be the disease risk factor in concern for detecting a given disease. Assume that there is an IC dataset $\{y(t_{ij}), j = 1, 2, \ldots, J_i, i = 1, 2, \ldots, m\}$ that contains observed longitudinal data of y of m non-disease people, where $\{t_{ij}, j = 1, 2, \ldots, J_i, i = 1, 2, \ldots, m\}$ are observation times in $[0, 1]$ and they could be unequally spaced within each person. Let

$$F(x; t) = P(y(t) \leq x), \qquad \text{for } x \in R.$$

Then, $F(x; t)$ is the cumulative distribution function (cdf) of $y(t)$ (cf., Section 2.1). In this section, we suggest *describing the regular longitudinal pattern of* y

by $F(x;t)$, instead of by the mean and variance functions $\mu(t)$ and $\sigma_y^2(t)$. For simplicity of presentation, let us assume that $F(x;t)$ is a continuous function of both x and t. This implies that the disease risk factor y has a continuous cdf at each t, and the cdf changes continuously over t, which should be reasonable in many applications including the Framingham heart study discussed in Example 4.1.

To estimate $F(x;t)$ from the IC data $\{y(t_{ij}), j = 1,2,\ldots,J_i, i = 1,2,\ldots,m\}$, one natural idea is to use the local kernel smoothing method (Fan et al., 1996; Yu and Jones, 1998). To this end, let $W(\cdot)$ be a pre-specified kernel function that has all the properties of a cdf, and $W_{h_w}(\cdot) = W(\cdot/h_w)$, where $h_w > 0$ is a bandwidth parameter. Then, for any $x \in R$, $F(x;t)$ can be estimated by

$$\widehat{F}(x;t) = \arg\min_{a \geq 0} \sum_{i=1}^{m} \sum_{j=1}^{J_i} \left[W_{h_w}(x - y(t_{ij})) - a\right]^2 K_{h_t}(t_{ij} - t), \tag{4.26}$$

where $K_{h_t}(\cdot) = K(\cdot/h_t)/h_t$, $K(\cdot)$ is a pre-specified density kernel function, and $h_t > 0$ is another bandwidth parameter. In (4.26), because there are two kernel functions $W(\cdot)$ and $K(\cdot)$ used, this estimation procedure is called a *double-kernel smoother* in the literature (Yu and Jones, 1998). For computing the estimator $\widehat{F}(x;t)$, the density kernel function $K(\cdot)$ can be chosen to be the Epanechnikov kernel function, namely, $K(u) = 0.75(1-u^2)I(|u| \leq 1)$, or other commonly used kernel functions mentioned in Subsection 2.5.4. To ensure that $\widehat{F}(x;t)$ can take values in the entire interval $(0,1)$, the kernel function $W(\cdot)$ should not have a compact support. To meet this requirement, the one suggested in Yu and Jones (1998) can be used, which is the cdf of the standard normal distribution, i.e.,

$$W(u) = \frac{1}{\sqrt{2\pi}} \int_{-\infty}^{u} \exp(-s^2/2)\, ds.$$

In the estimation procedure (4.26), there are two bandwidth parameters h_w and h_t to choose in advance. To this end, by the normal referencing rule suggested by Silverman (1986) and Fan and Gijbels (1995), h_w can be chosen by the formula

$$h_w = \int_0^1 \widehat{\sigma}_y(t)\, dt \left[\frac{8\pi^{1/2} \int_{-\infty}^{\infty} w^2(u)\, du}{3\left\{\int_{-\infty}^{\infty} u^2 w(u)\, du\right\}^2 \sum_{i=1}^{m} J_i}\right]^{1/5},$$

where $\widehat{\sigma}_y^2(t)$ is an estimate of $\sigma_y^2(t)$ (cf., Subsection 4.2.1), and $w(u) = W'(u)$ is the density function of $W(u)$. To choose the bandwidth parameter h_t, we can consider using the following residual squares criterion (RSC):

$$\text{RSC}(h_t) = \sum_{i=1}^{m} \sum_{j=1}^{J_i} U_0\left(y(t_{ij}), t_{ij}; h_t\right) \left[1 + \frac{3S_0(t_{ij})}{V_0^2(t_{ij})}\right],$$

where

$$\begin{aligned}
U_0(y,t;h_t) &= \frac{1}{V_0(t)-S_0(t)/V_0(t)}\sum_{i=1}^{m}\sum_{j=1}^{J_i}\left[W_{h_w}(y-y(t_{ij}))-\widehat{F}(y;t)\right]^2 \times \\
&\quad K_{h_t}(t_{ij}-t), \\
V_0(t) &= \sum_{i=1}^{m}\sum_{j=1}^{J_i} K_{h_t}(t_{ij}-t), \\
S_0(t) &= \sum_{i=1}^{m}\sum_{j=1}^{J_i} K_{h_t}(t_{ij}-t)^2.
\end{aligned}$$

Then, h_t can be chosen by minimizing RSC(h_t).

4.5.2 Online Monitoring of the Observed Disease Risk Factor

Next, we want to sequentially monitor the observed disease risk factor of a new patient for disease early detection. The patient's observations of the disease risk factor y are denoted as $\{y(t_j^*), j \geq 1\}$. The original univariate DySS method discussed in Section 4.2 uses the standardized observations $\widehat{\epsilon}(t_j^*) = [y(t_j^*) - \widehat{\mu}(t_j^*)]/\widehat{\sigma}(t_j^*)$, for $j \geq 1$, to compare the observed longitudinal pattern of y for the new patient with the estimated regular longitudinal pattern that is described by $\widehat{\mu}(t)$ and $\widehat{\sigma}^2(t)$, for $t \in [0,1]$. As discussed earlier in Subsection 4.5.1, the regular longitudinal pattern of y can be described properly by $\mu(t)$ and $\sigma^2(t)$ only in cases when the time-varying distribution of y is normal, which is rarely valid in practice. To overcome this limitation, You and Qiu (2021a) suggested describing the regular longitudinal pattern of y by the time-varying IC process distribution $F(x;t)$.

After $F(x;t)$ is estimated by $\widehat{F}(x;t)$ in (4.26), You and Qiu (2021a) suggested transforming the original observations $\{y(t_j^*), j \geq 1\}$ of the new patient into

$$z_j^* = \Phi^{-1}\left[\widehat{F}\left(y(t_j^*);t_j^*\right)\right], \qquad \text{for } j \geq 1, \tag{4.27}$$

where $\Phi(\cdot)$ is the cdf of the standard normal distribution (cf., Subsection 2.2.2). If the observed longitudinal pattern of the new patient is IC, then by the properties of the uniform distribution, the distribution of $F(y(t_j^*);t_j^*)$ would be close to $U[0,1]$ and the distribution of z_j^* in (4.27) would be approximately $N(0,1)$, for each j. In such cases, $\{z_j^*, j \geq 1\}$ could be regarded as a sequence of standard normal random variables.

In cases when the original process observations $\{y(t_j^*), j \geq 1\}$ are independent of each other at different time points, it is obvious that the transformed data $\{z_j^*, j \geq 1\}$ would be independent of each other at different time points as well. In such cases, it is natural to apply the conventional CUSUM chart to $\{z_j^*, j \geq 1\}$. For instance, to detect an upward mean shift in $\{y(t_j^*), j \geq 1\}$, the conventional CUSUM charting statistic is defined to be

$$\widetilde{C}_j^+ = \max\left(0, \widetilde{C}_{j-1}^+ + z_j^* - \widetilde{k}\right), \quad \text{for } j \geq 1, \tag{4.28}$$

where $\widetilde{C}_0^+ = 0$, and $\widetilde{k} > 0$ is an allowance constant. The chart gives a signal when

$$\widetilde{C}_j^+ > \widetilde{\rho}_C, \tag{4.29}$$

where $\widetilde{\rho}_C > 0$ is a properly chosen control limit. Control charts for detecting downward or arbitrary mean shifts can be constructed similarly (cf., Subsection 3.1.3).

In practice, the original process observations $\{y(t_j^*), j \geq 1\}$ are often serially correlated across different time points. Consequently, the transformed observations $\{z_j^*, j \geq 1\}$ would be serially correlated as well. As discussed in Section 4.3, the autocorrelation among $\{z_j^*, j \geq 1\}$ can be estimated from the IC dataset. To this end, let

$$z_{ij} = \Phi^{-1}\left(\widehat{F}(y_i(t_{ij}), t_{ij})\right), \quad \text{for } j = 1, 2, \ldots, J_i, i = 1, 2, \ldots, m$$

be the transformed observations of the IC data. For any $s, t \in [0, 1]$, let

$$Q(s,t) = \text{Cov}\left[\Phi^{-1}\left(\widehat{F}(y(s); s)\right), \Phi^{-1}\left(\widehat{F}(y(t); t)\right)\right]$$

be the covariance function of $\Phi^{-1}(\widehat{F}(y(t); t))$. Then, similar to (4.18), $Q(s,t)$ can be estimated by the following kernel estimator: for $s \neq t \in [0, 1]$,

$$\widehat{Q}(s,t) = \frac{\sum_{i=1}^m \sum_{1 \leq j_1 \neq j_2 \leq J_i} z_{ij_1} z_{ij_2} K_{h_\sigma}(t_{ij_1} - s) K_{h_\sigma}(t_{ij_2} - t)}{\sum_{i=1}^m \sum_{1 \leq j_1 \neq j_2 \leq J_i} K_{h_\sigma}(t_{ij_1} - s) K_{h_\sigma}(t_{ij_2} - t)}.$$

When $s = t$, define $\widehat{Q}(s,t) = 1$, since the transformed observations $\{z_{ij}, j = 1, 2, \ldots, J_i, i = 1, 2, \ldots, m\}$ would have asymptotic variances of 1. The bandwidth parameter h_σ in the above expression can be selected by the cross-validation procedure, as discussed in Subsection 4.3.1.

After $Q(s,t)$ is estimated from the IC dataset by $\widehat{Q}(s,t)$, the transformed data $\{z_j^*, j \geq 1\}$ of the new patient under monitoring can be decorrelated using the data decorrelation and standardization procedure discussed in Section 4.4. Here, we present a different data decorrelation procedure that was originally proposed in You and Qiu (2019), which was shown more computationally efficient than the one discussed Section 4.4.

- When $j = 1$, let $U_1 = [\widehat{Q}(t_1^*, t_1^*)]^{-1/2}$. Then, the first standardized observation is defined to be

$$e_1^* = U_1 z_1^*.$$

- When $j > 1$, the decorrelated and standardized observation of z_j^* is defined to be

$$e_j^* = \left[z_j^* - \mathbf{v}_j'(e_1^*, e_2^*, \ldots, e_{j-1}^*)'\right] / d_j,$$

where

$$\mathbf{v}_j = \mathbf{U}_{j-1}\Big(\widehat{Q}(t_1^*, t_j^*), \widehat{Q}(t_2^*, t_j^*), \ldots, \widehat{Q}(t_{j-1}^*, t_j^*)\Big)',$$
$$d_j = \left[\widehat{Q}(t_j^*, t_j^*) - \mathbf{v}_j'\mathbf{v}_j\right]^{1/2},$$
$$\mathbf{U}_j = \begin{pmatrix} \mathbf{U}_{j-1} & \mathbf{0} \\ -\mathbf{v}_j'\mathbf{U}_{j-1}/d_j & 1/d_j \end{pmatrix}.$$

After using the above data decorrelation procedure, it can be checked that the decorrelated observations $\{e_j^*, j \geq 1\}$ are asymptotically uncorrelated with each other and each of them has the asymptotic mean of 0 and the asymptotic variance of 1. Because the distribution of z_j^* is approximately $N(0,1)$, for each j, the distribution of e_j^* should be even closer to $N(0,1)$, since e_j^* is a linear combination of $\{z_1^*, z_2^*, \ldots, z_j^*\}$. After data decorrelation, to detect an upward mean shift in the original process observations, it is natural to use the following CUSUM chart:

$$C_j^+ = \max\left(0, C_{j-1}^+ + e_j^* - k\right), \qquad \text{for } j \geq 1, \tag{4.30}$$

where $C_0^+ = 0$, and $k > 0$ is an allowance constant. The chart gives a signal when

$$C_j^+ > \rho_C, \tag{4.31}$$

where $\rho_C > 0$ is a properly chosen control limit. CUSUM charts for detecting downward or arbitrary mean shifts can be constructed similarly.

For both CUSUM charts (4.28)–(4.29) and (4.30)–(4.31), their control limits $\widetilde{\rho}_C$ and ρ_C can be determined by Monte Carlo simulations, once the sampling rate d of the observation times is specified. That is because both charts are constructed from a sequence of (asymptotically) i.i.d. standard normal random variables when the process under monitoring is IC. See Subsection 4.2.3 for some related discussions.

4.6 Some Discussions

In this chapter, we have introduced some basic DySS methods for sequential monitoring of one or more disease risk factors in order to detect a disease in concern as quickly as possible. These methods combine cross-sectional comparison between a patient under monitoring and some non-diseased people in an IC data with regard to their observed disease risk factors, and a sequential decision-making mechanism so that historical data of the patient can be used efficiently. Numerical studies presented in some papers (e.g., Li and Qiu, 2016, 2017; Qiu and Xiang, 2014, 2015; You and Qiu, 2020a) have confirmed that they are effective for disease early detection.

To measure the performance of a DySS method, its ATS_0 and ATS_1 values can be used, as discussed in the previous sections. But, these metrics are for evaluating the performance of a control chart when monitoring a single sequential process (Qiu, 2014, Section 3.2). In the current disease early detection problem, the observed disease risk factors of a patient can be regarded as a sequential process, and there are many such processes involved since the DySS methods would be used for detecting the disease in concern for many patients. In the disease diagnosis literature, people often use the false positive rate (FPR), false negative rate (FNR), and the related receiver operating characteristic (ROC) curve to evaluate the overall performance of a disease diagnostic method (e.g., Obuchowski, 2003; Pepe, 2003; Qiu and Le, 2001; Zhou et al., 2002). But, these metrics alone cannot be good enough to measure the performance of the DySS methods because they do not take into account the signal times of the related control charts that are critically important for disease early detection. To overcome the limitations of the two types of performance metrics mentioned above, Qiu et al. (2020b) suggested a type of new performance metrics called *dynamic false positive rate* (DFPR), *dynamic true positive rate* (DTPR), and the related *process monitoring ROC* (PM-ROC) *curve* to measure the performance of the DySS methods. These metrics combine the signal times of the related control charts with the conventional FPR and FNR metrics in a proper way, so that they can reflect both false positive and false negative rates of the DySS methods and how fast the related control charts give signals.

It should be pointed out that besides disease early detection, DySS methods can be used in many other applications involving sequential monitoring of dynamic processes. For instance, durable goods (e.g., airplanes, computers) often need to be checked regularly or occasionally for certain performance variables. The distribution of such performance variables would change over time when the durable goods get older, even when they perform satisfactorily at their ages. The research problem to monitor the longitudinal performance of such dynamic processes is called *dynamic screening* (DS) in the literature (cf., Qiu and Xiang, 2014). So, the DySS methods can provide a powerful analytic tool for handling DS applications.

The DySS methods discussed in this chapter can only be used in cases when all disease risk factors are continuous numerical variables. In practice, however, some disease risk factors could be binary and/or categorical (e.g., smoking status). For such applications, methods for modeling longitudinal binary and/or categorical data (e.g., Parzen et al., 2011; Sutradhar, 2014) should be helpful for estimating the regular longitudinal pattern of the disease risk factors. More research is needed in this direction to construct appropriate DySS methods for handling cases with some or all disease risk factors being binary and/or categorical.

4.7 Exercises

4.1 Summarize the major features of the observed data in the disease screening problem discussed in Section 4.1. Give some reasons why the conventional longitudinal data analysis and statistical process control methods cannot solve the disease screening problem effectively.

4.2 Regarding Model (4.1),

(i) give an example to intuitively explain the meaning of the two components $\varepsilon_0(t)$ and $\varepsilon_1(t)$ of the error term $\varepsilon(t)$ discussed in the paragraph below Expression (4.1), and

(ii) derive a formula for $\sigma_y^2(t) := V(t,t)$ from Expression (4.2).

4.3 Explain why the standardized observations of a new patient defined in (4.7) can be used for disease early detection for the new patient.

4.4 The CUSUM chart (4.8)–(4.9) is used for detecting upward mean shifts in the observed data of the disease risk factor y.

(i) Define a CUSUM chart for detecting downward mean shifts in the observed data of y.

(ii) Define a CUSUM chart for detecting arbitrary mean shifts in the observed data of y.

4.5 (i) Give a tool example to explain why the metrics ARL_0 and ARL_1 are inappropriate to measure the performance of the CUSUM chart (4.8)–(4.9) in cases when observation times are unequally spaced.

(ii) When observation times are equally spaced, please explain that it is equivalent to use either the metrics ARL_0 and ARL_1 or the metrics ATS_0 and ATS_1 for measuring the performance of the CUSUM chart (4.8)–(4.9).

4.6 Derive Model (4.11) from the AR(1) model (4.10).

4.7 For the estimated mean function $\widehat{\boldsymbol{\mu}}(t;\widetilde{\Sigma})$ and the estimated covariance matrix function $\widehat{\Sigma}(s,t)$ discussed in Subsection 4.3.1, for $s,t \in [0,1]$, it has been proved in Qiu and Xiang (2015) that they converge to the true mean function $\boldsymbol{\mu}(t)$ and the true covariance matrix function $\Sigma(s,t)$, respectively, under some regularity conditions. Based on this result, verify that the means and covariance matrices of the standardized observations $\{\widehat{\boldsymbol{\epsilon}}(t_j^*), j \geq 1\}$ defined in (4.20) are asymptotically $\mathbf{0}$ and $I_{q\times q}$.

4.8 For the MEWMA charting statistic $\mathbf{E}_j$ defined in (4.21), verify that its IC covariance matrix has the expression

$$\Sigma_{0,\boldsymbol{E}_j} = \frac{\lambda}{2-\lambda}\left[1-(1-\lambda)^{2j}\right]\Sigma_{0,\widehat{\boldsymbol{\epsilon}}(t_j^*)}, \quad \text{for } j \geq 1.$$

4.9 The CUSUM chart (4.24)–(4.25) is designed for detecting upward mean shifts in the observed disease risk factor $\{y(t_j^*), j \geq 1\}$.

(i) Construct CUSUM charts for detecting downward and/or arbitrary mean shifts in the observed disease risk factor.

(ii) Construct an EWMA chart for detecting arbitrary mean shifts in the observed disease risk factor.

4.10 Derive a formula for $\widehat{F}(x;t)$ from Expression (4.26).

4.11 In Expression (4.27), if the estimated cdf $\widehat{F}(x;t)$ is replaced by the true cdf $F(x;t)$, verify that the distribution of $\Phi^{-1}[F(y(t_j^*); t_j^*)]$ is $N(0,1)$, for each j.

4.12 Regarding the transformed data defined in (4.27), verify that the transformed data $\{z_j^*, j \geq 1\}$ are independent of each other at different time points if the original process observations $\{y(t_j^*), j \geq 1\}$ are independent of each other at different time points.

5

Disease Screening by Online Disease Risk Monitoring

5.1 Introduction

The DySS methods introduced in the previous chapter try to detect a disease in concern for individual patients in three major steps. First, the regular longitudinal pattern of the related disease risk factors is estimated from an IC dataset. Second, for a given patient, the patient's observed disease risk factors is standardized using the estimated regular longitudinal pattern. Third, the standardized data of the given patient are then monitored sequentially by an SPC chart for disease early detection. These DySS methods have at least the following two limitations. First, for a given disease in concern, there could be many potential disease risk factors considered. Some of them may be more important than the others in predicting the occurrence of the disease, and some others may actually provide little useful information for disease early detection. In the DySS methods discussed in the previous chapter, however, all disease risk factors are treated equally in the sequential decision-making process. This may negatively affect the effectiveness of the related DySS methods, since the irrelevant disease risk factors can only increase the variability of the charting statistics of the related control charts, especially in cases when the number of disease risk factors considered is large. Second, besides the IC data that contain observed data of some non-diseased people, we often have observed data of some diseased people as well in practice, collected before disease screening for new patients. For instance, in some large observational studies, such as the Framingham Heart Study discussed in Example 4.1 of Section 4.2, many data about some important disease risk factors have been collected for both diseased and non-diseased people. Proper use of such data of both diseased and non-diseased people should be helpful in exploring the association between the disease risk factors and the likelihood of a disease in concern, and thus helpful for disease early detection. But, the DySS methods discussed in the previous chapter have ignored such useful information in the observed data of diseased people collected before disease screening.

To overcome the two major limitations mentioned above, Qiu and You (2022), You and Qiu (2020a) and You and Qiu (2020b) suggested several modified DySS methods based on *disease risk* quantification and sequential

DOI: 10.1201/9781003138150-5

monitoring of the quantified disease risk. The basic idea of these methods can be described as follows. Instead of monitoring the observed longitudinal pattern of the disease risk factors of a given patient directly for disease early detection, a predictive model in the survival data analysis literature (Klein and Moeschberger, 2003) is used for describing the longitudinal association between the incidence of a disease in concern and the disease risk factors, and this model is estimated based on a *training dataset* that contains the observed data of both diseased and non-diseased people. Then, disease risk is quantified at each observation time for the patient under monitoring, using the estimated predictive model and the patient's observed disease risk factors. In the quantified disease risk, the weights received by different disease risk factors depend on their relative importance in predicting the incidence of the disease in concern, and irrelevant disease risk factors can also be deleted from the quantified disease risk by using some variable selection methods (You and Qiu, 2020b). For disease screening, the regular longitudinal pattern of the disease risk can be estimated first from the training data, and the observed longitudinal pattern of the disease risk of the given patient can then be monitored sequentially for disease early detection, after the two longitudinal patterns are compared cross-sectionally at each observation time.

The remaining parts of this chapter are organized as follows. A basic method for quantification of the disease risk proposed in You and Qiu (2020a) is introduced in Section 5.2. Sequential monitoring of the quantified disease risk for disease early detection is discussed in Section 5.3. An improved version of the disease screening method discussed in Sections 5.2 and 5.3 is described in Section 5.4, which is based on the methods for joint modeling of survival and longitudinal data discussed in You and Qiu (2021b) and Qiu and You (2022). A method suggested in You and Qiu (2020b) for handling high-dimensional cases is discussed in Section 5.5. Finally, some concluding remarks are given in Section 5.6.

5.2 Quantification of Disease Risk

Assume that a training dataset containing the observed data of m individual people is available before disease screening for new patients. The training data are further assumed to contain observed data of both diseased and non-diseased people. From such training data, we can explore the numerical relationship between the incidence of a disease in concern and its disease risk factors, by building a predictive model. Based on the estimated predictive model, the risk for a given new patient to have the disease in concern at a specific time point can be quantified from the new patient's observed disease risk factors. Details of this disease risk quantification method discussed originally in You and Qiu (2020a) are given below.

For each individual person in the training data, the following survival and longitudinal data are assumed to be observed. First, let T_i be the last follow-up time of the ith person, δ_i be the indicator that indicates whether a disease in concern is observed at T_i and D_i be the true disease occurrence time, for $i = 1, 2, \ldots, m$. Then, define $T_i = \min\{D_i, C_i\}$ and $\delta_i = I(D_i \leq C_i)$, where C_i denotes the censoring time for the ith person. For non-diseased people, it is obvious that $T_i = C_i$ and $\delta_i = 0$. So, in this setup, it is actually assumed that an individual person will not be followed any more after the occurrence of the disease or censoring. In practice, if the disease in concern is not fatal, a diseased person usually continues to be followed. In such cases, the disease screening method discussed here can still be used, although the data collected after the occurrence of the disease are actually not used. Second, there are q time-dependent disease risk factors and their values at time t are denoted by the q-dimensional vector $\boldsymbol{x}_i(t)$. For these disease risk factors, assume that they are observed at times $\{t_{i1}, t_{i2}, \ldots, t_{iJ_i}\}$ for the ith person, which may not be equally spaced in the study period $[0, \mathcal{T}]$, for $i = 1, 2, \ldots, m$. In this setup, it is obvious that $t_{iJ_i} = T_i$ for each i. Finally, let $\boldsymbol{z}_i$ be a vector of p time-independent covariates (e.g., gender, race) of the ith individual person that explain the heterogeneity of the population. Then, the observed training data are assumed to follow the Cox proportional hazards model (Klein and Moeschberger, 2003) below:

$$\lambda_i(t) = \lambda_0(t) \exp\left[\boldsymbol{\beta}'\boldsymbol{x}_i(t) + \boldsymbol{\gamma}'\boldsymbol{z}_i\right], \qquad \text{for } t \in [0, \mathcal{T}],\ i = 1, 2, \ldots, m, \tag{5.1}$$

where $\lambda_i(t)$ is the hazard rate function of the ith individual person, $\lambda_0(t)$ is the baseline hazard rate function, and $\boldsymbol{\beta}$ and $\boldsymbol{\gamma}$ are respectively q-dimensional and p-dimensional vectors of coefficients. In Model (5.1), roughly speaking, the hazard rate function $\lambda_i(t)$ measures the likelihood (or hazard) for the ith individual person to have the disease occurring at time t given the observed values of $\boldsymbol{x}_i(t)$ and $\boldsymbol{z}_i$, and the baseline hazard rate function $\lambda_0(t)$ measures the likelihood of the event to have the disease occurring at time t when $\boldsymbol{x}_i(t)$ and $\boldsymbol{z}_i$ are all 0. It can be seen that the hazard ratio $\lambda_i(t)/\lambda_0(t)$ of the ith individual person has been modeled to be an increasing function of $\boldsymbol{\beta}'\boldsymbol{x}_i(t) + \boldsymbol{\gamma}'\boldsymbol{z}_i$, in which $\boldsymbol{\beta}'\boldsymbol{x}_i(t)$ represents the contribution of the time-dependent disease risk factors to the hazard ratio and $\boldsymbol{\gamma}'\boldsymbol{z}_i$ explains the heterogeneity among different population groups. Because our goal is to detect the disease in concern promptly by monitoring the longitudinal pattern of the observed disease risk factors of an individual person and the second part $\boldsymbol{\gamma}'\boldsymbol{z}_i$ does not change over time, we focus on the first part $\boldsymbol{\beta}'\boldsymbol{x}_i(t)$ for disease screening. Then, we have the following definition.

Definition of the Disease Risk Function

The disease risk function of the ith individual person in the training data is defined to be $r_i(t) := \boldsymbol{\beta}'\boldsymbol{x}_i(t)$, for each i.

For simplicity of presentation, let $R(t) = \{i : T_i \geq t\}$ denote the set of people in the training data who are at risk at time t, $y_i(t) = I(T_i \geq t)$ indicate whether the ith individual is at risk at time t, and $\boldsymbol{\theta} = (\boldsymbol{\beta}', \boldsymbol{\gamma}')'$ be the vector of all parameters in Model (5.1). Then, estimation of Model (5.1) is discussed below. Because the observation times $\{t_{i1}, t_{i2}, \ldots, t_{iJ_i}\}$ might be unequally spaced in $[0, \mathcal{T}]$ for each i, and $\boldsymbol{x}_i(t)$ is observed at $\{t_{i1}, t_{i2}, \ldots, t_{iJ_i}\}$ only, if Model (5.1) is estimated as usual by the conventional partial likelihood estimation procedure (Cox, 1972), then for a given patient, $\boldsymbol{x}_i(t)$ has to be interpolated or extrapolated at some observed disease occurrence times of other people in the training data. A naive solution of this problem is to impute $\boldsymbol{x}_i(t)$ by using the last-observation-carried-forward data imputation method, by which $\boldsymbol{x}_i(t)$ at an unobserved time is set to be its previous observed value. However, this method will not guarantee an unbiased estimate of $\boldsymbol{\beta}$ when $\boldsymbol{x}_i(t)$ is not piecewise constant and/or when $\{t_{i1}, t_{i2}, \ldots, t_{iJ_i}\}$ are sparsely distributed. In the literature, there are some existing discussions about different strategies to extrapolate $\boldsymbol{x}_i(t)$ (cf., Lin and Ying, 1993; Paik and Tsai, 1997). However, these methods need to assume that $\boldsymbol{x}_i(t)$ is observed completely in an interval, which is invalid in the current disease screening problem. When $\boldsymbol{x}_i(t)$ is assumed to follow a parametric longitudinal model, some model estimation methods have been suggested in the literature based on joint modeling of survival and longitudinal data (e.g., Dupuy et al., 2006). But, the assumed parametric longitudinal model is often difficult to justify in practice. As an alternative to the methods mentioned above, You and Qiu (2020a) suggested a kernel smoothing method for estimation of Model (5.1), without imposing any parametric form on $\boldsymbol{x}_i(t)$. In the literature, kernel smoothing methods have been found useful in estimating time-varying coefficients in a Cox proportional hazards model (e.g., Cai and Sun, 2003; Yu and Lin, 2010), where the related time-dependent covariates are usually assumed to be observable at any time in the study interval $[0, \mathcal{T}]$. Here, the kernel smoothing methods are extended to cases when the time-dependent covariates in $\boldsymbol{x}_i(t)$ are observed at some unequally spaced time points. Details of this model estimation procedure are given below.

In the conventional partial likelihood estimation procedure, the partial likelihood function is defined to be

$$\prod_{i:\delta_i=1} \frac{\exp\left[\boldsymbol{\beta}'\boldsymbol{x}_i(T_i) + \boldsymbol{\gamma}'\boldsymbol{z}_i\right]}{\sum_{l \in R(T_i)} \exp\left[\boldsymbol{\beta}'\boldsymbol{x}_l(T_i) + \boldsymbol{\gamma}'\boldsymbol{z}_i\right]}.$$

This function cannot be used here because many terms in $\{\boldsymbol{x}_l(T_i), l \in R(T_i)\}$ used in the denominator of the above expression are not observed, as discussed above. To overcome this difficulty, we suggest using the following local smoothing partial likelihood function:

$$L(\boldsymbol{\theta}) = \prod_{i:\delta_i=1} \frac{\exp\left[\boldsymbol{\beta}'\boldsymbol{x}_i(T_i) + \boldsymbol{\gamma}'\boldsymbol{z}_i\right]}{\sum_{l \in R(T_i)} \sum_{j=1}^{J_l} K_{h_\theta}(T_i - t_{lj}) \exp\left[\boldsymbol{\beta}'\boldsymbol{x}_l(t_{lj}) + \boldsymbol{\gamma}'\boldsymbol{z}_l\right]}, \tag{5.2}$$

where $K_{h_\theta}(s) = K(s/h_\theta)/h_\theta$, $K(s)$ is a density kernel function, and $h_\theta > 0$ is a bandwidth parameter. In (5.2), $\{\exp[\boldsymbol{\beta}'\boldsymbol{x}_l(t_{lj}) + \boldsymbol{\gamma}'\boldsymbol{z}_l], j = 1, 2, \ldots, J_l\}$ in the denominator are weightedly averaged for estimating $\exp[\boldsymbol{\beta}'\boldsymbol{x}_l(T_i) + \boldsymbol{\gamma}'\boldsymbol{z}_i]$, and the weights are determined by the kernel function and the bandwidth. To estimate $\boldsymbol{\theta}$, it is often more convenient to use the following logarithm of $L(\boldsymbol{\theta})$:

$$
\begin{aligned}
\ell(\boldsymbol{\theta}) &= \log(L(\boldsymbol{\theta})) \\
&= \sum_{i:\delta_i=1} \{\boldsymbol{\beta}'\boldsymbol{x}_i(T_i) + \boldsymbol{\gamma}'\boldsymbol{z}_i - \\
&\quad \log\left[\sum_{l \in R(T_i)} \sum_{j=1}^{J_l} K_{h_\theta}(T_i - t_{lj}) \exp\left(\boldsymbol{\beta}'\boldsymbol{x}_l(t_{lj}) + \boldsymbol{\gamma}'\boldsymbol{z}_l\right)\right]\Bigg\}.
\end{aligned}
$$

Then, the estimate of $\boldsymbol{\theta}$ is defined to be

$$
\widehat{\boldsymbol{\theta}} = \arg\max_{\boldsymbol{\theta}} \ \ell(\boldsymbol{\theta}). \tag{5.3}
$$

To compute $\widehat{\boldsymbol{\theta}}$ by (5.3), the following Newton-Raphson iterative algorithm can be used: for $j \geq 0$, let

$$
\widehat{\boldsymbol{\theta}}^{(k+1)} = \widehat{\boldsymbol{\theta}}^{(k)} - \left[\nabla^2 \ell(\widehat{\boldsymbol{\theta}}^{(k)})\right]^{-1} \nabla \ell(\widehat{\boldsymbol{\theta}}^{(k)}), \qquad \text{for } k \geq 0,
$$

where $\widehat{\boldsymbol{\theta}}^{(0)} = \mathbf{0}$, and

$$
\begin{aligned}
\nabla \ell(\boldsymbol{\theta}) &= \sum_{i:\delta_i=1} \left[\begin{pmatrix} \boldsymbol{x}_i(T_i) \\ \boldsymbol{z}_i \end{pmatrix} - \frac{\mathbf{S}_1(\boldsymbol{\theta}; T_i)}{S_0(\boldsymbol{\theta}; T_i)}\right], \\
\nabla^2 \ell(\boldsymbol{\theta}) &= -\sum_{i:\delta_i=1} \left[\frac{S_0(\boldsymbol{\theta}; T_i)\mathbf{S}_2(\boldsymbol{\theta}; T_i) - \mathbf{S}_1(\boldsymbol{\theta}; T_i)\mathbf{S}_1'(\boldsymbol{\theta}; T_i)}{[S_0(\boldsymbol{\theta}; T_i)]^2}\right], \\
S_0(\boldsymbol{\theta}; t) &= \frac{1}{m} \sum_{i \in R(t)} \sum_{j=1}^{J_i} K_{h_\theta}(t - t_{ij}) y_i(t) \exp\left[\boldsymbol{\beta}'\boldsymbol{x}_i(t_{ij}) + \boldsymbol{\gamma}'\boldsymbol{z}_i\right], \\
\mathbf{S}_1(\boldsymbol{\theta}; t) &= \frac{1}{m} \sum_{i \in R(t)} \sum_{j=1}^{J_i} K_{h_\theta}(t - t_{ij}) y_i(t) \exp\left[\boldsymbol{\beta}'\boldsymbol{x}_i(t_{ij}) + \boldsymbol{\gamma}'\boldsymbol{z}_i\right] \begin{pmatrix} \boldsymbol{x}_i(t_{ij}) \\ \boldsymbol{z}_i \end{pmatrix}, \\
\mathbf{S}_2(\boldsymbol{\theta}; t) &= \frac{1}{m} \sum_{i \in R(t)} \sum_{j=1}^{J_i} K_{h_\theta}(t - t_{ij}) y_i(t) \exp\left[\boldsymbol{\beta}'\boldsymbol{x}_i(t_{ij}) + \boldsymbol{\gamma}'\boldsymbol{z}_i\right] \begin{pmatrix} \boldsymbol{x}_i(t_{ij}) \\ \boldsymbol{z}_i \end{pmatrix}^{\otimes 2}.
\end{aligned}
$$

In the last expression, $\boldsymbol{x}^{\otimes 2}$ denotes the outer product of a vector $\boldsymbol{x}$ with itself (i.e., $\boldsymbol{x}\boldsymbol{x}'$). This iterative algorithm stops at the $(k+1)$-th iteration when $\|\widehat{\boldsymbol{\theta}}^{(k+1)} - \widehat{\boldsymbol{\theta}}^{(k)}\| \leq \epsilon$, where $\|\boldsymbol{x}\|$ denotes the L_2 norm of $\boldsymbol{x}$ (i.e., $\sqrt{\boldsymbol{x}'\boldsymbol{x}}$), and $\epsilon > 0$ is a pre-specified small number. After $\widehat{\boldsymbol{\theta}} = (\widehat{\boldsymbol{\beta}}', \widehat{\boldsymbol{\gamma}}')'$ is obtained from

(5.3), the estimated disease risk function of the ith individual in the training data is then defined to be $\widehat{r}_i(t) = \widehat{\boldsymbol{\beta}}'\boldsymbol{x}_i(t)$, for each i.

For the estimated disease risk function discussed above, we next discuss how to describe its longitudinal pattern by estimating its mean and variance functions. To this end, let $\mu(t) = \mathrm{E}[r_i(t)|T_i \geq t]$ be the mean disease risk at time t for all people at risk in the training dataset, and $\sigma^2(t) = \mathrm{Var}(r_i(t)|T_i \geq t)$ be the corresponding variance. They can be estimated by the local linear kernel smoothing procedure (cf., Subsection 2.5.5), and the corresponding estimators are

$$\widehat{\mu}(t) = \frac{R_0(t)W_{\mu,2}(t) - R_1(t)W_{\mu,1}(t)}{W_{\mu,0}(t)W_{\mu,2}(t) - W_{\mu,1}(t)^2}, \tag{5.4}$$

$$\widehat{\sigma}^2(t) = \frac{Q_0(t)W_{\sigma,2}(t) - Q_1(t)W_{\sigma,1}(t)}{W_{\sigma,0}(t)W_{\sigma,2}(t) - W_{\sigma,1}(t)^2}, \tag{5.5}$$

where for $l = 0, 1, 2$,

$$\begin{aligned}
W_{\mu,l}(t) &= \frac{1}{m}\sum_{i\in R(t)}\sum_{j=1}^{J_i} K_{h_\mu}(t_{ij}-t)\left(\frac{t_{ij}-t}{h_\mu}\right)^l, \\
R_l(t) &= \frac{1}{m}\sum_{i\in R(t)}\sum_{j=1}^{J_i} K_{h_\mu}(t_{ij}-t)\left(\frac{t_{ij}-t}{h_\mu}\right)^l \widehat{r}_i(t_{ij}), \\
W_{\sigma,l}(t) &= \frac{1}{m}\sum_{i\in R(t)}\sum_{j=1}^{J_i} K_{h_\sigma}(t_{ij}-t)\left(\frac{t_{ij}-t}{h_\sigma}\right)^l, \\
Q_l(t) &= \frac{1}{m}\sum_{i\in R(t)}\sum_{j=1}^{J_i} K_{h_\sigma}(t_{ij}-t)\left(\frac{t_{ij}-t}{h_\sigma}\right)^l \widehat{\epsilon}_i^2(t_{ij}),
\end{aligned}$$

$\widehat{\epsilon}_i(t_{ij}) = \widehat{r}_i(t_{ij}) - \widehat{\mu}(t_{ij})$, for each i and j, and $h_\mu, h_\sigma > 0$ are two bandwidth parameters. Under some regularity conditions, You and Qiu (2020a) proved that the estimators $\widehat{\boldsymbol{\theta}}$, $\widehat{\mu}(t)$ and $\widehat{\sigma}^2(t)$ are all consistent in probability (cf., Subsection 2.4.1).

When computing the estimators $\widehat{\boldsymbol{\theta}}$, $\widehat{\mu}(t)$ and $\widehat{\sigma}^2(t)$ by (5.3)–(5.5), the kernel function $K(s)$ can be chosen to be the Epanechnikov kernel function $K(s) = 0.75(1-s^2)I(|s| \leq 1)$, for $s \in R$ (cf., Subsection 2.5.4). The bandwidths h_θ, h_μ and h_σ can be chosen by the cross-validation (CV) procedures (cf., Subsection 2.5.5), described below. To choose h_θ, we suggest using the following leave-one-out CV score modified from the one suggested by Tian et al. (2005):

$$CV_\theta(h_\theta) = \sum_{i=1}^{m} PE_i^2(h_\theta),$$

where $PE_i(h_\theta)$ is the leave-one-out prediction error for the ith individual, defined to be

$$PE_i(h_\theta) = \delta_i - \sum_{\substack{k\neq i,\, \delta_k=1 \\ T_k \leq T_i}} \frac{\sum_{j=1}^{J_i} K_{h_\theta}(T_k - t_{ij}) \exp\left[\widehat{\boldsymbol{\beta}}'_{-i}\boldsymbol{x}_i(t_{ij}) + \widehat{\boldsymbol{\gamma}}'_{-i}\boldsymbol{z}_i\right]}{\sum_{\substack{d\in R(T_k) \\ d\neq k}} \sum_{j=1}^{J_d} K_{h_\theta}(T_k - t_{dj}) \exp\left[\widehat{\boldsymbol{\beta}}'_{-i}\boldsymbol{x}_d(t_{dj}) + \widehat{\boldsymbol{\gamma}}'_{-i}\boldsymbol{z}_d\right]},$$

where $\widehat{\boldsymbol{\beta}}_{-i}$ and $\widehat{\boldsymbol{\gamma}}_{-i}$ are the estimates of $\boldsymbol{\beta}$ and $\boldsymbol{\gamma}$ when the observed data of the ith individual are excluded from estimation. For choosing h_μ and h_σ, the following CV scores that are similar to those discussed in Qiu and Xiang (2014) can be used:

$$CV_\mu(h_\mu) = \sum_{i=1}^{m}\sum_{j=1}^{J_i} \left[\widehat{\epsilon}_i(t_{ij}) - \widehat{\mu}_{-i}(t_{ij})\right]^2,$$

$$CV_\sigma(h_\sigma) = \sum_{i=1}^{m}\sum_{j=1}^{J_i} \left[\widehat{\epsilon}_i^2(t_{ij}) - \widehat{\sigma}^2_{-i}(t_{ij})\right]^2,$$

where $\widehat{\mu}_{-i}(t)$ and $\widehat{\sigma}^2_{-i}(t)$ denote the leave-one-out estimates of $\mu(t)$ and $\sigma^2(t)$, respectively, when the observations of the ith individual are excluded from estimation. Then, h_θ, h_μ and h_σ are chosen by minimizing $CV_\theta(h_\theta)$, $CV_\mu(h_\mu)$ and $CV_\sigma(h_\sigma)$, respectively.

It should be pointed out that Model (5.1) assumes that the impact of the disease risk factors in $\boldsymbol{x}_i(t)$ and the covariates in $\boldsymbol{z}_i$ does not change over time since their coefficients do not depend on time t. If it is believed that such impact could change over time, then the following time-varying coefficient model might be more appropriate (cf., Hastie and Tibshirani, 1993; Zucker and Karr, 1990):

$$\lambda_i(t) = \lambda_0(t)\exp\left[\boldsymbol{\beta}'(t)\boldsymbol{x}_i(t) + \boldsymbol{\gamma}'(t)\boldsymbol{z}_i\right], \qquad \text{for } t \in [0, \mathcal{T}], \tag{5.6}$$

where $\boldsymbol{\beta}(t)$ and $\boldsymbol{\gamma}(t)$ are time-varying coefficients. Let $\boldsymbol{\theta}(t) = (\boldsymbol{\beta}'(t), \boldsymbol{\gamma}'(t))'$. Then, there are some existing discussions about estimation of $\boldsymbol{\theta}(t)$ in Model (5.6), using the generalized additive modeling procedures (e.g., Hastie and Tibshirani, 1993), smoothing splines (e.g., Zucker and Karr, 1990), or local likelihood estimation (e.g., Cai and Sun, 2003) in cases when both the covariates and the disease risk factors do not change over time or are continuously observed in a time interval. By using the same idea as that for estimating Model (5.1) discussed above, we suggest using a kernel estimation procedure for estimating Model (5.6), which can accommodate unequally spaced observation times and time-varying coefficients. To this end, we first define the following local log-likelihood function:

$$\begin{aligned}\ell(\boldsymbol{\theta},t) &= \sum_{i:\delta_i=1} K_{h_\theta}(T_i-t)\left\{\boldsymbol{\beta}'\boldsymbol{x}_i(T_i)+\boldsymbol{\gamma}'\boldsymbol{z}_i-\right.\\ &\left.\log\left[\sum_{l\in R(T_i)}\sum_{j=1}^{J_l} K_{h_\theta}(T_i-t_{lj})\exp\left(\boldsymbol{\beta}'\boldsymbol{x}_l(t_{lj})+\boldsymbol{\gamma}'\boldsymbol{z}_l\right)\right]\right\},\end{aligned}$$

where some related quantities are the same as those in (5.2). Then, the Newton-Raphson algorithm can be used to minimize the above function. The resulting estimator of $\boldsymbol{\theta}(t)$ is defined to be

$$\widehat{\boldsymbol{\theta}}(t) = \arg\max_{\boldsymbol{\theta}} \ \ell(\boldsymbol{\theta},t),$$

where $\widehat{\boldsymbol{\theta}}(t) = (\widehat{\boldsymbol{\beta}}'(t), \widehat{\boldsymbol{\gamma}}'(t))'$. The disease risk function in such cases is defined to be $r_i(t) = \boldsymbol{\beta}'(t)\boldsymbol{x}_i(t)$, and the estimated disease risk function is $\widehat{r}_i(t) = \widehat{\boldsymbol{\beta}}'(t)\boldsymbol{x}_i(t)$. After these modifications, the estimates of $\mu(t)$ and $\sigma^2(t)$ can still be computed by Equations (5.4) and (5.5).

5.3 Disease Screening by Online Monitoring of Quantified Disease Risks

In this section, we discuss disease early detection for individual people by sequentially monitoring their disease risks quantified from the observed disease risk factors. To this end, assume that the q disease risk factors in $\boldsymbol{x}(t)$ of a new patient are observed at times $\{t_j^*, j \geq 1\}$. Then, the patient's estimated disease risks at these time points are $\widehat{r}(t_j^*) = \widehat{\boldsymbol{\beta}}'\boldsymbol{x}(t_j^*)$, for $j \geq 1$, where $\widehat{\boldsymbol{\beta}}$ is computed in advance by (5.3) from a training data. The *standardized disease risks* are defined to be

$$\widehat{e}(t_j^*) = \frac{\widehat{r}(t_j^*) - \widehat{\mu}(t_j^*)}{\widehat{\sigma}(t_j^*)}, \qquad \text{for } j \geq 1, \tag{5.7}$$

where $\widehat{\mu}(t)$ and $\widehat{\sigma}^2(t)$ are computed in advance from the training data by (5.4) and (5.5), respectively.

In (5.7), $\widehat{\mu}(t)$ and $\widehat{\sigma}(t)$ describe the estimated longitudinal pattern of the quantified disease risks for people in the population that the training dataset represents, and $\{\widehat{e}(t_j^*), j \geq 1\}$ are the standardized disease risks of the new patient under monitoring, after cross-sectional comparison between the observed longitudinal pattern of the disease risks of the new patient and the estimated longitudinal pattern of the people in the population represented by the training data. So, a larger value of $\widehat{e}(t_j^*)$ implies a larger chance for the new patient to have the disease in concern at time t_j^*. This approach to define the standardized disease risks for the new patient was suggested in You and Qiu (2020a). An alternative approach is to compare the disease risks of the new patient with those of the non-diseased people in the training data only, as discussed in the DySS methods described in Chapter 4. By this alternative approach, $\widehat{\mu}(t)$ and $\widehat{\sigma}(t)$ should be computed from the observed data of the non-diseased people in the training data only, which can still be accomplished by (5.4) and (5.5) when the computation is constrained within the subset of the training data that contains the observed data of all non-diseased people. Between the two approaches, the alternative one could be more effective in detecting the disease in concern.

To sequentially monitor the standardized disease risks $\{\widehat{e}(t_j^*), j \geq 1\}$, we should take into account the fact that the observation times $\{t_j^*, j \geq 1\}$ are often unequally spaced. The conventional control charts in the literature are designed for cases with equally spaced observation times only (cf., Qiu, 2014). To overcome this difficulty and accommodate unequally spaced observation times, You and Qiu (2020a) suggested a modified EWMA chart described below. Let $\omega > 0$ be the basic time unit (cf., Subsection 4.2.3) that all observation times are its integer multiples. Then, $\{n_j^* = t_j^*/\omega, j \geq 1\}$ are the observation times in the basic time unit. The modified EWMA charting statistic is defined to be

$$\begin{aligned} E_1 &= \upsilon_\lambda(t_1^*)\widehat{e}(t_1^*) \\ E_j &= \left[1 - \upsilon_\lambda(t_j^*)\right] E_{j-1} + \upsilon_\lambda(t_j^*)\widehat{e}(t_j^*), \qquad \text{for } j \geq 2, \end{aligned} \tag{5.8}$$

where

$$\begin{aligned} \upsilon_\lambda(t_1^*) &= 1 - (1-\lambda)^{\bar{\Delta}}, \\ \upsilon_\lambda(t_j^*) &= \upsilon_\lambda(t_{j-1}^*)/[(1-\lambda)^{\Delta_j} + \upsilon_\lambda(t_{j-1}^*)], \qquad \text{for } j \geq 2, \end{aligned}$$

$\bar{\Delta}$ is the mean of $\Delta_j = n_j^* - n_{j-1}^*$, for all j, that can be estimated from the training data by the related sample mean, and $\lambda \in [0, 1)$ is a weighting parameter. It can be checked that the charting statistic E_j in (5.8) is a weighted average of $\{\widehat{e}(t_j^*), \widehat{e}(t_{j-1}^*), \ldots, \widehat{e}(t_2^*), \widehat{e}(t_1^*)\}$, and the weights are proportional to

$$1, (1-\lambda)^{n_j^* - n_{j-1}^*}, \ldots, (1-\lambda)^{n_j^* - n_2^*}, (1-\lambda)^{n_j^* - n_1^*},$$

respectively. Therefore, the weights are controlled by λ and by how far away a previous observation time is from the current observation time in the basic time unit. Thus, unequal observation times have been accommodated properly in E_j. This weighting scheme was also recommended in Qiu et al. (2018) and Wright (1986). In cases when observation times are equally spaced, the charting statistic E_j becomes the conventional EWMA charting statistic (cf., Subsection 3.1.4), since $\{\upsilon_\lambda(t_j^*)\}$ become a constant in such cases. Then, the modified EWMA chart gives a signal when

$$E_j > \rho_E, \tag{5.9}$$

where $\rho_E > 0$ is a control limit.

It should be mentioned that the modified EWMA chart (5.8)–(5.9) is designed for detecting upward mean shifts in the quantified disease risks of the new patient under monitoring. Because the quantified disease risks are related to the hazard rates of the new patient at different time points (cf., (5.1)) and a larger hazard rate would usually imply a larger chance for the new patient to have the disease in concern, the upward form of the chart is reasonable to use here. However, in some other applications, a downward or two-sided chart might be more reasonable to use. Such alternative charts can be constructed in a similar way. See the related discussion in Subsection 3.1.4 about three different forms of an EWMA chart.

To evaluate the performance of the modified EWMA chart (5.8)–(5.9), the metrics ATS_0 and ATS_1 can be used, as discussed in Subsection 4.2.3. To this end, ATS_0 is usually pre-specified, and the chart performs better for detecting a given shift in the longitudinal pattern of the quantified disease risk if its ATS_1 value is smaller. In the chart, the weighting parameter λ and the control limit ρ_E should be chosen in advance. To this end, λ is usually pre-specified and ρ_E is chosen to achieve a given value of ATS_0. To choose ρ_E, we can use a block bootstrap procedure similar to the one discussed in Subsection 4.2.3, where the block bootstrap is considered because the within-subject observations are often correlated.

The modified EWMA chart (5.8)–(5.9) should be reliable to use when its control limit ρ_E is determined from the training data by the block bootstrap procedure. However, construction of the chart does not take into account possible serial correlation in the observed data, although unequally spaced observation times have been accommodated. A possible improvement of the disease screening method discussed above is to first apply the data decorrelation and standardization procedure described in Section 4.4 to the quantified disease risks $\{\widehat{r}(t_j^*), j \geq 1\}$ of the new patient, and then apply the modified EWMA chart (5.8)–(5.9) to the decorrelated and standardized disease risks.

Example 5.1 *In the dataset considered in Example 4.1 from the SHARe Framingham Heart Study, there were a total of 1055 people involved, among which 27 people experienced strokes during the study period and the remaining 1028 people did not. Each person was followed 7 times, and three medical indices, including the systolic blood pressure (mmHg), diastolic blood pressure (mmHg), and total cholesterol level (mg/100ml) were recorded at each time. The observed data of these three indices are shown in Figure 5.1. To apply the disease screening method discussed above, we randomly select two-thirds of the stroke people and two-thirds of the non-stroke people, and their observed data are used as the training data and the remaining data are used as the test data for disease early detection. In the test data, there are a total of 9 stroke people and 342 non-stroke people involved. In the entire dataset, all observation times are between 16 and 83 years old, and the mean interval length between two consecutive observation times is* $\bar{\Delta} = 4.37$ *(in years).*

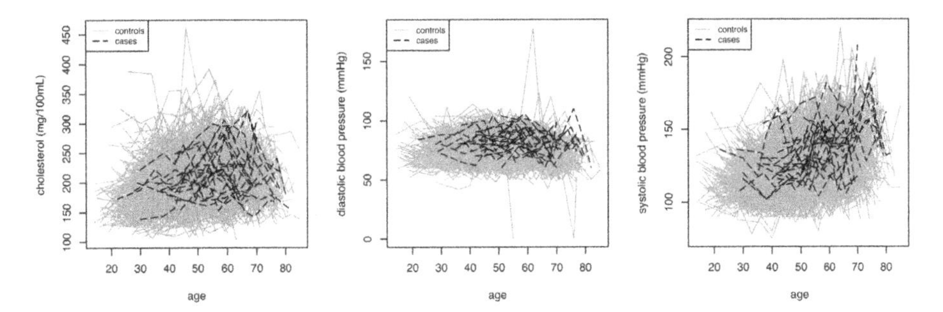

FIGURE 5.1
Three risk factors in the stroke data: systolic blood pressure (mmHg), diastolic blood pressure (mmHg), and total cholesterol level (mg/100ml). The solid gray lines denote the longitudinal observations of the non-stroke people, and the black dashed lines denote the longitudinal observations of the stroke people.

The goodness-of-fit test discussed in Park and Qiu (2014) is first applied to the training data, which confirms that the Cox proportional hazards model (5.1) is appropriate to use for describing the observed survival data. Then, Model (5.1) can be estimated from the training data, and the estimated regression coefficients are $\widehat{\boldsymbol{\beta}} = (0.0001, 0.0047, 0.0269)'$. *Consequently,* $\widehat{\mu}(t)$ *and* $\widehat{\sigma}^2(t)$ *can be obtained by (5.4) and (5.5). In the modified EWMA chart (5.8)–(5.9),* λ *is chosen to be 0.1, and* ATS_0 *is chosen to be 10 or 15 years. As a comparison, the multivariate DySS method discussed in Section 4.3 (cf., Expressions (4.21) and (4.23)) is also considered here, in which* λ *and* ATS_0 *are chosen to be the same as those of the modified EWMA chart (5.8)–(5.9). The results of the two methods are summarized in Table 5.1. From the table, it can be seen that when* $ATS_0 = 10$, *both methods give signals to all 9 stroke people, but the modified EWMA chart (5.8)–(5.9) gives less signals to non-stroke people and its* ATS_1 *value is also smaller than that of the multivariate DySS method. Thus, in this case, it is obvious that the modified EWMA chart (5.8)–(5.9) performs better. In the case when* $ATS_0 = 15$ *and* $\lambda = 0.1$, *it is difficult to compare the two methods directly because the multivariate DySS method gives less signals to both stroke and non-stroke people. To overcome this difficulty, we adjust the* λ *value in the multivariate DySS method to be 0.027, and keep the* λ *value in the modified EWMA chart (5.8)–(5.9) to be 0.01. After this adjustment, both methods give 7 signals to stroke people. But, the multivariate DySS method give signals to more non-stroke people and its* ATS_1 *value is larger. So, the modified EWMA chart (5.8)–(5.9) performs better in this case as well.*

TABLE 5.1
Numbers of signals and calculated ATS_1 values of the modified EWMA chart (5.8)–(5.9) (denoted as "Method 1") and the multivariate DySS method discussed in Section 4.3 (denoted as "Method 2") in the stroke data example when they are applied to the 351 people contained in the test data.

ATS_0	λ	Method	ATS_1	# Signals to Stroke People	# Signals to Non-Stroke People
10	0.1	Method 1	7.56	9	187
	0.1	Method 2	8.56	9	202
15	0.1	Method 1	11.57	7	125
	0.1	Method 2	17.50	2	52
	0.027	Method 2	15.71	7	142

5.4 Disease Screening by Joint Modeling of Survival and Longitudinal Data

The disease screening method discussed in Section 5.3 tries to make use of helpful information in the observed data of both non-diseased and diseased people contained in the training data. To this end, it first builds a functional relationship between the observed longitudinal data of the disease risk factors and the survival outcomes that are related to the occurrence of the disease in concern for people in the training data, by estimating a Cox proportional hazards model (i.e., Model (5.1)). From the estimated model, disease risks of a patient at different observation times can be quantified based on the observed disease risk factors. Then, the quantified disease risks can be monitored sequentially by a control chart for disease early detection. In the statistical literature, it has been well demonstrated that joint modeling of the survival and longitudinal data is usually more effective than the corresponding modeling of the survival outcomes alone that includes the related longitudinal data as covariates (cf., Wulfsohn and Tsiatis, 1997). Based on this intuition, Qiu and You (2022) developed a new disease early detection method using the joint modeling approach, which is introduced below.

5.4.1 Joint Modeling of Survival and Longitudinal Data

Assume that there is a training dataset containing longitudinal observations of q disease risk factors and survival outcomes related to the occurrence of a disease in concern of m individuals. For the ith individual, longitudinal observations of the kth disease risk factor are obtained at times $\{t_{ik1}, t_{ik2}, \ldots, t_{ikJ_{ik}}\}$, for $i = 1, 2, \ldots, m$ and $k = 1, 2, \ldots, q$, where the observation times of different disease risk factors and/or different individuals could be different. The corresponding observations of the kth disease risk factor are denoted as

$\{x_{ik}(t_{ik1}), x_{ik}(t_{ik2}), \ldots, x_{ik}(t_{ikJ_{ik}})\}$. The survival outcome of the ith individual is denoted as (T_i, δ_i), where T_i represents the last follow-up time and δ_i is the indicator of the event that the ith individual has the disease at T_i, as discussed in Section 5.2. Let $N_i(t) = \delta_i I(T_i \leq t)$ be the right-continuous counting process of the survival status for the ith individual, $R(t) = \{i : T_i \geq t\}$ be the set of individuals who are still at risk at time t, and $[0, \mathcal{T}]$ be the study period that contains all observation times. Then, the longitudinal observations of the disease risk factors are assumed to follow the multivariate nonparametric mixed-effects model below:

$$\begin{aligned} x_{ik}(t_{ikj}) &= \mu_k^{(0)}(t_{ikj}) + \delta_i \Delta_k(t_{ikj}) + v_{ik}(t_{ikj}) + \varepsilon_{ik}(t_{ikj}), \\ & \quad \text{for } j = 1, 2, \ldots, J_{ik}, i = 1, 2, \ldots, m, k = 1, 2, \ldots, q, \end{aligned} \tag{5.10}$$

where

$$\mu_k^{(0)}(t) = \mathrm{E}\left[x_{ik}(t) | T_i \geq t, \delta_i = 0\right]$$

is the population mean function of the kth disease risk factor for non-diseased individuals,

$$\mu_k^{(1)}(t) = \mu_k^{(0)}(t) + \Delta_k(t) = \mathrm{E}\left[x_{ik}(t) | T_i \geq t, \delta_i = 1\right]$$

is the population mean function of the kth disease risk factor for diseased individuals, $v_{ik}(t)$ is the zero-mean random-effects function for describing the person-to-person variation from the population mean function $\mu_k^{(0)}(t) + \delta_i \Delta_k(t)$, and $\{\varepsilon_{ik}(t_{ikj})\}$ are the i.i.d. zero-mean measurement errors with $\mathrm{Var}(\varepsilon_{ik}(t_{ikj})) = \sigma_k^2(t_{ikj})$, for all i, j and k. Let

$$\begin{aligned} \boldsymbol{v}_i(t) &= \left(v_{i1}(t), v_{i2}(t), \ldots, v_{iq}(t)\right)', \\ \boldsymbol{\varepsilon}_i(t) &= \left(\varepsilon_{i1}(t), \varepsilon_{i2}(t), \ldots, \varepsilon_{iq}(t)\right)', \\ \boldsymbol{\mu}^{(0)}(t) &= \left(\mu_1^{(0)}(t), \mu_2^{(0)}(t), \ldots, \mu_q^{(0)}(t)\right)', \\ \boldsymbol{\Delta}(t) &= \left(\Delta_1(t), \Delta_1(t), \ldots, \Delta_q(t)\right)'. \end{aligned}$$

Then,

$$\boldsymbol{m}_i(t) = (m_{i1}(t), m_{i2}(t), \ldots, m_{iq}(t))' = \boldsymbol{\mu}^{(0)}(t) + \delta_i \boldsymbol{\Delta}(t) + \boldsymbol{v}_i(t)$$

denotes the latent trajectories of the disease risk factors after the measurement errors are removed from their longitudinal observations. To describe the association between these latent trajectories and the observed survival outcomes, the following Cox proportional hazards model is considered:

$$\lambda_i(t) = \lambda_0(t) \exp\left[\boldsymbol{\beta}' \boldsymbol{m}_i(t)\right], \qquad \text{for } i = 1, 2, \ldots, m, \tag{5.11}$$

where $\lambda_i(t)$ is the hazard rate function of the ith individual, $\lambda_0(t)$ is the baseline hazard rate function, and $\boldsymbol{\beta}$ is the q-dimensional coefficient vector.

By comparing Models (5.11) and (5.1), it can be seen that the vector $\boldsymbol{z}_i$ of the time-independent covariates is not included in Model (5.11). This is just for convenience of discussion about Model (5.11). Actually, all discussions in this section can go through if $\boldsymbol{z}_i$ is included explicitly in Model (5.11). Alternatively, $\boldsymbol{z}_i$ can be regarded as a part of $\boldsymbol{x}_i(t) = (x_{i1}(t), x_{i2}(t), \ldots, x_{iq}(t))'$, and thus has been included in Model (5.11) implicitly.

From Model (5.11), it can be seen that the disease risk factors of the ith individual are associated with the hazard rate function through the *disease risk function* $r_i(t) = \boldsymbol{\beta}'\boldsymbol{m}_i(t)$, for each i. For $r_i(t)$, it can be checked that its mean among all non-diseased people who are at risk at time t is

$$\mu_r^{(0)}(t) = \mathrm{E}[r_i(t)|T_i \geq t, \delta_i = 0] = \boldsymbol{\beta}'\boldsymbol{\mu}^{(0)}(t),$$

and its mean among all diseased people who are at risk at time t is

$$\mu_r^{(1)}(t) = \mathrm{E}[r_i(t)|T_i \geq t, \delta_i = 1] = \boldsymbol{\beta}'\boldsymbol{\mu}^{(1)}(t),$$

where $\boldsymbol{\mu}^{(1)}(t) = \boldsymbol{\mu}^{(0)}(t) + \boldsymbol{\Delta}(t)$.

Next, we discuss estimation of the joint models (5.10) and (5.11). To this end, Qiu and You (2022) developed a multivariate local polynomial mixed-effects model estimation procedure that was extended from the univariate version discussed in Wu and Zhang (2002), which is described below. At a given time point $t \in [0, \mathcal{T}]$, consider a small neighborhood $[t-h, t+h]$, where h is a bandwidth parameter. In that neighborhood, $\boldsymbol{\mu}^{(0)}(s)$, $\boldsymbol{\Delta}(s)$ and $\boldsymbol{v}_i(s)$, for any $s \in [t-h, t+h]$, can be approximated by their lth-order Taylor's expansions:

$$\boldsymbol{\mu}^{(0)}(s) \approx \sum_{k=0}^{l} \frac{(s-t)^k}{k!}\boldsymbol{\mu}^{(0k)}(t) = \boldsymbol{X}(s-t)\begin{bmatrix} \boldsymbol{\mu}^{(0)}(t) \\ \vdots \\ \frac{1}{l!}\boldsymbol{\mu}^{(0l)}(t) \end{bmatrix},$$

$$\boldsymbol{\Delta}(s) \approx \sum_{k=0}^{l} \frac{(s-t)^k}{k!}\boldsymbol{\Delta}^{(k)}(t) = \boldsymbol{X}(s-t)\begin{bmatrix} \boldsymbol{\Delta}(t) \\ \vdots \\ \frac{1}{l!}\boldsymbol{\Delta}^{(l)}(t) \end{bmatrix},$$

$$\boldsymbol{v}_i(s) \approx \sum_{k=0}^{l} \frac{(s-t)^k}{k!}\boldsymbol{v}_i^{(k)}(t) = \boldsymbol{X}(s-t)\begin{bmatrix} \boldsymbol{v}_i(t) \\ \vdots \\ \frac{1}{l!}\boldsymbol{v}_i^{(l)}(t) \end{bmatrix},$$

where $\boldsymbol{X}(t) = (I_{q\times q}, tI_{q\times q}, \ldots, t^l I_{q\times q})$, $I_{q\times q}$ is the $q \times q$ identity matrix, and $\boldsymbol{\mu}^{(0k)}(t), \boldsymbol{\Delta}^{(k)}(t)$ and $\boldsymbol{v}_i^{(k)}(t)$ are the kth order derivatives of $\boldsymbol{\mu}^{(0)}(t), \boldsymbol{\Delta}(t)$ and $\boldsymbol{v}_i(t)$, respectively, for $k = 1, 2, \ldots, l$. By these local function approximations, $\boldsymbol{m}_i(s)$, for $s \in [t-h, t+h]$, can be approximated by

$$\boldsymbol{X}(s-t)\left[\boldsymbol{c}(t) + \delta_i \boldsymbol{d}(t) + \boldsymbol{a}_i(t)\right],$$

where

$$\begin{aligned}
\boldsymbol{c}(t) &= \left[\left(\boldsymbol{\mu}^{(0)}(t)\right)', \left(\boldsymbol{\mu}^{(01)}(t)\right)', \ldots, \frac{1}{l!}\left(\boldsymbol{\mu}^{(0l)}(t)\right)'\right]', \\
\boldsymbol{d}(t) &= \left[(\boldsymbol{\Delta}(t))', \left(\boldsymbol{\Delta}^{(1)}(t)\right)', \ldots, \frac{1}{l!}\left(\boldsymbol{\Delta}^{(l)}(t)\right)'\right]', \\
\boldsymbol{a}_i(t) &= \left[(\boldsymbol{v}_i(t))', \left(\boldsymbol{v}_i^{(1)}(t)\right)', \ldots, \frac{1}{l!}\left(\boldsymbol{v}_i^{(l)}(t)\right)'\right]', \text{ for each } i.
\end{aligned}$$

Consequently, Model (5.10) can be approximated by the following linear mixed-effects model: for $t_{ikj} \in [t-h, t+h]$,

$$x_{ik}(t_{ikj}) = \boldsymbol{e}_k' \boldsymbol{X}(t_{ikj} - t)\left[\boldsymbol{c}(t) + \delta_i \boldsymbol{d}(t) + \boldsymbol{a}_i(t)\right] + \varepsilon_{ik}(t_{ikj}), \tag{5.12}$$

where $\boldsymbol{e}_k$ is a q-dimensional vector with its kth element being 1 and all other elements being 0, $\boldsymbol{c}(t)+\delta_i\boldsymbol{d}(t)$ is the fixed-effects term, and $\boldsymbol{a}_i(t)$ is the random-effects term. To simply the notation, let $\boldsymbol{b}_i(t) = \boldsymbol{c}(t) + \delta_i\boldsymbol{d}(t) + \boldsymbol{a}_i(t)$, and its covariance matrix is denoted as $\boldsymbol{\Sigma}_b(t)$. Then, $\boldsymbol{X}(s-t)\boldsymbol{b}_i(t)$ is an approximation of $\boldsymbol{m}_i(s)$, for $s \in [t-h, t+h]$.

To estimate $\boldsymbol{m}_i(s)$ and other quantities in Model (5.12), let $K(u)$ be a symmetric density kernel function with the support $[-1, 1]$. For instance, $K(u)$ can be chosen to be the Epanechnikov kernel function $K(u) = 0.75(1-u^2)I(|u| \leq 1)$. Then, a two-stage procedure for estimating the time-varying parameters $\boldsymbol{c}(t)$, $\boldsymbol{d}(t)$, $\boldsymbol{\Sigma}_b(t)$ and $\sigma_k^2(t)$, and the time-independent parameter vector $\boldsymbol{\beta}$ in the joint models (5.11) and (5.12) is described below. Assume that the ith individual is in $R(t)$ (i.e., it is at risk at time t). In the neighborhood $[t-h, t+h]$, if it is assumed that $x_{ik}(t_{ikj})$ follows a normal distribution with mean $\boldsymbol{e}_k'\boldsymbol{X}(t_{ikj} - t)\boldsymbol{b}_i(t)$ and variance $\sigma_k^2(t)$, then conditional on $\boldsymbol{b}_i(t)$, the log local-weighted probability density of $\mathcal{X}_i = \{x_{ik}(t_{ikj}), j = 1, 2, \ldots, J_{ik}, k = 1, 2, \ldots, q\}$ at time t is

$$\begin{aligned}
\log f_t(\mathcal{X}_i|\boldsymbol{b}_i(t)) &= -\frac{1}{2}\sum_{k=1}^{q}\sum_{j=1}^{J_{ik}} \log\left[2\pi\sigma_k^2(t)\right] K_h(t_{ikj} - t) \\
&\quad -\frac{1}{2}\sum_{k=1}^{q}\sum_{j=1}^{J_{ik}} \frac{\left[x_{ik}(t_{ikj}) - \boldsymbol{e}_k'\boldsymbol{X}(t_{ikj} - t)\boldsymbol{b}_i(t)\right]^2}{\sigma_k^2(t)} K_h(t_{ikj} - t),
\end{aligned} \tag{5.13}$$

where $K_h(s) = K(s/h)/h$. The quantity $-2\log f_t(\mathcal{X}_i|\boldsymbol{b}_i(t))$ can also be regarded as a penalized local-weighted least squares objective function with the penalty term $\sum_{k=1}^{q}\sum_{j=1}^{J_{ik}} \log\{2\pi\sigma_k^2(t)\}K_h(t_{ikj} - t)$. Thus, the normality assumption mentioned above is not essential for the suggested model estimation procedure. It is used mainly for the convenience in deriving the objective function. Similarly, the log probability density function of the random-effects term $\boldsymbol{b}_i(t)$ is

$$\log f_t(\boldsymbol{b}_i(t)) =$$
$$-\frac{1}{2}\log|2\pi\boldsymbol{\Sigma}_b(t)| - \frac{1}{2}\left[\boldsymbol{b}_i(t) - \boldsymbol{c}(t) - \delta_i\boldsymbol{d}(t)\right]' \boldsymbol{\Sigma}_b^{-1}(t)\left[\boldsymbol{b}_i(t) - \boldsymbol{c}(t) - \delta_i\boldsymbol{d}(t)\right].$$

Then, for a given $t \in [0, \mathcal{T}]$, the time-varying parameters $\boldsymbol{c}(t)$, $\boldsymbol{d}(t)$, $\boldsymbol{\Sigma}_b(t)$ and $\sigma_k^2(t)$ can be estimated by maximizing the following local likelihood function:

$$L\left(\boldsymbol{c}(t), \boldsymbol{d}(t), \boldsymbol{\Sigma}_b(t), \sigma_k^2(t)\right) = \prod_{i: t \leq T_i} \int f_t(\mathcal{X}_i | \boldsymbol{b}_i(t)) f_t(\boldsymbol{b}_i(t))\, d\boldsymbol{b}_i(t).$$

To solve the above local maximization problem, a local version of the expectation–maximization (EM) algorithm was suggested by Qiu and You (2022). Similar to the conventional EM algorithm (Dempster et al., 1977), the local version proceeds by iterating between the expectation and maximization steps. In the expectation step, the expectation of the log-likelihood is evaluated conditional on the observed data. Then, in the maximization step, parameter estimates are updated by maximizing the conditional expectation of the log-likelihood. Different from the conventional EM algorithm, the local EM algorithm works with the local likelihood function and thus the conditional expectation in the EM algorithm is taken with respect to the local probability density function. To save space, detailed description of the local EM algorithm is omitted here. Interested readers can find its details in Qiu and You (2022).

After the time-varying parameters are estimated using the local EM algorithm, we can proceed to the second stage for estimating the time-independent coefficient vector $\boldsymbol{\beta}$ in the survival model (5.11). Let $\widehat{\boldsymbol{c}}(t)$, $\widehat{\boldsymbol{d}}(t)$, $\widehat{\boldsymbol{\Sigma}}_b(t)$, and $\widehat{\sigma}_k^2(t)$ be the local maximum likelihood estimators of $\boldsymbol{c}(t)$, $\boldsymbol{d}(t)$, $\boldsymbol{\Sigma}_b(t)$ and $\sigma_k^2(t)$, respectively, obtained by the local EM algorithm discussed above. Then, $\boldsymbol{\mu}^{(0)}(t)$, $\boldsymbol{\Delta}(t)$ and $\boldsymbol{\Sigma}_m(t) = \text{Var}(\boldsymbol{m}_i(t))$ can be estimated by $\boldsymbol{X}(0)\widehat{\boldsymbol{c}}(t)$, $\boldsymbol{X}(0)\widehat{\boldsymbol{d}}(t)$ and $\boldsymbol{X}(0)\widehat{\boldsymbol{\Sigma}}_b(t)\boldsymbol{X}(0)'$, respectively. The random-effects term $\boldsymbol{b}_i(t)$ can be estimated by its corresponding best linear unbiased predictor (BLUP), defined to be $\widehat{\boldsymbol{b}}_i(t) = \widehat{\text{E}}[\boldsymbol{b}_i(t)|\mathcal{X}_i] = \widehat{\boldsymbol{m}}_{b,i}(t)$, where $\widehat{\boldsymbol{m}}_{b,i}(t)$ was defined in Qiu and You (2022). Because the expression of $\widehat{\boldsymbol{m}}_{b,i}(t)$ is quite complex, it is omitted here. Then, the quantity $\boldsymbol{m}_i(t)$ can be estimated similarly by $\boldsymbol{X}(0)\widehat{\boldsymbol{b}}_i(t)$, for each i. To estimate $\boldsymbol{\beta}$, we can first plug in the estimated values of $\{\boldsymbol{m}_i(t)\}$ into the following Cox partial likelihood function:

$$\text{pl}(\boldsymbol{\beta}) = \sum_{i=1}^{m} \delta_i \left[\boldsymbol{\beta}'\boldsymbol{m}_i(T_i) - \log\left\{\sum_{l=1}^{m} \exp\left[\boldsymbol{\beta}'\boldsymbol{m}_l(T_i)\right] I(T_l \geq T_i)\right\}\right]. \quad (5.14)$$

Then, $\boldsymbol{\beta}$ can be estimated by the maximizer of (5.14), denoted as $\widehat{\boldsymbol{\beta}}$, which can be computed by the Newton-Raphson algorithm (cf., the related discussion in Section 5.2).

In the local EM algorithm discussed above (cf., Expression (5.13)), the bandwidth parameter h should be chosen properly. To this end, a multivariate version of the modified cross-validation (MCV) criterion discussed in Altman (1990) can be used. Let $\tau_1 < \tau_2 < \cdots < \tau_G$ be G distinct time points in the set $\{t_{ikj}, j = 1, 2, \ldots, J_{ik}, i = 1, 2, \ldots, m, k = 1, 2, \ldots, q\}$, and $\widehat{m}_{ik}^{(-g)}(t)$ be the estimate of $m_{ik}(t)$ when all observations at τ_g are excluded, where $m_{ik}(t)$

is the kth component of $\boldsymbol{m}_i(t)$, for $k = 1, 2, \ldots, q$. Then, the MCV score is defined to be

$$\text{MCV}(h) = \sum_{g=1}^{G} \sum_{\{(i,k,j), t_{ikj} = \tau_g\}} \left[x_{ik}(t_{ikj}) - \widehat{m}_{ik}^{(-g)}(t_{ikj}) \right]^2.$$

Obviously, $\text{MCV}(h)$ measures the difference between the predicted values of $m_{ik}(t_{ikj})$ and the observed disease risk factors at t_{ikj}, for all i, j and k. Then, the bandwidth h is selected by minimizing the MCV score $\text{MCV}(h)$. To use this bandwidth selection procedure, in cases when the scales of x_{ik} are very different for different k, it is suggested to re-scale the data in advance so that the rescaled disease risk factors have similar spreads.

5.4.2 Dynamic Disease Screening

After the joint models (5.10) and (5.11) are estimated from a training data as discussed in the previous subsection, we can use the estimated models for detecting the disease in concern for a new patient, as described below. Assume that the new patient's kth disease risk factor $x_k^*(t)$ is observed at times $\{t_{kj}^*, j \geq 1\}$, for $k = 1, 2, \ldots, q$, where the superscript "*" is used to distinguish the quantities of the new patient from those in the training data (cf., Model (5.10)). The observed disease risk factors of the new patient is assumed to follow the model

$$x_k^*(t_{kj}^*) = m_k^*(t_{kj}^*) + \varepsilon_k^*(t_{kj}^*), \qquad \text{for } j \geq 1,\ k = 1, 2, \ldots, q,$$

where $m_k^*(t)$ is the latent longitudinal trajectory of the kth disease risk factor, and $\varepsilon_k^*(t)$ is the random error term. If the new patient does not have the disease in concern, then his/her disease risk function can be defined to be $\widehat{r}^*(t) = \widehat{\boldsymbol{\beta}}'\boldsymbol{m}^*(t)$, where $\widehat{\boldsymbol{\beta}}$ is obtained from the training dataset, as discussed in Subsection 5.4.1 (cf., (5.14)), and $\boldsymbol{m}^*(t) = (m_1^*(t), m_2^*(t), \ldots, m_q^*(t))'$.

To detect the disease in concern for the new patient, a natural idea is to compare his/her disease risk function with the estimated mean disease risk function of non-diseased people computed from the training data, namely, with $\widehat{\mu}_r^{(0)}(t) = \widehat{\boldsymbol{\beta}}'\widehat{\boldsymbol{\mu}}^{(0)}(t)$ discussed in Subsection 5.4.1. Based on that idea, let us consider the following statistic:

$$U(t) = \frac{\widehat{r}^*(t) - \widehat{\mu}_r^{(0)}(t)}{\sqrt{\widehat{\boldsymbol{\beta}}'\widehat{\boldsymbol{\Sigma}}_m(t)\widehat{\boldsymbol{\beta}}}} = \frac{\widehat{\boldsymbol{\beta}}'\boldsymbol{m}^*(t) - \widehat{\mu}_r^{(0)}(t)}{\sqrt{\widehat{\boldsymbol{\beta}}'\widehat{\boldsymbol{\Sigma}}_m(t)\widehat{\boldsymbol{\beta}}}}, \tag{5.15}$$

where $\widehat{\boldsymbol{\beta}}$, $\widehat{\mu}_r^{(0)}(t)$ and $\widehat{\boldsymbol{\Sigma}}_m(t)$ are obtained by the joint modeling approach discussed in Subsection 5.4.1. The statistic $U(t)$ in (5.15) has $\boldsymbol{m}^*(t)$ involved, which should be estimated in advance. To this end, let us consider the following objective function:

$$L(\boldsymbol{m}^*(t)) = -\frac{1}{2}\sum_{k=1}^{q}\sum_{j:t_{kj}^*\le t}\frac{\left[x_k^*(t_{kj}^*)-m_k^*(t)\right]^2}{\sigma_k^2(t)}(1-\lambda)^{(t-t_{kj}^*)/\bar{d}} -\frac{1}{2}\left[\boldsymbol{m}^*(t)-\boldsymbol{\mu}^{(0)}(t)\right]'\boldsymbol{\Sigma}_m^{-1}(t)\left[\boldsymbol{m}^*(t)-\boldsymbol{\mu}^{(0)}(t)\right],$$

where $\bar{d}$ is the average distance between two consecutive observation times that can be estimated from the training dataset, and λ is a weighting parameter. It can be seen that the expression of $L(\boldsymbol{m}^*(t))$ is similar to that of (5.13), with $\boldsymbol{X}(t_{ikj}-t)$ being replaced by $\boldsymbol{X}(0)$ and $K_h(t_{ikj}-t)$ replaced by $(1-\lambda)^{(t-t_{kj}^*)/\bar{d}}$. Thus, $L(\boldsymbol{m}^*(t))$ can also be regarded as a local weighted likelihood with an exponential weighting function. In $L(\boldsymbol{m}^*(t))$, past observations of the disease risk factors, $\{x_k^*(t_{kj}^*), t_{kj}^*\le t, k=1,2,\ldots,q\}$, have been used. They receive the weights $(1-\lambda)^{(t-t_{kj}^*)/\bar{d}}$ that decrease exponentially fast as $t-t_{kj}^*$ increase. Namely, older observations would receive exponentially smaller weights. The estimator of $\boldsymbol{m}^*(t)$ is then defined to be the maximizer of $L(\boldsymbol{m}^*(t))$. Since $L(\boldsymbol{m}^*(t))$ has a quadratic form of $\boldsymbol{m}^*(t)$, the estimator for $\boldsymbol{m}^*(t)$ can be derived to be

$$\widehat{\boldsymbol{m}}^*(t) = \left[\sum_{k=1}^{q}\sum_{j:t_{kj}^*\le t}\frac{\boldsymbol{e}_k\boldsymbol{e}_k'}{\widehat{\sigma}_k^2(t)}(1-\lambda)^{(t-t_{kj}^*)/\bar{d}}+\widehat{\boldsymbol{\Sigma}}_m^{-1}(t)\right]^{-1} \times\left[\sum_{k=1}^{q}\sum_{j:t_{kj}^*\le t}\frac{x_k^*(t_{kj}^*)\boldsymbol{e}_k}{\widehat{\sigma}_k^2(t)}(1-\lambda)^{(t-t_{kj}^*)/\bar{d}}+\widehat{\boldsymbol{\Sigma}}_m^{-1}(t)\widehat{\boldsymbol{\mu}}^{(0)}(t)\right],$$

where $\boldsymbol{e}_k$ is the q-dimensional vector with the kth element being 1 and all other elements being 0, and $\boldsymbol{\Sigma}_m(t)$, $\sigma_k^2(t)$ and $\boldsymbol{\mu}^{(0)}(t)$ have been replaced by $\widehat{\boldsymbol{\Sigma}}_m(t)$, $\widehat{\sigma}_k^2(t)$ and $\widehat{\boldsymbol{\mu}}^{(0)}(t)$, respectively, in the above expression. After $\boldsymbol{m}^*(t)$ is replaced by $\widehat{\boldsymbol{m}}^*(t)$ in (5.15), the resulting charting statistic is

$$\widehat{U}(t) = \frac{\widehat{\boldsymbol{\beta}}'\widehat{\boldsymbol{m}}^*(t)-\widehat{\mu}_r^{(0)}(t)}{\sqrt{\widehat{\boldsymbol{\beta}}'\widehat{\boldsymbol{\Sigma}}_m(t)\widehat{\boldsymbol{\beta}}}}. \tag{5.16}$$

Then, the chart gives a signal at time t if $\widehat{U}(t) > \rho$, where $\rho > 0$ is a control limit.

In the control chart (5.16), the weighting parameter λ controls the amount of historical data used in process monitoring at the current time point t. If λ is chosen larger, then more weight is assigned to the observed data at the current observation time and less weights are assigned to the previous observations. Next, we describe a method to determine λ based on the training data. For a given value of λ, consider the following loss function for the ith individual in the training data:

$$\begin{aligned}\widetilde{L}(\boldsymbol{m}_i(t)) &= -\frac{1}{2}\sum_{k=1}^{q}\sum_{j:t_{ikj}<t}^{J_{ik}} \left[x_{ik}(t_{ikj}) - m_{ik}(t)\right]^2 (1-\lambda)^{(t-t_{ikj})/\bar{d}} \\ &\quad -\frac{1}{2}\left[\boldsymbol{m}_i(t) - \boldsymbol{\mu}^{(0)}(t)\right]' \boldsymbol{\Sigma}_m^{-1}(t)\left[\boldsymbol{m}_i(t) - \boldsymbol{\mu}^{(0)}(t)\right].\end{aligned}$$

It can be seen that $\widetilde{L}(\boldsymbol{m}_i(t))$ is the same as $L(\boldsymbol{m}_i(t))$, except that observations at the current time point t have been excluded when computing $\widetilde{L}(\boldsymbol{m}_i(t))$. Let $\widetilde{\boldsymbol{m}}_{i,\lambda}(t)$ be the minimizer of $\widetilde{L}(\boldsymbol{m}_i(t))$ after certain unknown quantities are replaced by their estimators. Then, $\widetilde{\boldsymbol{m}}_{i,\lambda}(t)$ can be regarded as a prediction of $\boldsymbol{m}_i(t)$ based on the historical data, and the prediction error can be measured by

$$\mathrm{PE}(\lambda) = \sum_{i=1}^{m}\sum_{k=1}^{q}\sum_{j=1}^{J_{ik}} \left[x_{ik}(t_{ikj}) - \boldsymbol{e}_k'\widetilde{\boldsymbol{m}}_{i,\lambda}(t_{ikj})\right]^2.$$

Then, the value of λ can be chosen by minimizing $\mathrm{PE}(\lambda)$.

As discussed in Section 5.3 about the EWMA chart (5.8)–(5.9), the performance of the control chart (5.16) can be evaluated by the metrics ATS_0 and ATS_1. Usually, the value of ATS_0 is pre-specified. Then, the control limit ρ of the chart (5.16) can be chosen from the training data by a block bootstrap procedure similar to the one discussed in Subsection 4.2.3 so that the pre-specified ATS_0 value is reached.

Example 5.2 *Qiu and You (2022) presented some simulation results about the numerical performance of the disease screening method (5.16) described above, which is denoted as "New" in this example. In the simulation study, the training dataset contains observations of* $m = 500$ *individuals with* $q = 4$ *disease risk factors. The basic time unit is assumed to be* $\omega = 0.001$*, and the study time period is* $[0, 2]$*. The following five cases are considered. In cases (I) and (II), IC longitudinal observations of the disease risk factors are generated from the following mixed-effects model: for* $i = 1, 2, \ldots, m$ *and* $k = 1, 2, \ldots, q$*,*

$$\begin{aligned}x_{ik}(t) &= m_{ik}(t) + \varepsilon_{ik}(t) \\ &= 2 + \sin(\pi t) + \xi_{ik1}\phi_1(t) + \xi_{ik2}\phi_2(t) + \xi_{ik3}\phi_3(t) + \varepsilon_{ik}(t),\end{aligned}$$

where $\phi_1(t) = (t-1)^2$, $\phi_2(t) = \sin(2\pi t)$, $\phi_3(t) = \cos(2\pi t)$, $\{\xi_{ikl}, l = 1, 2, 3\}$ *are i.i.d. random numbers generated from the* $N(0, 1)$ *distribution, and the random errors* $\{\varepsilon_{ik}(t)\}$ *at different observation times are i.i.d. and follow the* $N(0, 1)$ *distribution and the t-distribution with 3 degrees of freedom, respectively, in cases (I) and (II), for all* i *and* k*. So, in the above model,* $\xi_{ik1}\phi_1(t)+\xi_{ik2}\phi_2(t)+\xi_{ik3}\phi_3(t)$ *is the random-effects part (i.e.,* $v_{ik}(t)$ *in Model (5.10)). For simplicity, it is assumed that different disease risk factors of a given patient are observed at the same observation times. More precisely,* $t_{i1j} = t_{i2j} = t_{i3j} = t_{i4j}$*, for all* i *and* j*, and* t_{i1j} *is generated from the uniform* *distribution in the interval* $[(j-1)/200, j/200]$, *for each* i *and* j. *To study the impact of the percentage of diseased people in the training dataset on the performance of the proposed method, the three scenarios when the baseline hazard function in Model (5.11) is* $\lambda_0(t) = 0.03$, 0.02 *and* 0.01 *are considered, so that the percentages of diseased people in the second and third scenarios are approximately* $2/3$ *and* $1/3$ *of the one in the first scenario. In cases (III)–(V), IC longitudinal observations of the disease risk factors are generated from the following model:*

$$\begin{aligned} x_{ik}(t) &= m_{ik}(t) + \varepsilon_{ik}(t) \\ &= 2 + \sin(\pi t/2) + g_{ik}(t) + \varepsilon_{ik}(t), \end{aligned}$$

where $\{g_{ik}(t)\}$ *are i.i.d. Gaussian processes with the covariance function* $\sigma(s,t) = 2\exp\{-10(s-t)^2\}$, *and* $\{\varepsilon_{ik}(t)\}$ *are i.i.d. random errors from the* $N(0, \sigma^2)$ *distribution. It is further assumed that* $\sigma^2 = 1, 0.5$ *and* 0, *respectively, in cases (III)–(V). The survival outcomes in these three cases are generated in the same way as that in cases (I) and (II).*

Besides the method "New", the DySS methods suggested by Qiu and Xiang (2015) and You and Qiu (2020a) are also considered, which are discussed in Sections 4.3 and 5.3, respectively. The method by Qiu and Xiang (2015) has two versions: the one using a multivariate EWMA chart and the one combining multiple univariate control charts, which are denoted respectively as "DySS-M" and "DySS-C". The risk monitoring method by You and Qiu (2020a) is denoted as "Risk-Mnt". Among the four methods, "DySS-M" and "DySS-C" use the longitudinal observations of the non-diseased people in the training dataset only for estimating the regular longitudinal patterns of the disease risk factors, while "Risk-Mnt" and "New" first quantify the disease risk and then monitor the quantified disease risk of individual people for disease screening. The major difference between "New" and "Risk-Mnt" is that the former uses a joint modeling framework when quantifying the disease risk while the latter uses a survival model alone.

To evaluate the performance of the four methods, we compare their ATS_1 *values. To this end, we first simulate 1000 IC longitudinal processes of* $\boldsymbol{m}_i(t) = (m_{i1}(t), m_{i2}(t), m_{i3}(t), m_{i4}(t))'$ *from the IC models described above for the five different cases. Then, we add shifts to these processes in the direction of* $\boldsymbol{\beta} = (0.5, 0.4, -0.3, -0.2)'$ *to obtain the following OC longitudinal processes:*

$$\boldsymbol{m}_{i,OC}^{\delta}(t) = \boldsymbol{m}_i(t) + \delta\boldsymbol{\beta},$$

where $\delta\boldsymbol{\beta}$ *is the vector of shift sizes in the four disease risk factors. Then, the* ATS_1 *values of the four methods are computed in all cases considered, when* δ *changes from 0 to 6 and when the* ATS_0 *values of all methods are set to be* 370×0.001. *The results are shown in Figure 5.2. From the figure, we can have the following conclusions. First, all methods can reach the pre-specified* ATS_0 *value when the shift is 0. Second, "New" has the smallest* ATS_1 *values in all cases, compared to the other three methods. Because the*

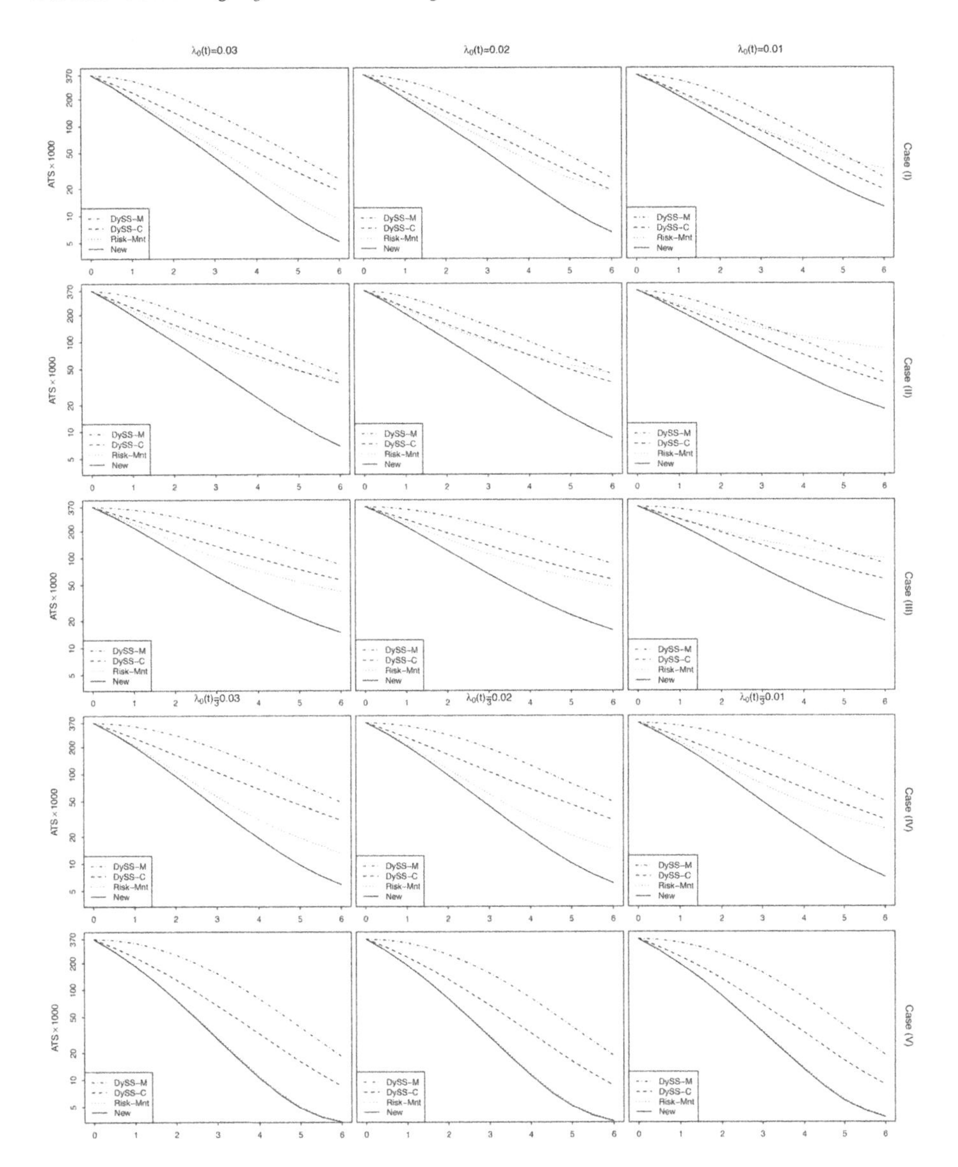

FIGURE 5.2
Calculated ATS_1 values of the four methods "DySS-M", "DySS-C", "Risk-Mnt", and "New" in cases (I)–(V) when ATS_0 is set to be 370×0.001 and the shift sizes in the disease risk factors are $\delta\boldsymbol{\beta}$, where $\boldsymbol{\beta} = (0.5, 0.4, -0.3, -0.2)'$ and δ is the x-axes of the plots that changes from 0 to 6.

longitudinal observations of the disease risk factors contain random errors in most cases considered, the estimate of $\boldsymbol{\beta}$ *used by "Risk-Mnt" cannot be perfect in such cases (i.e., the estimate would not be the same as* $\boldsymbol{\beta}$*), which explains why "Risk-Mnt" performs worse than "New" in these cases. In Case (V) when the longitudinal observations do not have random errors involved, "Risk-Mnt" and "New" have almost the same performance. Third, when the baseline hazard decreases, the number of diseased people in the training dataset would decrease as well. Consequently, both "Risk-Mnt" and "New" become less effective, as seen from Figure 5.2 that their* ATS_1 *values increase from Column 1 to Column 3. As a comparison, the perfromance of "DySS-M" and "DySS-C" does not change much because they do not rely on the survival information in the training dataset. Fourth, by comparing cases (III)–(V) when the noise level gets smaller and smaller, it can be seen that all four methods perform better and better, which is intuitively reasonable.*

5.5 Disease Screening by Variable Selection

The disease screening methods introduced in the previous sections consist of two major steps. First, a survival model is estimated from a training dataset and the estimated model is used for quantifying disease risks for individual people. Second, the quantified disease risks of an individual are monitored sequentially by a control chart for disease early detection. In these methods, the quantified disease risks are linear combinations of the observed disease risk factors (cf., Section 5.2) or their latent trajectories (cf., Section 5.4). More important disease risk factors would receive more weights in the linear combinations, making the corresponding disease screening methods effective. However, these methods still include all disease risk factors in the quantified disease risks. Intuitively, if certain disease risk factors contain little useful information about the disease in concern, then they should be removed from disease screening. In practice, in order to detect/predict the occurrence of a disease effectively, many potential disease risk factors would be considered, especially when we do not know which disease risk factors are important and which ones are not for a given disease. So, removal of unimportant disease risk factors in such cases becomes important, because inclusion of such disease risk factors in model estimation can only increase the variability of the quantified disease risks and reduce the effectiveness of the corresponding disease screening methods. Based on these considerations, You and Qiu (2020b) developed a disease screening method in which variable selection by the least absolute shrinkage and selection operator (LASSO) (Tibshirani, 1996) was incorporated in survival data modeling, so that the redundant disease risk factors could be removed during survival model estimation. The idea of this method can be applied to most disease screening methods discussed in Chapter 4 and the previous sections of this chapter. Next, it is described in the same setup as that in Sections 5.2 and 5.3.

As in Section 5.2, assume that a training dataset is available in advance, which contains the observed disease risk factors and survival outcomes of m individuals. The survival outcomes of the ith individual are described by (T_i, δ_i), where $T_i = \min\{D_i, C_i\}$ is the last follow-up time, D_i is the true disease occurrence time, C_i is the censoring time, and $\delta_i = I(D_i \leq C_i)$ is the survival indicator with $\delta_i = 1$ indicating the occurrence of the disease in concern at T_i and 0 otherwise. The q longitudinal disease risk factors of the ith individual are denoted as the q-dimensional vector $\boldsymbol{x}_i(t)$. It is observed at times $t_{i1}, t_{i2}, \ldots, t_{iJ_i}$, where these observation times could be unequally spaced in the study time period $[0, \mathcal{T}]$ and $t_{iJ_i} = T_i$, for each i. The observed survival data are assumed to follow the Cox proportional hazards model below:

$$\lambda_i(t) = \lambda_0(t) \exp\left[\boldsymbol{\beta}' \boldsymbol{x}_i(t)\right], \qquad \text{for } i = 1, 2, \ldots, m, \tag{5.17}$$

where $\boldsymbol{\beta}$ is a q-dimensional vector of coefficients, and $\lambda_0(t)$ is the baseline hazard function. Compared to Model (5.1), the time-independent covariate vector $\boldsymbol{z}_i$ is not included in Model (5.17) for simplicity. Actually, $\boldsymbol{z}_i$ can be considered as a part of $\boldsymbol{x}_i(t)$. In that sense, Model (5.17) is as flexible as Model (5.1).

As discussed in Section 5.2, the disease risk function of the ith individual is defined to be $r_i(t) = \boldsymbol{\beta}' \boldsymbol{x}_i(t)$. To estimate $r_i(t)$, we need to estimate Model (5.17). To this end, You and Qiu (2019) suggested using the following kernel-smoothed likelihood function:

$$L(\boldsymbol{\beta}) = \prod_{i:\delta_i=1} \frac{\exp\left[\boldsymbol{\beta}' \boldsymbol{x}_i(T_i)\right]}{\sum_{l \in R(T_i)} \sum_{j=1}^{J_l} K_h(T_i - t_{lj}) \exp\left[\boldsymbol{\beta}' \boldsymbol{x}_l(t_{lj})\right]},$$

where $R(t) = \{i, T_i \geq t\}$, $K_h(s) = K(s/h)/h$, $K(s)$ is a density kernel function, and $h > 0$ is a bandwidth. The corresponding log kernel-smoothed likelihood function is

$$\ell(\boldsymbol{\beta}) = \sum_{i:\delta_i=1} \left\{ \boldsymbol{\beta}' \boldsymbol{x}_i(T_i) - \log\left[\sum_{l \in R(T_i)} \sum_{j=1}^{J_l} K_h(T_i - t_{lj}) \exp(\boldsymbol{\beta}' \boldsymbol{x}_l(t_{lj})) \right] \right\}. \tag{5.18}$$

Then, $\boldsymbol{\beta}$ can be estimated by the maximizer of (5.18), denoted as $\widetilde{\boldsymbol{\beta}}$, which can be obtained by the Newton-Raphson algorithm discussed in Section 5.2.

For the estimator $\widetilde{\boldsymbol{\beta}}$, all its elements are usually non-zero, even when some disease risk factors are unimportant or even irrelevant for predicting the disease in concern. Thus, if $\widetilde{\boldsymbol{\beta}}$ is used for estimating the disease risk function $r_i(t)$ of the ith individual, for each i, then all disease risk factors will be used, including the unimportant ones. To properly select important disease risk factors and exclude unimportant ones, we need to identify zero elements in the coefficient vector $\boldsymbol{\beta}$, which can be achieved by using the LASSO method (Tibshirani, 1996). The main idea of LASSO is to add a penalty term to the related objective function for estimating the coefficient vector, in order to shrink the coefficients of unimportant disease risk factors toward zero. To this end, the following adaptive LASSO penalty (cf., Zou, 2006) is considered:

$$p_\gamma(\boldsymbol{\beta}) = \gamma \sum_{k=1}^{q} w_k |\beta_k|,$$

where γ is a non-negative regularization parameter, $\{w_k = 1/|\widetilde{\beta}_k|, k = 1, 2, \ldots, q\}$ are adaptive weights, and $\widetilde{\boldsymbol{\beta}} = (\widetilde{\beta}_1, \widetilde{\beta}_2, \ldots, \widetilde{\beta}_q)$. The adaptive LASSO estimate of $\boldsymbol{\beta}$, denoted as $\widehat{\boldsymbol{\beta}}$, is then defined to be the minimizer of the following penalized log-likelihood function:

$$-\ell(\boldsymbol{\beta}) + p_\gamma(\boldsymbol{\beta}). \tag{5.19}$$

Minimization of the objective function in (5.19) can be achieved by the coordinate optimization algorithm discussed in Friedman et al. (2007) and Simon et al. (2011).

For the adaptive LASSO estimate $\widehat{\boldsymbol{\beta}}$, if a disease risk factor has nothing to do with the disease in concern, then the related element of $\widehat{\boldsymbol{\beta}}$ would be 0. Thus, if $\widehat{\boldsymbol{\beta}}$ is used for estimating the disease risk function $r_i(t)$ of the ith individual, for each i, then the disease risk factors that contribute little in predicting the disease in concern would actually not be used. For this reason, You and Qiu (2020b) suggested estimating the disease risk function of the ith individual by

$$\widehat{r}_i(t) = \widehat{\boldsymbol{\beta}}' \boldsymbol{x}_i(t).$$

After $\widehat{\boldsymbol{\beta}}$ is obtained by the adaptive LASSO approach and the disease risk functions of different people are estimated accordingly, the mean disease risk function $\mu(t) = \mathrm{E}[r_i(t)|T_i \geq t]$ and the related variance function $\sigma^2(t) = \mathrm{Var}[r_i(t)|T_i \geq t]$ can be estimated by $\widehat{\mu}(t)$ and $\widehat{\sigma}^2(t)$ defined in (5.4) and (5.5), respectively. Then, the disease screening method described in Section 5.3 can be used for disease early detection for individual people.

In the adaptive LASSO objective function defined in (5.19), the regularization parameter γ needs to be chosen properly in advance. To this end, the Akaike information criterion (AIC) approach (Akaike, 1992; Tibshirani, 1997) can be used. Let $c(\boldsymbol{a})$ denote the number of non-zero elements of a vector $\boldsymbol{a}$. Then, the AIC criterion for the survival model (5.17) is defined to be

$$\mathrm{AIC}(\gamma) = -2\ell(\widehat{\boldsymbol{\beta}}) + 2c(\widehat{\boldsymbol{\beta}}),$$

where $\widehat{\boldsymbol{\beta}}$ is the adaptive LASSO estimate of $\boldsymbol{\beta}$ when the regularization parameter is γ. Then, γ is chosen to be the minimizer of $\mathrm{AIC}(\gamma)$.

Example 5.3 *For the stroke data considered in Example 5.1, the training data and test data are selected as discussed in that example. So, the test data contain 9 stroke participants and 342 non-stroke participants, although the test data and training data in the current example may not be the same as* *those in Example 5.1 since these two datasets are selected randomly from the stroke and non-stroke participants of the whole stroke dataset, respectively. The estimate of* $\boldsymbol{\beta}$ *obtained by minimizing the objective function in (5.18) is* $\widetilde{\boldsymbol{\beta}} = (-0.0013, 0.0178, 0.0099)'$*, and the adaptive LASSO estimate of* $\boldsymbol{\beta}$ *obtained by minimizing the objective function in (5.19) is* $\widehat{\boldsymbol{\beta}} = (0.0000, 0.0169, 0.0092)'$*, where the parameter* γ *in (5.19) is chosen by AIC to be 0.05. It can be seen that the first element of the adaptive LASSO estimate has been shrunk to 0.*

We then use the following three disease screening methods to detect stroke for people in the test data. The first one is the multivariate DySS method discussed in Section 4.3, denoted as MDySS, that is based on direct sequential monitoring of the observed disease risk factors. The second and third ones are the methods discussed in Section 5.3 and this section, denoted as DySS-DR and DySS-DR-LASSO, respectively, where "DR" denotes "disease risk", and "LASSO" denotes "variable selection by adaptive LASSO". So, both DySS-DR and DySS-DR-LASSO are based on disease risk quantification, and their major difference is that DySS-DR-LASSO uses variable selection in disease risk quantification while DySS-DR does not. When $\lambda = 0.2$ *and* $ATS_0 = 10$ *years in all three methods, a summary of their disease screening results is presented in Table 5.2. From the table, we can see that i) all three methods give signals to 8 out of 9 stroke participants in the test data, ii) DySS-DR gives signals to 132 out of 342 non-stroke participants, iii) DySS-DR-LASSO gives signals to 123 non-stroke participants, and iv) MDySS gives signals to 167 non-stroke participants. Thus, while their sensitivities are kept the same, the specificity of DySS-DR-LASSO is the best and the specificity of DySS is the worst among the three methods in this example.*

TABLE 5.2
Summary of disease screening results of the three disease screening methods when they are used to detect stroke for 9 stroke participants and 342 non-stroke participants in the test data considered in Example 5.3.

	MDySS		DySS-DR		DySS-DR-LASSO	
Participants	Signal	No Signal	Signal	No Signal	Signal	No Signal
Stroke	8	1	8	1	8	1
Non-Stroke	167	175	132	210	123	219

5.6 Some Discussions

In this chapter, we have introduced some disease screening methods based on disease risk quantification and sequential monitoring of quantified disease risks. These methods have two major differences from the DySS methods described in Chapter 4. The first major difference is that the former methods make use of helpful information of both non-diseased and diseased people in a training dataset while the latter methods use the observed data of non-diseased people only. By exploring the numerical association between the observed disease risk factors and the hazard rate of the disease in concern using a survival modeling approach, the former methods can use the observed disease risk factors in a way that is associated with the disease to detect. The second major difference between the two types of methods is that the disease screening methods introduced in this chapter try to detect the disease in concern for a given individual by sequentially monitoring the individual's longitudinal pattern of the quantified disease risks, which is a linear combination of the observed disease risk factors, while the basic DySS methods described in Chapter 4 monitor the observed disease risk factors of the given individual directly. So, in the former methods, disease risk factors that are more important for predicting the disease would receive more weights in the quantified disease risks, the less important ones would receive less weights, and the irrelevant ones can even be eliminated from disease screening after a variable selection method is used in disease risk quantification (cf., Section 5.5). As a comparison, all disease risk factors are treated equally important in the latter methods. Numerical studies in Qiu and You (2022), You and Qiu (2020a) and You and Qiu (2020b) have shown that the former methods would have a better performance in various cases considered.

In each disease screening method introduced in this chapter, a parametric Cox proportional hazards model (e.g., Model (5.1)) is used for describing the functional association between the observed disease risk factors and the hazard rate of the disease in concern. Some generalizations of this model have been discussed in Qiu and You (2022) and You and Qiu (2020a). For instance, one generalization is to allow time-varying coefficients in the related model. But, all generalized models discussed in these papers are still in the Cox proportional hazards model framework. Validity of these models needs to be checked carefully in practice.

The modified EWMA chart (5.8)–(5.9) discussed in Section 5.3 depends on the weighting parameter λ. In the SPC literature, this parameter is usually pre-specified, and it has been demonstrated that a large λ value is good for detecting a large shift in the related process and a small λ value is good for detecting a small shift (cf., Qiu, 2014, Chapter 5). In many applications, however, it is often unknown whether a future shift is large or small. So, pre-specification of λ becomes difficult in such cases. In the literature, there are two approaches to overcome this difficulty. One is to use the so-called adaptive EWMA chart (cf., Subsection 3.2.2), in which the shift size is estimated sequentially during online process monitoring and then the λ value is adjusted accordingly (cf., Qiu, 2014, Section 5.4). Another strategy is to use a set of λ values and the charting statistic at each time point is defined to be the maximum of the charting statistics with the individual λ values (cf., Qiu et al.,

2018). Both strategies can be considered in practice when using the disease screening methods discussed in this chapter and Chapter 4.

The disease screening methods introduced in this chapter are designed for detecting a single disease. In practice, a patient could have multiple diseases simultaneously, especially when chronic diseases are concerned. For instance, a cancer patient could suffer stroke or other cardiovascular diseases. In cases when detection of multiple diseases is our interest, new DySS methods need to be developed, which should take into account the association among different diseases, the association between a disease and its risk factors, and the association among different disease risk factors. In the literature, when multimorbidity is a concern, some analytic methods for survival data analysis with competing risks have been developed (e.g., Austin et al., 2016; Fine and Gray, 1999). But, such methods are designed mainly for analyzing time-to-event data, while the current disease screening problem is for disease early detection by sequentially monitoring the observed disease risk factors. Thus, they cannot be used for handling the disease screening problem directly.

5.7 Exercises

5.1 Let T be the time to an event (e.g., occurrence of a given disease) of a patient. Then, the hazard rate function $\lambda(t)$ used in Section 5.2 is defined as follows:

$$\lambda(t) = \lim_{\Delta t \to 0} \frac{\mathrm{P}(t \leq T < t + \Delta t | T \geq t)}{\Delta t}.$$

From the formal definition above, it can be seen that the hazard rate function $\lambda(t)$ measures the instantaneous rate of occurrence of the event in concern at time t among all people who have not experienced the event by time t. Based on this intuition about the hazard rate function $\lambda(t)$, answer the following questions:

(i) In Model (5.1), if $q = 1$ (i.e., there is a single disease risk factor), $x_i(t)$ increases by one unit (i.e., $x_i(t)$ changes to $x_i(t) + 1$, and $\boldsymbol{z}_i$ keeps unchanged, what will be the resulting change in $\lambda_i(t)$? Provide an intuitive explanation about the coefficient β based on the answer to this question.

(ii) In Model (5.1), if $p = 1$ (i.e., there is a single time-independent covariate), the ith and i'th individuals have the same observed values of the disease risk factors at t (i.e., $\boldsymbol{x}_i(t) = \boldsymbol{x}_{i'}(t)$), but $z_i = z_{i'} + 2$, what is the ratio $\lambda_i(t)/\lambda_{i'}(t)$? Provide an intuitive explanation about the result.

5.2 In an observed survival dataset, assume that there are 10 people involved and their observed survival times (i.e., the values of T_i) in the study period $[0, 2]$ are

$$0.5, 0.75, 0.8, 0.8, 1.0, 1.1, 1.3, 1.3, 1.5, 1.9$$

Find $R(t) = \{i : T_i \geq t\}$, for $t \in [0, 2]$.

5.3 Verify formulas (5.4) and (5.5), using the expressions in (2.53) in Subsection 2.5.5.

5.4 In the second paragraph of Section 5.3, an alternative aproach to define standardized disease risks is discussed, which uses the observed data of the non-diseased people in the training data only to compute $\widehat{\mu}(t)$ and $\widehat{\sigma}(t)$.

(i) Discuss the pros and cons of this alternative approach and the approach of (5.7) suggested by You and Qiu (2020a) for disease early detection.

(ii) Discuss in details how to implement the alternative approach in a given application.

5.5 The charting statistic E_j in (5.8) is a wighted average of $\{\widehat{e}(t_j^*), \widehat{e}(t_{j-1}^*), \ldots, \widehat{e}(t_2^*), \widehat{e}(t_1^*)\}$, for $j \geq 2$. Provide analytic expressions for the weights and verify that they are proportional to $1, (1-\lambda)^{n_j^*-n_{j-1}^*}, \ldots, (1-\lambda)^{n_j^*-n_2^*}, (1-\lambda)^{n_j^*-n_1^*}$, respectively.

5.6 The standardized disease risks $\{\widehat{e}(t_j^*), j \geq 1\}$ defined in (5.7) could be serially correlated, and construction of the modified EWMA chart (5.8)–(5.9) does not take into account such serial correlation. A possible improvement of the disease screening method discussed in Section 5.3 is to first apply the data decorrelation and standardization procedure described in Section 4.4 to the quantified disease risks $\{\widehat{r}(t_j^*), j \geq 1\}$ of an individual under monitoring, and then apply the modified EWMA chart (5.8)–(5.9) to the decorrelated and standardized disease risks. Discuss in details how to implement this alternative disease screening method.

5.7 The multivariate nonparametric mixed-effects model (5.10) is for describing the observed disease risk factors of both diseased and non-diseased individuals in the training data.

(i) Derive separate models from Model (5.10) for describing the observed disease risk factors of the diseased and non-diseased individuals in the training data, respectively.

(ii) Provide an intuitive explanation about the quantities $\mu_k^{(0)}(t)$, $\Delta_k(t)$ and $v_{ik}(t)$ in the two models, for each i and k.

5.8 If the time-independent vector of covariates $\boldsymbol{z}_i$ is included in Model (5.11) explicitly, discuss in details how the model estimation procedure described in Subsection 5.4.1 can be modified accordingly.

5.9 For the control chart (5.16), explain how the previous observations of the disease risk factors have actually been used in the charting statistic $\widehat{U}(t)$.

5.10 For the disease screening method described in Section 5.5, discuss in details how disease screening can proceed after $\widehat{\boldsymbol{\beta}}$ is obtained by the adaptive LASSO approach (cf., (5.19)) and the related disease risk functions are estimated accordingly.

6

R Package **DySS** *for Dynamic Disease Screening*

6.1 Introduction

In the previous two chapters, we have introduced some recent statistical methods, called dynamic screening system (DySS) methods, developed mainly for disease screening of individual people. These DySS methods aim to detect a disease in concern as early as possible by sequentially monitoring the observed disease risk factors using a properly designed statistical process control (SPC) chart. One major feature of such DySS methods is that they take into account the longitudinal pattern of the observed disease risk factors when detecting a disease, instead of just the observed disease risk factors at the current or a few nearby observation times as in the traditional medical diagnoses. A DySS method proceeds in three general steps. First, the regular longitunal pattern (cf., Section 4.2) of the disease risk factors is estimated from an IC dataset that contains the observed data of some non-diseased people. Second, to detect the disease for a specific patient, the patient's observed longitunal pattern of the disease risk factors is compared to the estimated regular longitunal pattern by a sequential data decorrelation and standardization procedure. This step actually compares the patient's observed disease risk factors with those of the non-diseased people in the IC dataset cross-sectionally at each observation time. Finally, the patient's decorrelated and standardized data are monitored sequentially by an SPC chart, so that all historical data of the patient have been used efficiently for disease screening. Numerical results presented in the previous two chapters and/or the related research papers (e.g., Qiu and Xiang, 2014; You and Qiu, 2020a) show that the DySS methods are effective for disease screening.

For readers' convenience to implement the DySS methods introduced in the previous two chapters, an *R* package named **DySS** has been developed recently (You and Qiu, 2022). This chapter introduces this package in two sections. Major functions built in the package are first introduced in Section 6.2, and then these functions and the related statistical methods are demonstrated using the stroke data (cf., Example 4.1) in Section 6.3.

DOI: 10.1201/9781003138150-6

6.2 Major Functions in the *R* Package DySS

There are two ways to use the *R* Package **DySS**. First, we can install it on our own computer by i) downloading the archive file **DySS_1.0.tar.gz** from the comprehensive *R* archive network (CRAN) webpage with the following address

https://cran.r-project.org/web/packages/DySS/index.html

to the current directory on our computer, and ii) installing the package by running the following commands in the *R* environment:

```
> install.packages("DySS_1.0.tar.gz")
> library("DySS")
```

Note that the sequence of numbers "1.0" in the archive file name **DySS_1.0.tar.gz** represents the version of the package. Usually, the package is updated once a year. So, in order to use the latest version of the package, we need to download the archive file regularly.

Second, in the *R* environment, we can run the following command:

```
> install.packages("DySS")
```

Then, a window will pop up, providing us a list of secure CRAN mirror sites. We can choose a site that is close to our physical location. After the selection, the package will be installed on our computer, and we can run the following command in order to use the related functions in the package:

```
> library("DySS")
```

By comparing with the first way of package installation, we do not specify the package version in this installation. Actually, the latest version is always used in this way of package installation.

After the package is installed, we are ready to use its built-in functions and datasets. To have an access to the package description, use the following *R* command:

```
> help(package="DySS")
```

To have an access to the description about a specific built-in function or dataset (e.g., the built-in function **monitor_long_1d()**), use the following *R* command:

```
> ?monitor_long_1d
```

All built-in functions and datasets in the *R* package **DySS** are described below. Demonstration on how to use them for real data analysis is given in the next section.

calculate_ATS() This function is for calculating the average time to signal (ATS) of a given control chart, where ATS is defined to be the average time from the start of process monitoring to the signal time given by the chart. This function can be used in the *R* environment as follows.

```
> calculate_ATS(chart_matrix,time_matrix,nobs,starttime,
  endtime,design_interval,n_time_units,time_unit,CL,
  no_signal_action = "omit")
```

The arguments of the above *R* command are explained below.

chart_matrix	A numeric matrix containing the charting statistic values, where chart_matrix[i,j] is the jth charting statistic value for the ith person.
time_matrix	A numeric matrix containing the observation times, arranged in the same way as that of chart_matrix.
nobs	An integer vector specifying the numbers of observations of all people in the observed data. Thus, nobs[i] is the number of observations of the ith person.
starttime	A numeric vector that specifies the starting times (e.g., ages) of process monitoring for different people.
endtime	A numeric vector that specifies the ending times of process monitoring for different people.
design_interval	A numeric vector of length two that gives the time interval of all observation times. By default, design_interval=range(time_matrix,na.rm=TRUE).
n_time_units	An integer value that gives the total number of basic time units in the design interval. The design interval is thus seq(design_interval[1],design_interval[2], length.out=n_time_units).
time_unit	An optional argument specifying the basic time unit that is used when n_time_units is missing. The design interval can be written as seq(design_interval[1],design_interval[2], by=time_unit).
CL	A numeric value specifying the control limit of the chart.

no_signal_action A character specifying the method to use when a signal is not given by the chart. If no_signal_action="omit", then processes with no signals will be omitted when computing ATS. If no_signal_action="maxtime", then the signal times of the processes with no signals are set to be the right end of design_interval. If no_signal_action="endtime", then the signal times of the processes with no signals are set to be the ending times.

This function returns the ATS value of the control chart.

calculate_signal_times() This function records the time to the signal given by a control chart to each person under monitoring. It can be used in the *R* environment as follows.

```
> calculate_signal_times(chart_matrix,time_matrix,nobs,
  starttime,endtime,design_interval,n_time_units,time_unit,
  CL)
```

The arguments of the above *R* command are explained below.

chart_matrix A numeric matrix containing the charting statistic values, where chart_matrix[i,j] is the jth charting statistic value for the ith person.

time_matrix A numeric matrix containing the observation times, arranged in the same way as that of chart_matrix.

nobs An integer vector specifying the numbers of observations of all people in the observed data. Thus, nobs[i] is the number of observations of the ith person.

starttime A numeric vector that specifies the starting times (e.g., ages) of process monitoring for different people.

endtime A numeric vector that specifies the ending times of process monitoring for different people.

design_interval A numeric vector of length two that gives the time interval of all observation times. By default, design_interval=range(time_matrix,na.rm=TRUE).

n_time_units An integer value that gives the total number of basic time units in the design interval. The design interval is thus seq(design_interval[1],design_interval[2], length.out=n_time_units).

time_unit — An optional argument specifying the basic time unit that is used when n_time_units is missing. The design interval can be written as seq(design_interval[1],design_interval[2], by=time_unit).

CL — A numeric value specifying the control limit of the chart.

This function returns a list with the following values.

signal_times — A numerical vector giving the recorded signal times for all people under monitoring.

signals — A logical vector specifying whether each person receives a signal.

data_example_long_1d() This function generates a simulated univariate longitudinal dataset for demonstrating certain DySS methods. It can be used in the *R* environment as follows.

```
> data(data_example_long_1d)
```

After running the above command, an *R* data frame is generated to store a simulated univariate longitudinal dataset, which is named "data_example_long_1d" with 9 variables. This dataset contains 200 non-diseased people and 200 diseased people with 200 observations of a disease risk factor for each person in the dataset. A brief description of all its 9 variables is given below.

data_matrix_IC — A matrix of dimensions 200×200 that contains the generated data of 200 non-diseased people with 200 observations of a disease risk factor for each non-diseased person.

time_matrix_IC — A matrix of dimensions 200×200 that contains the corresponding observation times of the non-diseased people.

nobs_IC — A numerical vector giving the number of observations for each non-diseased person.

data_matrix_OC — A matrix of dimensions 200×200 that contains the generated data of 200 diseased people with 200

	observations of a disease risk factor for each diseased person.
time_matrix_OC	A matrix of dimensions 200 × 200 that contains the corresponding observation times of the diseased people.
nobs_OC	A numerical vector giving the number of observations for each diseased person.
design_interval	A numeric vector of length two that gives the time interval of all observation times. In this simulated dataset, the time interval is [0,1].
n_time_units	An integer value that gives the total number of basic time units in design_interval.
time_unit	A numeric value specifying the basic time unit, which is 0.001 in this example.

data_example_long_md() This function generates a simulated multivariate longitudinal dataset for demonstrating certain DySS methods. It can be used in the *R* environment as follows.

```
> data(data_example_long_md)
```

After running the above command, an *R* data frame is generated to store a simulated multivariate longitudinal dataset, which is named "data_example_long_md" with 9 variables. This dataset contains 200 non-diseased people and 200 diseased people with 100 observations of 3 disease risk factors for each non-diseased person. A brief description of all its 9 variables is given below.

data_array_IC	An array of dimensions 200 × 100 × 3 that contains the generated data of 200 non-diseased people with 100 observations of 3 disease risk factors for each non-diseased person.
time_matrix_IC	A matrix of dimensions 200 × 100 that contains the corresponding observation times of the non-diseased people.
nobs_IC	A numerical vector giving the number of observations for each non-diseased person.

data_array_OC	An array of dimensions $200 \times 100 \times 3$ that contains the generated data of 200 diseased people with 100 observations of 3 disease risk factors for each diseased person.
time_matrix_OC	A matrix of dimensions 200×100 that contains the corresponding observation times of the diseased people.
nobs_OC	A numerical vector giving the number of observations for each diseased person.
design_interval	A numeric vector of length two that gives the time interval of all observation times. In this simulated dataset, the time interval is [0,1].
n_time_units	An integer value that gives the total number of basic time units in design_interval.
time_unit	A numeric value specifying the basic time unit, which is 0.001 in this example.

data_example_long_surv() This function generates a simulated multivariate longitudinal dataset for demonstrating certain DySS methods based on the joint modeling of survival and longitudinal data. It can be used in the *R* environment as follows.

```
> data(data_example_long_surv)
```

After running the above command, an *R* data frame is generated to store a simulated multivariate longitudinal dataset, which is named "data_example_long_surv" with 15 variables. This dataset contains 500 non-diseased people and 500 diseased people with 100 observations of 3 disease risk factors for each person in the dataset. A brief description of all its 15 variables is given below.

data_array_IC	An array of dimensions $500 \times 100 \times 3$ that contains the generated data of 500 non-diseased people with 100 observations of 3 disease risk factors for each non-diseased person.
time_matrix_IC	A matrix of dimensions 500×100 that contains the corresponding observation times of the non-diseased people.

nobs_IC	A numerical vector giving the number of observations for each non-diseased person.
starttime_IC	A numeric vector specifying the ages of non-diseased people at the first observation time.
survtime_IC	A numeric vector specifying non-diseased people's survival times.
survevent_IC	A logic vector indicating whether an event is observed for each non-diseased person. The event is observed for the ith person if survevent_IC[i]=TRUE, and not observed otherwise.
data_array_OC	An array of dimensions $500 \times 100 \times 3$ that contains the generated data of 500 diseased people with 100 observations of 3 disease risk factors for each diseased person.
time_matrix_OC	A matrix of dimensions 500×100 that contains the corresponding observation times of the diseased people.
nobs_OC	A numerical vector giving the number of observations for each diseased person.
starttime_OC	A numeric vector specifying the ages of diseased people at the first observation time.
survtime_OC	A numeric vector specifying diseased people's survival times.
survevent_OC	A logic vector indicating whether an event is observed for each diseased person. The event is observed for the ith person if survevent_OC[i]=TRUE, and not observed otherwise.
design_interval	A numeric vector of length two that gives the time interval of all observation times. In this simulated dataset, the time interval is $[0,1]$.
n_time_units	An integer value that gives the total number of basic time units in design_interval.
time_unit	A numeric value specifying the basic time unit, which is 0.001 in this example.

data_stroke() This function provides the stroke dataset described in Example 4.1. In the dataset, there are longitudinal observations of 27 stroke people and 1028 non-stroke people. For each person, observations of the three disease risk factors systolic blood pressure, diastolic blood pressure, and cholesterol level, are collected at 7 different time points. The dataset can be retrieved in the *R* environment as follows.

```
> data(data_stroke)
```

After running the above command, an *R* data frame named "data_stroke" with 8 variables is retrieved for our use. For instance, the variable systolic_ctrl contains the observed systolic blood pressure data of all 1028 non-stroke people, arranged as a 1028×7 matrix. Thus, the following command

```
> data_stroke$systolic_ctrl[1,]
```

gives the 7 longitudinal observations of the systolic blood pressure of the first non-stroke person. A brief description of all 8 variables in the dataset is given below.

systolic_ctrl	A 1028×7 matrix that contains the observed systolic blood pressure data of all 1028 non-stroke people.
diastolic_ctrl	A 1028×7 matrix that contains the observed diastolic blood pressure data of all 1028 non-stroke people.
cholesterol_ctrl	A 1028×7 matrix that contains the observed cholesterol level data of all 1028 non-stroke people.
age_ctrl	A 1028×7 matrix that contains the age information of all 1028 non-stroke people when their longitudinal observations are obtained.
systolic_case	A 1028×7 matrix that contains the observed systolic blood pressure data of all 27 stroke people.
diastolic_case	A 1028×7 matrix that contains the observed diastolic blood pressure data of all 27 stroke people.
cholesterol_case	A 1028×7 matrix that contains the observed cholesterol level data of all 27 stroke people.
age_case	A 1028×7 matrix that contains the age information of all 27 stroke people when their longitudinal observations are obtained.

estimate_pattern_long_1d() This function estimates the regular longitudinal pattern of a univariate disease risk factor based on an in-control (IC) dataset. This is usually used as the first step for dynamic disease screening. The regular longitudinal pattern can be described by the IC mean, variance, covariance, and distribution functions, depending on the estimation method. This function can be used in the *R* environment as follows.

```
> estimate_pattern_long_1d(data_matrix,time_matrix,nobs,
  design_interval,n_time_units,time_unit,estimation_method,
  smoothing_method = "local linear",bw_mean,bw_var,bw_cov,
  bw_t,bw_y)
```

The arguments of the above *R* command are explained below.

data_matrix	A matrix of the observed disease risk factor in the IC data. data_matrix[i,j] is the jth observation of the ith person.
time_matrix	A matrix of the observation times arranged in the same way as data_matrix.
nobs	A numerical vector giving the number of observations for each person in the IC data.
design_interval	A numeric vector of length two that gives the left and right endpoints of the design interval. By default, design_interval=range(time_matrix,na.rm=TRUE).
n_time_units	An integer value giving the total number of basic time units in design_interval. The design interval is descretized to be seq(design_interval[1],design_interval[2], length.out=n_time_units).
time_unit	An optional argument specifying the basic time unit used when n_time_units is missing. The design interval is descretized to be seq(design_interval[1],design_interval[2], by=time_unit).
estimation_method	A characteristic variable specifying the estimation method as described below. i) If estimation_method="meanvar", then the mean and variance functions of the disease risk factor will be estimated as discussed in Qiu and Xiang (2014).

ii) If estimation_method="meanvarcov", then the mean, variance and covariance functions will be estimated by the method discussed in Li and Qiu (2016).
iii) If estimation_method="meanvarcovmean", then the mean, variance and covariance functions will be estimated by the method in Li and Qiu (2016) with the mean function estimate updated using the estimated covariance function.
iv) If estimation_method="distribution", then the distribution function will be estimated as in You and Qiu (2021a).
v) If estimation_method="distributionvarcov", then the distribution and covariance functions of the related standardized observations will be estimated by the method in You and Qiu (2021a).

smoothing_method A characteristic variable specifying the smoothing method as described below.
i) If smoothing_method="local constant", then the local constant kernel smoothing method is used.
ii) If smoothing_method="local linear", then the local linear kernel smoothing method is used.

bw_mean The bandwidth for estimating the mean function.

bw_var The bandwidth for estimating the variance function.

bw_cov The bandwidth for estimating the covariance function.

bw_t The bandwidth in time for estimating the distribution function.

bw_y The bandwidth in y for estimating the distribution function.

This function returns a list with the following labels:

- If estimation_method="meanvar", then the list label is pattern_long_1d_meanvar;
- If estimation_method="meanvarcov", then the list label is pattern_long_1d_meanvarcov;
- If estimation_method="distribution", then the list label is pattern_long_1d_distribution;
- If estimation_method="distributionvarcov", then the list label is pattern_long_1d_distributionvarcov.

The related estimated values are saved in the following variables of the list.

grid	A grid of the design time interval.
mean_est	Estimated mean values at the grid points.
var_est	Estimated variance values at the grid points.
cov_est	Estimated covariance values at the grid points.

estimate_pattern_long_md() This function estimates the regular longitudinal pattern of multiple disease risk factors based on an in-control (IC) dataset. This is usually used in the first step of dynamic disease screening. The regular longitudinal pattern can be described by the IC mean, variance, covariance, and distribution functions, depending on the estimation method. This function can be used in the *R* environment as follows.

```
> estimate_pattern_long_md(data_array,time_matrix,nobs,
  design_interval,n_time_units,time_unit,estimation_method,
  bw_mean,bw_var,bw_cov)
```

The arguments of the above *R* command are explained below.

data_array	An array of the observed disease risk factors of the IC data. data_array[i,j,k] is the jth observation of the kth disease risk factor of the ith person.
time_matrix	A matrix of the observation times arranged in the way according to the first two dimensions of data_array.
nobs	A numerical vector giving the number of observations for each person in the IC data.
design_interval	A numeric vector of length two that gives the left and right endpoints of the design interval. By default, design_interval=range(time_matrix,na.rm=TRUE).
n_time_units	An integer value giving the total number of basic time units in design_interval. The design interval is descretized to be seq(design_interval[1],design_interval[2], length.out=n_time_units).
time_unit	An optional argument specifying the basic time unit

	used when n_time_units is missing. The design interval is descretized to be seq(design_interval[1],design_interval[2], by=time_unit).
estimation_method	A characteristic variable specifying the estimation method. i) If estimation_method="meanvar", then the mean and variance functions of the disease risk factors will be estimated by the method in Qiu and Xiang (2015). ii) If estimation_method="meanvarcov", then the mean, variance and covariance functions will be estimated as discussed in Li and Qiu (2017).
bw_mean	The bandwidth for estimating the mean function.
bw_var	The bandwidth for estimating the variance function.
bw_cov	The bandwidth for estimating the covariance function.

The values of this function are saved in a list with the following labels:

- If estimation_method="meanvar", then the list label is pattern_long_md_meanvar;
- If estimation_method="meanvarcov", then the list label is pattern_long_md_meanvarcov.

The related estimated values are saved in the following variables of the list.

grid	A grid of the design time interval.
mean_est	Estimated mean values at the grid points.
var_est	Estimated variance values at the grid points.
cov_est	Estimated covariance values at the grid points.

estimate_pattern_long_surv() This function estimates the joint models of the survival and longitudinal data based on a training dataset. This is usually used as the first step for dynamic disease screening. The risk of a new patient to monitor can be quantified by a linear combination of the patient's observed disease risk factors according to the estimated survival model. This function can be used in the *R* environment as follows.

```
> estimate_pattern_long_surv(data_array,time_matrix,nobs,
```

```
starttime,survtime,survevent,design_interval,n_time_units,
time_unit,estimation_method = "risk",smoothing_method =
"local linear",bw_beta,bw_mean,bw_var)
```

The arguments of the above *R* command are explained below.

data_array	An array of the observed disease risk factors of the people in the training data. data_array[i,j,k] is the jth observation of the kth disease risk factor of the ith person.
time_matrix	A matrix of the observation times arranged in the way according to the first two dimensions of data_array.
nobs	A numerical vector giving the number of observations for each person in the training data.
starttime	A numeric vector specifying the ages of people at the first observation time.
survtime	A numeric vector specifying people's survival times.
survevent	A logic vector indicating whether an event is observed for people in the training data. The event is observed for the ith person if survevent[i]==TRUE, and not observed otherwise.
design_interval	A numeric vector of length two that gives the left and right endpoints of the design interval. By default, design_interval=range(time_matrix,na.rm=TRUE).
n_time_units	An integer value that gives the total number of basic time units in the design time interval. The design time interval is descretized to be seq(design_interval[1],design_interval[2], length.out=n_time_units).
time_unit	An optional argument specifying the basic time unit used when n_time_units is missing. The design time interval is descretized to be seq(design_interval[1],design_interval[2], by=time_unit).
estimation_method	A logic variable specifying the estimation method. In the current version of the package, only the method "risk" discussed in You and Qiu (2020a) is available.

smoothing_method A characteristic variable specifying the smoothing method as described below.
i) If smoothing_method="local constant", then the local constant kernel smoothing method is used.
ii) If smoothing_method="local linear", then the local linear kernel smoothing method is used.

bw_beta The bandwidth for estimating the IC survival model.

bw_mean The bandwidth for estimating the mean of the quantified risk.

bw_var The bandwidth for estimating the variance of the quantified risk.

The values of this function are saved in a list with the label pattern_long_surv_risk. The related estimated values are saved in the following variables of the list.

grid A grid of the design time interval.

beta_est Estimated regression coefficients.

mean_risk_est Estimated mean risk values at the grid points.

var_risk_est Estimated variance values of the risk at the grid points.

evaluate_control_chart_one_group() This function evaluates the performance of a control chart for disease screening when its charting statistic values for both the diseased and non-diseased people in a given dataset are provided in a single matrix. This function can be used in the *R* environment as follows.

```
> evaluate_control_chart_one_group(chart_matrix,time_matrix,
  nobs,starttime,endtime,status,design_interval,n_time_units,
  time_unit,no_signal_action = "omit")
```

The arguments of the above *R* command are explained below.

chart_matrix A numeric matrix containing the charting statistic values, where chart_matrix[i,j] is the jth charting statistic value for the ith person in a given dataset.

time_matrix	A numeric matrix containing the observation times, arranged in the same way as that of chart_matrix.
nobs	An integer vector giving the numbers of observations for all people. Thus, nobs[i] is the total number of observations collected for the *i*th person.
starttime	A numeric vector that specifies the starting times of process monitoring for all different people.
endtime	A numeric vector that specifies the ending times of process monitoring for all different people.
status	A logic vector indicating the disease status of each person. The *i*th person is non-diseased if status[i]=FALSE, and diseased if status[i]=TRUE.
design_interval	A numeric vector of length two that gives the left and right endpoints of the design time interval. By default, design_interval=range(time_matrix,na.rm=TRUE).
n_time_units	An integer value that gives the total number of basic time units in the design time interval. The design time interval is descretized to be seq(design_interval[1],design_interval[2], length.out=n_time_units).
time_unit	An optional argument specifying the basic time unit used when n_time_units is missing. The design time interval is descretized to be seq(design_interval[1],design_interval[2], by=time_unit).
no_signal_action	A characteristic variable specifying the way to handle cases with no signals. If no_signal_action="omit", then cases with no signals will be omitted when computing the performance metrics. If no_signal_action="maxtime", then the right endpoint of the design interval is used as the signal times for cases with no signals. If no_signal_action="endtime", then the last observation times of the people who do not receive signals would be used as the signal times.

This function returns a list with the following values.

thres	A numeric vector of control limits for the chart.

FPR A numeric vector of false positive rates.

TPR A numeric vector of true positive rates.

ATS0 A numeric vector of IC ATS values.

ATS1 A numeric vector of OC ATS values.

evaluate_control_chart_two_groups() This function evaluates the performance of a control chart for disease screening when its charting statistic values for the diseased and non-diseased people in a given dataset are provided in two separate matrices. This function can be used in the *R* environment as follows.

```
> evaluate_control_chart_two_groups(chart_matrix_IC,
  time_matrix_IC,nobs_IC,starttime_IC,endtime_IC,
  chart_matrix_OC,time_matrix_OC,nobs_OC,starttime_OC,
  endtime_OC,design_interval,n_time_units,time_unit,
  no_signal_action = "omit")
```

The arguments of the above *R* command are explained below.

chart_matrix_IC A numeric matrix containing the charting statistic values of non-diseased people, where chart_matrix_IC[i,j] is the jth charting statistic value for the ith non-diseased person.

time_matrix_IC A numeric matrix containing the observation times of non-diseased people, arranged in the same way as that of chart_matrix_IC.

nobs_IC An integer vector giving the numbers of observations for all non-diseased people. Thus, nobs_IC[i] is the number of observations of the ith non-diseased person.

starttime_IC A numeric vector that specifies the starting times of process monitoring for all non-diseased people.

endtime_IC A numeric vector that specifies the ending times of process monitoring for all non-diseased people.

chart_matrix_OC A numeric matrix containing the charting statistic values of diseased people, where chart_matrix_OC[i,j] is the jth charting statistic value for the ith diseased person.

time_matrix_OC A numeric matrix containing the observation times of diseased people, arranged in the same way as that of chart_matrix_OC.

nobs_OC An integer vector giving the numbers of observations of all diseased people. Thus, nobs_OC[i] is the number of observations of the ith diseased person.

starttime_OC A numeric vector that specifies the starting times of process monitoring for all diseased people.

endtime_OC A numeric vector that specifies the ending times of process monitoring for all diseased people.

design_interval A numeric vector of length two that gives the left and right endpoints of the design time interval. By default, design_interval=range(time_matrix,na.rm=TRUE).

n_time_units An integer value that gives the total number of basic time units in the design time interval. The design time interval is descretized to be seq(design_interval[1],design_interval[2], length.out=n_time_units).

time_unit An optional argument specifying the basic time unit used when n_time_units is missing. The design time interval is descretized to be seq(design_interval[1],design_interval[2], by=time_unit).

no_signal_action A characteristic variable specifying the way to handle cases with no signals. If no_signal_action="omit", then cases with no signals will be omitted when computing the performance metrics. If no_signal_action="maxtime", then the right endpoint of the design interval is used as the signal times for cases with no signals. If no_signal_action="endtime", then the last observation times of the people who do not receive signals would be used as the signal times.

This function returns a list with the following values.

thres A numeric vector of control limits for the chart.

FPR A numeric vector of false positive rates.

TPR	A numeric vector of true positive rates.
ATS0	A numeric vector of IC ATS values.
ATS1	A numeric vector of OC ATS values.

monitor_long_1d() This function calculates the charting statistic values for disease screening when monitoring a single disease risk factor of some new patients. It can be used in the *R* environment as follows.

```
> monitor_long_1d(data_matrix_new,time_matrix_new,nobs_new,
  pattern,side="upward",chart="CUSUM",method="standard",
  parameter = 0.5,CL = Inf)
```

The arguments of the above *R* command are explained below.

data_matrix_new	A matrix of the observed disease risk factor of some new patients to monitor. data_matrix_new[i,j] is the jth observation of the ith new patient.
time_matrix_new	A matrix of the observation times arranged in the same way as data_matrix_new.
nobs_new	A numerical vector giving the number of observations for each new patient.
pattern	The estimated regular longitudinal pattern obtained by the *R* function estimate_pattern_long_1d().
side	A characteristic variable specifying the direction for process monitoring. It has three choices: "upward", "downward" and "both", representing detection of upward, downward and arbitrary shifts in the disease risk factor, respectively.
chart	A characteristic variable specifying the type of control chart to use, where chart="CUSUM" is to use a CUSUM chart and chart="EWMA" is to use an EWMA chart.
method	A characteristic variable specifying the method for process monitoring. i) If method="standard", then the method discussed

in Qiu and Xiang (2014) is used.
ii) If method="decorrelation", then the method discussed in Li and Qiu (2016) is used.
iii) If method="spring", then the method in You and Qiu (2019) is used.
iv) If method="distribution and standard", then the method in You and Qiu (2021a) is used.
v) If method="distribution and decorrelation", then the method in You and Qiu (2021a) is used after the transformed data are decorrelated.
vi) If method="distribution and sprint", then the method in You and Qiu (2021a) is used after the transformed data are decorrelated within the sprint length of the current observation time.

parameter — A numerical value to specify the allowance constant k when chart="CUSUM", and the weighting parameter λ when chart="EWMA".

CL — A numeric value speficying the control limit of the control chart.

This function returns a list with the following values.

chart_matrix — A numeric matrix of charting statistic values, where chart_matrix[i,j] is the jth charting statistic value of the ith patient.

standardized_values — A numeric matrix of the standardized observations, where standardized_values[i,j] is the jth standardized observation of the ith patient.

monitor_long_md() This function calculates the charting statistic values for disease screening when monitoring multiple disease risk factors of some new patients. It can be used in the R environment as follows.

```
> monitor_long_md(data_array_new,time_matrix_new,nobs_new,
  pattern,side="both",method="multivariate EWMA",
  parameter = 0.5,CL = Inf)
```

The arguments of the above R command are explained below.

data_array_new — An array of the observed disease risk factors of some new patients to monitor. data_matrix_new[i,j,k] is the jth observation of the kth disease risk factor of the

	ith new patient.
time_matrix_new	A matrix of the observation times arranged in the way according to data_array_new.
nobs_new	A numerical vector giving the number of observations for each new patient.
pattern	The estimated regular longitudinal pattern obtained by the *R* function estimate_pattern_long_md().
side	A characteristic variable specifying the direction for process monitoring. It has three choices: "upward", "downward" and "both", representing detection of upward, downward and arbitrary shifts in the disease risk factors, respectively.
method	A characteristic variable specifying the method for process monitoring, as described below. Six methods can be chosen: "simultaneous CUSUM", "simultaneous EWMA", "multivariate CUSUM", "multivariate EWMA", "decorrelation CUSUM" and "decorrelation EWMA". Their description can be found in You et al. (2020). Description of "multivariate EWMA", "decorrelation CUSUM" and "decorrelation EWMA" can also be found in Qiu and Xiang (2015) and Li and Qiu (2017).
parameter	A numerical value to specify the allowance constant k when method is a CUSUM chart, and the weighting parameter λ when method is an EWMA chart.
CL	A numeric value speficying the control limit of the control chart.

This function returns a list with the following values.

chart_matrix	A numeric matrix of charting statistic values, where chart_matrix[i,j] is the jth charting statistic value of the ith patient.
SSijk	A numeric array of the charting statistic values for monitoring individual disease risk factors separately.
standardized_values	A numeric array of the standardized observations.

	standardized_values[i,j,k] is the jth standardized observation of the kth risk factor of the ith patient.

monitor_long_surv() This function calculates the charting statistic values for disease screening when monitoring quantified disease risks of some new patients based on the survival modeling approach discussed in You and Qiu (2020a). It can be used in the *R* environment as follows.

```
> monitor_long_surv(data_array_new,time_matrix_new,
  nobs_new,pattern,method,parameter = 0.5,CL = Inf)
```

The arguments of the above *R* command are explained below.

data_array_new	An array of the observed disease risk factors of some new patients to monitor. data_matrix_new[i,j,k] is the jth observation of the kth disease risk factor of the ith new patient.
time_matrix_new	A matrix of the observation times arranged in the way according to data_array_new.
nobs_new	A numerical vector giving the number of observations for each new patient.
pattern	The estimated regular longitudinal pattern obtained by the *R* function estimate_pattern_long_surv().
method	A characteristic variable specifying the method for process monitoring. Currently, only the method "risk" discussed in You and Qiu (2020a) is available.
parameter	A numerical value to specify the weighting parameter λ of the related EWMA chart.
CL	A numeric value speficying the control limit of the control chart.

This function returns a list with the following values.

chart_matrix	A numeric matrix of charting statistic values, where chart_matrix[i,j] is the jth charting statistic value of the ith patient.
standardized_values	A numeric array of the standardized observations. standardized_values[i,j,k] is the jth standardized observation of the kth risk factor of the ith patient.

plot_evaluation() This function makes the ROC curves to evaluate the performance of disease screening methods, as discussed in Qiu et al. (2020b). It can be used in the *R* environment as follows.

```
> plot_evaluation(evaluate_control_chart)
```

In the above command, the argument evaluate_control_chart is the output of the *R* function **evaluate_control_chart_one_group()** or **evaluate_control_chart_two_group()**.

plot_PMROC() This function makes the PMROC curves to evaluate the performance of disease screening methods, as discussed in Qiu et al. (2020b). It can be used in the *R* environment as follows.

```
> plot_PMROC(evaluate_control_chart)
```

In the above command, the argument evaluate_control_chart is the output of the *R* function **evaluate_control_chart_one_group()** or **evaluate_control_chart_two_group()**.

search_CL() This function searches for the control limit (CL) of a control chart from the charting statistic values calculated in advance, so that a pre-specified IC average time to signal value (i.e., ATS_0) is reached. It can be used in the *R* environment as follows.

```
> search_CL(chart_matrix,time_matrix,nobs,starttime,
  endtime,design_interval,n_time_units,time_unit,
  ATS_nominal,CL_lower,CL_step,CL_upper,no_signal_action
  ="omit",ATS_tol,CL_tol)
```

The arguments of the above *R* command are explained below.

chart_matrix	A numeric matrix containing the charting statistic values, where chart_matrix[i,j] is the jth charting statistic value for the ith person.
time_matrix	A numeric matrix containing the observation times, arranged in the same way as that of chart_matrix.
nobs	An integer vector giving the numbers of observations for all people. Thus, nobs[i] is the number of observations of the ith person.

starttime	A numeric vector that specifies the starting times of process monitoring for all different people.
endtime	A numeric vector that specifies the ending times of process monitoring for all different people.
design_interval	A numeric vector of length two that gives the left and right endpoints of the design time interval. By default, design_interval=range(time_matrix,na.rm=TRUE).
n_time_units	An integer value giving the total number of basic time units in design_interval. The design interval is descretized to be seq(design_interval[1],design_interval[2], length.out=n_time_units).
time_unit	An optional argument specifying the basic time unit used when n_time_units is missing. The design interval is descretized to be seq(design_interval[1],design_interval[2], by=time_unit).
ATS_nominal	A numeric value specifying the pre-specified ATS_0 value.
CL_lower	Left endpoint of a pre-specified interval to search for CL.
CL_step	Step size to search for CL in the pre-specified interval [CL_lower, CL_upper].
CL_upper	Right endpoint of a pre-specified interval to search for CL.
no_signal_action	A characteristic variable specifying the way to handle cases with no signals. If no_signal_action="omit", then cases with no signals will be omitted when computing the performance metrics. If no_signal_action="maxtime", then the right endpoint of the design interval is used as the signal times for cases with no signals. If no_signal_action="endtime", then the last observation times of the people who do not receive signals would be used as the signal times.
ATS_tol	A tolerance value for ATS_0 used in searching for CL.
CL_tol	A tolerance value for CL used in searching for CL.

This function returns the control limit of the related control chart obtained by the built-in searching algorithm.

6.3 Some Demonstrations

Let us use the stroke dataset from the Framingham Heart Study that was described in Examples 4.1 and 5.1 to demonstrate how to use different built-in functions in the R package **DySS**. In the dataset, there are longitudinal observations of three disease risk factors "systolic blood pressures", "diastolic blood pressures", and "cholesterol levels" for a total of 1055 people. Among these people, 1028 of them never experienced any strokes and 27 of them experienced strokes for at least once during the study period. The dataset can be retrieved using the following *R* command after the package **DySS** is installed:

```
> data(data_stroke)
```

After running the above command, a data frame named "data_stroke" with the following 8 variables would be retrieved for our use: systolic_ctrl, diastolic_ctrl, cholesterol_ctrl, age_ctrl, systolic_case, diastolic_case, cholesterol_case, and age_case. See Section 6.2 for a description of these variables. For instance, the following command will give the observed cholesterol levels (mg/100ml) of the first 5 non-stroke people in the dataset:

```
> data_stroke$cholesterol_ctrl[1:5,]
     [,1] [,2] [,3] [,4] [,5] [,6] [,7]
[1,]  185  199  195  203  206  175  180
[2,]  257  229  232  203  200  174  219
[3,]  183  156  234  196  243  268  280
[4,]  167  207  182  204  192  185  212
[5,]  252  242  288  241  238  268  254
```

The whole dataset, including observations of the three disease risk factors of all 1055 people, is shown in Figure 5.1 in Section 5.3.

6.3.1 Estimation of the Regular Longitudinal Pattern of the Disease Risk Factors

To detect stroke early by monitoring its disease risk factors, we first need to estimate the regular longitudinal pattern of the three disease risk factors "systolic blood pressures", "diastolic blood pressures", and "cholesterol levels" from the IC data (i.e., the data of all 1028 non-stroke people in this case) by using the R function **estimate_pattern_long_md()**. See Section 6.2 for a description about this function. To use this function, we first need to prepare the stroke data in a proper way. For instance, the IC data of the three disease risk factors should be combined into an array and so forth. Then, the function **estimate_pattern_long_md()** can be implemented accordingly. The following R commands provide an example for this analysis.

```
> data(data_stroke)
> nrow=length(data_stroke$systolic_ctrl[,1])
> ncol=length(data_stroke$systolic_ctrl[1,])
> Estimated_Regular_Pattern = estimate_pattern_long_md(
  data_array=array(c(data_stroke$systolic_ctrl,
                     data_stroke$diastolic_ctrl,
                     data_stroke$cholesterol_ctrl),
                   dim=c(nrow,ncol,3)),
  time_matrix=data_stroke$age_ctrl,
  nobs=rep(ncol,nrow),
  time_unit=1,
  estimation_method="meanvar",
  bw_mean=10,
  bw_var=10)
```

The results about the estimated regular longitudinal pattern of the disease risk factors are saved in the list Estimated_Regular_Pattern. More specifically, the estimated mean and variance functions are saved in the variables Estimated_Regular_Pattern$mean_est and Estimated_Regular_Pattern$var_est, respectively. These results are shown in Figure 6.1, where the solid dark line in each plot denotes the estimated mean function, the dashed dark lines denote the pointwise 95% confidence intervals of the true mean function, and the small dots denote the related observed disease risk factors of all non-stroke patients. The estimated regular longitudinal pattern can be described by the estimated mean and variance functions in this example. From the figure, it can be seen that the estimated mean functions and the pointwise 95% confidence intervals can describe the longitudinal trend of the observed data well.

Implementation of the functions **estimate_pattern_long_1d()** and **estimate_pattern_long_surv()** is similar. Thus, they are not demonstrated here.

6.3.2 Disease Screening by Sequentially Monitoring the Observed Disease Risk Factors

In this part, we demonstrate the disease screening method discussed in Qiu and Xiang (2015) by sequentially monitoring the observed disease risk factors directly. This method can be accomplished by using the function **monitor_long_md()** in the R package **DySS**. To use this function, we first need to determine the control limit of the related control chart so that a pre-specified ATS_0 value can be achieved. To this end, let us first compute the charting statistic values when monitoring the 1028 no-stroke people in the stroke data

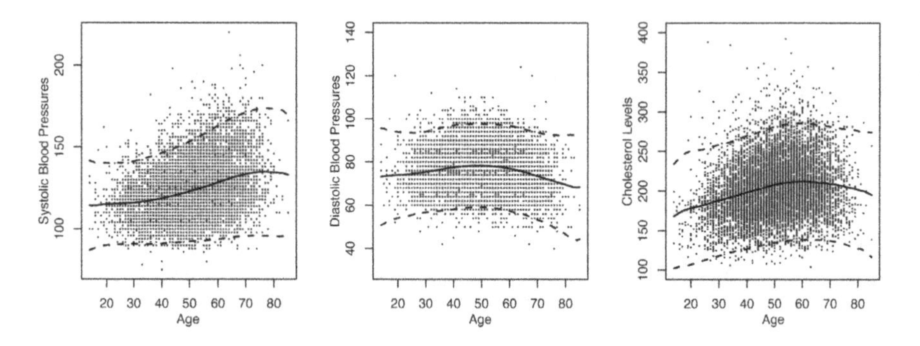

FIGURE 6.1
Three disease risk factors in the stroke data: systolic blood pressure (mmHg), diastolic blood pressure (mmHg), and total cholesterol level (mg/100ml). The solid dark line in each plot denotes the estimated mean function, the dashed dark lines denote the pointwise 95% confidence intervals of the true mean function, and the small dots denote the observed disease risk factor of all non-stroke patients.

and the weighting parameter in the chart is chosen to be $\lambda = 0.2$, by running the following R commands:

```
> data(data_stroke)
> nrow=length(data_stroke$systolic_ctrl[,1])
> ncol=length(data_stroke$systolic_ctrl[1,])
> Monitoring_Results_IC = monitor_long_md(
  data_array_new=array(c(data_stroke$systolic_ctrl,
                         data_stroke$diastolic_ctrl,
                         data_stroke$cholesterol_ctrl),
                       dim=c(nrow,ncol,3)),
  time_matrix_new=data_stroke$age_ctrl,
  nobs_new=rep(ncol,nrow),
  pattern=Estimated_Regular_Pattern,
  side="upward",
  method="multivariate EWMA",
  parameter=0.2)
```

In the above commands, the argument pattern=Estimated_Regular_Pattern has been used when running the R function **monitor_long_md()**, where Estimated_Regular_Pattern should have been computed in advance by running the R function **estimate_pattern_long_md()**. See Subsection 6.3.1 for details.

From the description of the R function **monitor_long_md()** in Section 6.2, it can be seen that the charting statistic values of the chart discussed in Qiu and Xiang (2015) for monitoring the disease risk factors of the 1028 no-stroke people in the stroke data are saved in the matrix Monitoring_Results_IC$chart_matrix. Next, we can use the built-in R function **search_CL()** to determine the control limit of the chart from the computed IC charting statistic values saved in Monitoring_Results_IC$chart_matrix such that a pre-specified ATS_0 value (e.g., 15 years) is reached. To this end, the following R commands can be implemented:

```
> CL=search_CL(
  chart_matrix=Monitoring_Results_IC$chart_matrix,
  time_matrix=data_stroke$age_ctrl,
  nobs=rep(ncol,nrow),
  starttime=data_stroke$age_ctrl[,1],
  endtime=data_stroke$age_ctrl[,ncol],
  time_unit=1,
  ATS_nominal=15)
> CL
[1] 1.774969
```

Again, the results in Monitoring_Results_IC and some other quantities used in the above R commands are assumed to be computed in advance by the R commands discussed earlier.

So, the control limit of the chart proposed in Qiu and Xiang (2015) is determined to be 1.775 in order to reach the pre-specified ATS_0 value of 15 years. Next, we can use the control chart to detect stroke for individual people. For that purpose, suppose we want to monitor the three observed disease risk factors of the 27 stroke people for disease screening. Then, the following R commands can be first implemented to compute the charting statistic values for monitoring the 27 stroke people:

```
> nrow_case=dim(data_stroke$systolic_case)[1]
> ncol_case=dim(data_stroke$systolic_case)[2]
> Monitoring_Results_OC=monitor_long_md(
  data_array_new=array(c(data_stroke$systolic_case,
                         data_stroke$diastolic_case,
                         data_stroke$cholesterol_case),
                       dim=c(nrow_case,ncol_case,3)),
  time_matrix_new=data_stroke$age_case,
  nobs_new=rep(ncol_case,nrow_case),
  pattern=Estimated_Regular_Pattern,
  side="upward",
  method="multivariate EWMA",
  parameter=0.2)
```

Then, the signal times can be recorded for all 27 stroke people by using the built-in R function **calculate_signal_times()** as follows:

```
> Signal_Times=calculate_signal_times(
```

```
chart_matrix=Monitoring_Results_OC$chart_matrix,
time_matrix=data_stroke$age_case,
nobs=rep(ncol_case,nrow_case),
starttime=data_stroke$age_case[,1],
endtime=data_stroke$age_case[,ncol_case],
time_unit=1,
CL=CL)

> Signal_Times$signal_times
 [1] 20 15 20 19  7 19 12  7 NA 28  8  8  7  8 13 NA 16 15
[19] NA NA 13 11 20 NA NA NA
> data_stroke$age_case[,1]
 [1] 43 44 22 44 43 57 44 51 35 28 37 51 55 51 42 29 36 30
[19] 50 30 53 42 42 40 50 37 45
```

From the above results, it can be seen that among the 27 stroke people, 20 of them receive signals from the control chart. The variable Signal_Times$signal_times gives the time from the beginning of process monitoring for each person to the signal time, and the variable data_stroke$age_case[,1] gives the age of each person at the beginning of process monitoring. So, for instance, the first stroke patient started to be monitored at the age of 43 and got the signal at the age of $43 + 20 = 63$ years old. The control charts for monitoring all these 27 stroke patients are shown in Figure 6.2.

6.3.3 Evaluation of the Disease Screening Methods

For a given disease screening method, we can evaluate its performance by computing its sensitivity, specificity and the related receiver operating characteristic (ROC) curve (e.g., Pepe, 2003). Sensitivity is the proportion of diseased people who receive signals from the related control chart and are diagnosed to be diseased people by the disease screening method. It is also called true positive rate (TPR). Specificity is the proportion of non-diseased people who do not receive signals from the related control chart and are diagnosed to be non-diseased people by the disease screening method. (1-specificity) is also called false positive rate (FPR). Then, for a given disease screening method, its TPR and FPR values can be determined from a training dataset if the control limit of the related control chart is specified. Similarly, the values of (ATS_0, ATS_1) of the control chart with a given control limit can also be computed. When the control limit changes, the curve formed by the pair (FPR,TPR) is the ROC curve. For the stroke data and the disease screening method considered in the previous two subsections, the values of (FPR,TPR) and (ATS_0, ATS_1) corresponding to various control limit values can be computed by the following R commands:

```
> Evaluation=evaluate_control_chart_two_groups(
  chart_matrix_IC=Monitoring_Results_IC$chart_matrix,
```

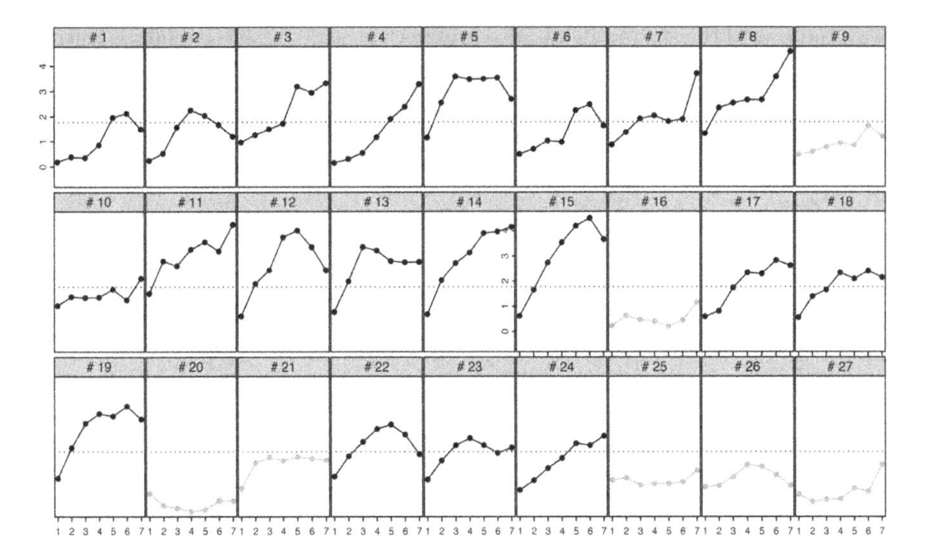

FIGURE 6.2
Multivariate EWMA charts proposed in Qiu and Xiang (2015) for monitoring the 27 stroke patients when $ATS_0 = 15$ and $\lambda = 0.2$. The dotted horizontal line in each plot denotes the control limit of the chart.

```
  time_matrix_IC=data_stroke$age_ctrl,
  nobs_IC=rep(ncol,nrow),
  starttime_IC=data_stroke$age_ctrl[,1],
  endtime_IC=data_stroke$age_ctrl[,ncol],
  chart_matrix_OC=Monitoring_Results_OC$chart_matrix,
  time_matrix_OC=data_stroke$age_case,
  nobs_OC=rep(ncol_case,nrow_case),
  starttime_OC=data_stroke$age_case[,1],
  endtime_OC=data_stroke$age_case[,ncol_case],
  time_unit=1,
  no_signal_action="maxtime")
```

Then, the ROC curve and the curve formed by the pair (ATS_0, ATS_1) can be generated by the following R command:

```
> plot_evaluation(Evaluation)
```

These two curves are shown in Figure 6.3. From the left panel, it can be seen that TPR is always larger than FPR in this example, implying that disease diagnosis by the disease screening method is better than a random guess. From the right panel, it can be seen that i) ATS_1 increases when ATS_0 increases, and ii) ATS_0 is always larger than ATS_1. The first result is intuitively reasonable and the second result also implies that the disease screening method is effective.

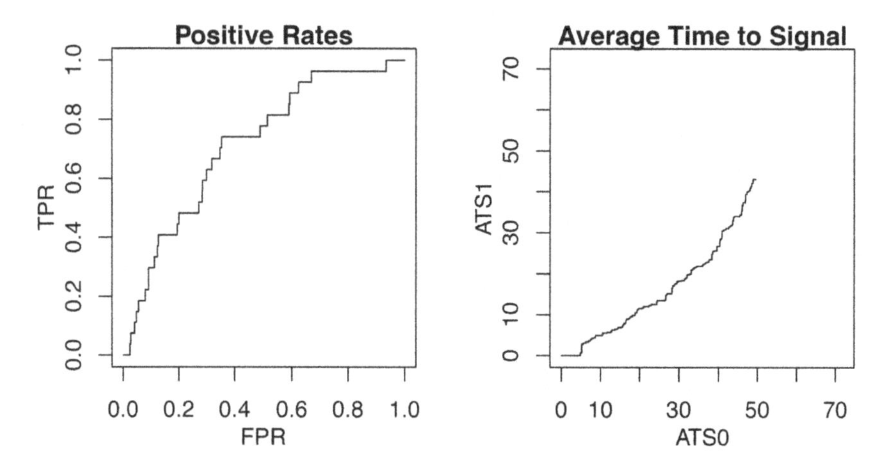

FIGURE 6.3
(a) ROC curve of the disease screening method considered in Subsections 6.3.1 and 6.3.2 for analyzing the stroke data. (b) The curve formed by (ATS_0, ATS_1) when the control limit of the related control chart changes.

The sensitivity, specificity and the related ROC curve do not take into account the signal times of the disease screening method. To overcome this limitation, Qiu et al. (2020b) suggested the dynamic true positive rate (DTPR), dynamic false positive rate (DFPR) and the related process monitoring ROC (PM-ROC) curve. See Section 4.6 for some related discussions. These quantities are proper combinations of (FPR,TPR) and (ATS_0, ATS_1) values. The PM-ROC curve can be generated by the following R command:

```
> plot_PMROC(Evaluation)
```

It is shown in Figure 6.4. From the plot, it can be seen that that DTPR is always larger than DFPR, which implies that the disease screening method is effective in terms of these alternative performance metrics.

6.4 Exercises

6.1 As described in Section 6.2, the simulated dataset data_example_long_md in the R package **DySS** contains observed data of 3 disease risk factors of 200 non-diseased people and 200 diseased people. For

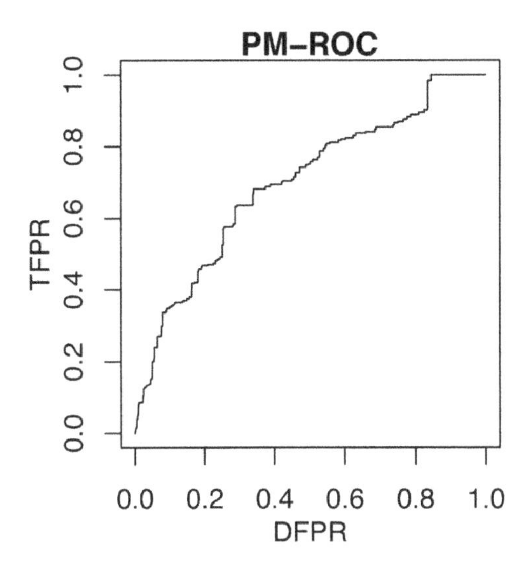

FIGURE 6.4
PM-ROC curve of the disease screening method considered in Subsections 6.1 and 6.2 for analyzing the stroke data.

each person, there are 100 three-dimensional longitudinal observation vectors generated at 100 observation times.

(i) Use the following R commands to obtain an overall description about the 9 variables saved in the dataset:

```
> data(data_example_long_md)
> summary(data_example_long_md)
```

(ii) The variable data_example_long_md$data_array_IC is an array of dimensions $200 \times 100 \times 3$ and contains the simulated IC data of 200 non-diseased people. Show the first 10 observed vectors of the first non-diseased person in R.

6.2 For the simulated dataset data_example_long_md, estimate the regular longitudinal pattern of the disease risk factors using the R function **estimate_pattern_long_md()** in the following three setups, respectively:

(i) estimation_method="meanvar", bw_mean=0.1 and bw_var=0.1;

(ii) estimation_method="meanvar", bw_mean=0.3 and bw_var=0.3;

(iii) estimation_method="meanvar", bw_mean=0.5 and bw_var=0.5.

For each choice of the bandwidths bw_mean and bw_var, make a figure similar to Figure 6.1 and discuss the impact of the bandwidths on the estimated mean functions.

6.3 For the simulated dataset data_example_long_md and the estimated regular longitudinal pattern of the disease risk factors discussed in Exercise 6.2 when bw_mean=0.3 and bw_var=0.3, monitor the observed disease risk factors of the 200 diseased people for disease screening by using the built-in function **monitor_long_md()** with method="multivariate EWMA", side="upward", and the following three setups, respectively:

(i) $ATS_0 = 50$ and parameter=0.5;

(ii) $ATS_0 = 100$ and parameter=0.5;

(iii) $ATS_0 = 100$ and parameter=0.1.

In the above process monitoring, you also need to use the built-in function **search_CL()** to determine the control limit of the related control chart, as discussed in Subsection 6.3.2, and then use the built-in function **calculate_signal_times()** to find the signal times of the 200 diseased people. Compare the results in the three setups described above.

6.4 For the disease screening method discussed in Exercise 6.3 when $ATS_0 = 50$ and parameter=0.5, make its ROC curve and PM-ROC curve, as discussed in Subsection 6.3.3.

7

Disease Surveillance by Some Retrospective Methods

7.1 Introduction

The disease screening methods discussed in the previous three chapters are developed mainly for detecting a disease in concern as early as possible for individual people in order to improve their health conditions. As discussed in Section 1.2, in order to make effective public health policies to handle certain urgent public health challenges (e.g., outbreak of an infectious disease) in a timely manner, it is also important to track the incidence of a disease in a population and check whether the disease incidence changes more dramatically than what is expected over time and/or spatial locations. This is the *disease surveillance* problem that is especially relevant in today's environment for detecting outbreaks of some deadly infectious diseases, such as COVID-19, Ebola, SARS and more. Thus, disease screening focuses mainly on individual people while disease surveillance is for tracking the spatio-temporal pattern of disease incidence in a population. In this and the next two chapters, we will introduce some basic statistical methods developed for handling the disease surveillance problem.

Because of the importance of the disease surveillance problem, there have been many discussions about it in the literature. Early methods for disease surveillance include the Knox, local Knox, Mantel, and k-nearest neighbor methods (Jacquez, 1996; Knox and Bartlett, 1964; Kulldorff and Hjalmars, 1999; Mantel, 1967; Rogerson, 2001). These methods try to detect disease clusters by identifying irregular space-time patterns in the observed disease incidence data. Some other popular methods for solving the disease surveillance problem are based on the spatial and/or spatio-temporal scan statistics (Kulldorff, 1997, 2001; Takahashi et al., 2008; Weinstock, 1981). These methods try to identify spatial and/or spatio-temporal disease clusters by testing whether the number of observed disease cases in different windows of circular or other more flexible shapes is significantly higher than the expected number of disease cases under the null hypothesis that there are no disease outbreaks in the observed data. Other existing disease surveillance methods include the ones based on generalized linear modeling (Jung, 2009; Kleinman et al., 2004; Zhang and Lin, 2009), Bayesian spatial modeling (Besag et al.,

DOI: 10.1201/9781003138150-7

1991; Best et al., 2005; Lawson et al., 2000; Zhou and Lawson, 2008), parametric and semi-parametric regression modeling (Pelat et al., 2007; Stern and Lightfoot, 1999; Stroup et al., 1999), time series modeling (Heisterkamp et al., 2006; Ngo et al., 1996; Reis and Mandl, 2003), point process modeling (Diggle et al., 2005), and some other data modeling approaches.

Most existing methods mentioned above are *retrospective* in the sense that the time interval of the observed disease incidence data should be given in advance in order to use these methods. However, the disease surveillance problem is *prospective* in nature, in the sense that the observation time of the disease incidence data keeps increasing, new observed data keep being collected, and we are expected to make a decision regarding whether there is a disease outbreak after the observed data is collected at the current observation time. Thus, the disease surveillance problem is essentially a sequential decision-making problem that is similar to the ones discussed in the previous three chapters about disease screening, although the related process here is usually spatial because disease incidence at multiple spatial locations is usually concerned in disease surveillance while many sequential processes are involved in disease screening about disease risk factors of different individuals and such processes are usually non-spatial. Because of this reason and the fact that most existing retrospective methods require various model assumptions that are rarely valid in practice, the existing methods discussed in the previous paragraph cannot generally handle the disease surveillance problem effectively (Marshall et al., 2007; Woodall et al., 2008; Yang and Qiu, 2020).

In this chapter, we introduce several basic retrospective methods discussed in the literature for disease surveillance. More specifically, the Knox test for detecting disease clusters is described in Section 7.2. The basic idea to use a scan statistic for disease surveillance is introduced in Section 7.3. The connection between the scan test and the generalized linear modeling (GLM) procedure is discussed in Section 7.4, along with some generalizations of the scan test by using the GLM framework. Some concluding remarks are given in Section 7.5. In the next chapter, some prospective disease surveillance methods developed recently based on sequential monitoring of spatial processes will be discussed. Their accompanying *R* package will be introduced in Chapter 9.

7.2 Detection of Space-Time Interaction by the Knox Test

The first *Knox test* was suggested by Knox and Bartlett (1964) for detecting space-time interaction in the observed spatio-temporal disease incidence data. More specifically, assume that there are n cases of a given disease observed in the region Ω within the time interval $[0, T]$. If there is no space-time interaction in the observed data, then the spatial distributions of the data in different small time intervals within $[0, T]$ should be all similar, and the temporal distributions of the data in different small regions within Ω should be similar as well. On the other hand, if the spatial distributions of the observed data in different small time intervals are quite different and/or the temporal distributions of the data in different small regions are quite different, then there could be a space-time interaction in the observed data and this information is often important to study the infectious etiology and/or transmissions of the disease. The Knox test is designed specifically for detecting space-time clusters (i.e., clusters of disease cases in the three-dimensional space-time domain) in the observed disease incidence data, which are a type of special space-time interactions.

The Knox test considers all $N = n(n-1)/2$ pairs of the n disease cases in the region Ω and the time interval $[0, T]$. Among these pairs, let N_{d_x} be the number of pairs that the Euclidean distance between two case locations in a pair is less than or equal to d_x, N_{d_t} be the number of pairs that the disease occurrence times of two cases in a pair is within d_t and N_{d_x,d_t} be the number of pairs that the Euclidean distance between two case locations in a pair is less than or equal to d_x and the occurrence times of the two related disease cases is within d_t as well. Then, the test statistic of the Knox test is N_{d_x,d_t}. It is obvious that N_{d_x,d_t} has the following expression:

$$N_{d_x,d_t} = \sum_{1 \le i < j \le n} I\left(d_E(\boldsymbol{s}_i, \boldsymbol{s}_j) \le d_x\right) I(|t_i - t_j| \le d_t), \tag{7.1}$$

where $\boldsymbol{s}_i$ and $\boldsymbol{s}_j$ denote the locations of the ith and jth disease cases, respectively, t_i and t_j are their disease occurrence times, $d_E(\cdot, \cdot)$ is the Euclidean distance and $I(a)$ is the indicator function that equals 1 when "a=True" and 0 otherwise.

Example 7.1 *As a tool example, consider a scenario with $n = 5$ disease cases occurred at the spatial locations $\boldsymbol{s}_i = (x_i, y_i) \in [0,1] \times [0,1]$ and the times $t_i \in [0, 1]$, for $i = 1, 2, 3, 4, 5$. The specific values of $\{((t_i; x_i, y_i), i = 1, 2, 3, 4, 5\}$ are given below:*

(0.206; 0.266, 0.898), (0.177; 0.372, 0.945), (0.687; 0.573, 0.661), (0.384; 0.908, 0.629), (0.770; 0.202, 0.062).

As a matter of fact, the values of x, y and t listed above are all generated randomly from the $U[0, 1]$ distribution. Thus, there should not be any space-time clusters in this dataset. The five disease cases are also shown in Figure 7.1.

In the scenario considered above, there are a total of $N = n(n-1)/2 = 10$ pairs of disease cases. For the (i, j)th pair, denoted as (C_i, C_j), the spatial distance of the two paired disease cases is defined to be $d_E(\boldsymbol{s}_i, \boldsymbol{s}_j)$, and the temporal distance is defined to be $|t_i - t_j|$, for $1 \le i < j \le 5$. The spatial and temporal distances for all 10 pairs are listed in Table 7.1. So, if $d_x = 0.5$ and $d_t = 0.2$, then $N_{d_x} = 4$, $N_{d_t} = 3$ and $N_{d_x,d_t} = 1$.

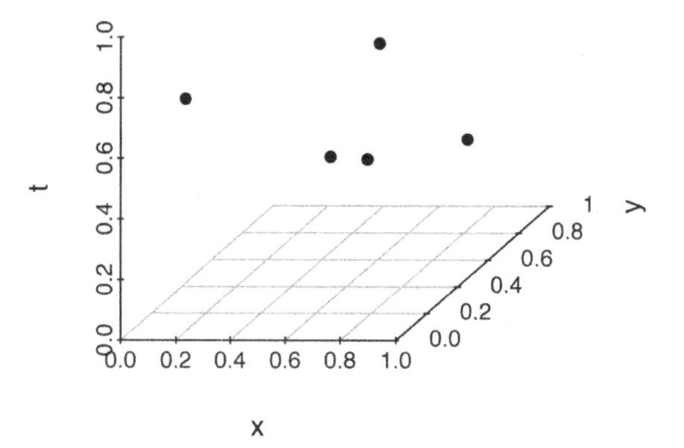

FIGURE 7.1
Five disease cases considered in Example 7.1.

TABLE 7.1
Spatial and temporal distances of the 10 pairs of disease cases in the example considered in Example 7.1.

Pair	Spatial Distance	Temporal Distance
(C_1, C_2)	0.116	0.029
(C_1, C_3)	0.388	0.481
(C_1, C_4)	0.697	0.178
(C_1, C_5)	0.839	0.564
(C_2, C_3)	0.348	0.510
(C_2, C_4)	0.622	0.208
(C_2, C_5)	0.899	0.593
(C_3, C_4)	0.337	0.303
(C_3, C_5)	0.705	0.083
(C_4, C_5)	0.906	0.386

From Equation (7.1), under the null hypothesis "H_0: there is no space-time interaction in the observed data" and other regularity conditions, a reasonable estimate of $\mathrm{E}(N_{d_x,d_t})$ is

$$\widehat{\mu}_{N_{d_x,d_t}} = N \times \frac{N_{d_x}}{N} \times \frac{N_{d_t}}{N} = \frac{N_{d_x} N_{d_t}}{N}.$$

Knox and Bartlett (1964) conjectured that the null distribution (i.e., the distribution under H_0) of the test statistic N_{d_x,d_t} would be Poisson, which was confirmed later by Barton and David (2006) in cases when both N_{d_x} and N_{d_t} are small relative to N. Barton and David (2006) also provided a formula for computing the variance of N_{d_x,d_t}, which is quite complicated and thus omitted here.

To perform the Knox test, people often approximate the null distribution of N_{d_x,d_t} by a Poisson or normal distribution. But, it has been found in the literature that such approximations are often biased due to data complexity (Kulldorff and Hjalmars, 1999). So, nonparametric tests, such as the *permutation tests* (Good, 2005; Jacquez, 1994), are often used in practice to perform the Knox test. For instance, to perform a permutation test based on disease occurrence times, we can proceed as follows. Let us consider a scenario with n disease cases observed in the time-space domain $[0,T] \times \Omega$ whose disease occurrence times and locations are denoted as $\{(t_i, \boldsymbol{s}_i), i = 1, 2, \ldots, n\}$. Then, the observed value of N_{d_x,d_t}, denoted as $N^*_{d_x,d_t}$, can be computed by Equation (7.1) from these original observed data. To perform the Knox test, we need to compute the p-value of the test, which can be estimated by the permutation procedure described below. Assume that $\{\widetilde{t}_i, i = 1, 2, \ldots, n\}$ is a permutation of all disease occurrence times $\{t_i, i = 1, 2, \ldots, n\}$. Let us consider the following time-permuted data $\{(\widetilde{t}_i, \boldsymbol{s}_i), i = 1, 2, \ldots, n\}$, from which the value of N_{d_x,d_t} can also be computed. Intuitively, if H_0 is true and there is no space-time interaction, then the value of N_{d_x,d_t} computed from the time-permuted data and its value computed from the original observed data (i.e., $N^*_{d_x,d_t}$) should have the same distribution. To estimate this distribution, we can consider all $n!$ possible permutations of $\{t_i, i = 1, 2, \ldots, n\}$. Then, $n!$ values of N_{d_x,d_t} can be computed from the corresponding $n!$ time-permuted datasets. The p-value of the Knox test can then be estimated by the proportion of these $n!$ values of N_{d_x,d_t} that are larger than $N^*_{d_x,d_t}$. If the p-value is smaller than or equal to a pre-specified significance level α whose default value is 0.05 (cf., Subsection 2.4.3), then we reject H_0 and conclude that the observed data have provided a significant evidence for space-time interaction. Otherwise, we fail to reject H_0.

In cases when the value of n is large, the total number of permutations, $n!$, would be too large for the permutation test described above to be used in practice, because of the heavy computing burden involved. For instance, if $n = 10$, then $n! = 3,628,800$. If $n = 20$, then $n!$ is already the huge number 2.432902×10^{18}. In practice, n could be 100 or larger. In such cases, $n!$ would be too large to handle. To overcome this difficulty, Dwass (1957) suggested a modified permutation test, by which only a pre-specified number of randomly selected permutations was considered. See Turnbull et al. (1990) for a related application of this method for detecting disease clusters.

As a side note, the permutation test described above is based on permuting the disease occurrence times. Of course, we can also perform the test by permuting the disease occurrence locations. As a matter of fact, these two approaches are equivalent. In addition, besides the permutation test, the bootstrap method introduced in Subsection 2.4.4 can also be used here to compute an estimate of the p-value of the Knox test.

To implement the Knox test, the *R* package **surveillance** has been developed, and its function **knox()** can be used to perform the knox test by using either the Poisson approximation to the null distribution of N_{d_x,d_t} or the (modified) permutation test discussed above. One example to use this *R* package is given below.

Example 7.2 *In Example 7.1, if we performance the Knox test using the R function* **knox()** *and the permutation approach for computing the p-value, then the p-value is computed to be 0.785. If the p-value is computed based on the Poisson approximation discussed above, then the estimated mean of* N_{d_x,d_t} *is 1.2 and the corresponding p-value is computed to be 0.337. In either case,* H_0 *cannot be rejected, and we conclude that there is no significance evidence of space-time clusters in the observed data. This conclusion is reasonable because we know that there is no space-time interaction in this simulated example since the observed data of disease occurrence times and disease occurrence locations are generated independently.*

In the literature, some modifications and/or generalizations of the Knox test have been proposed. See, for instance, Baker (2004), Kulldorff and Hjalmars (1999) and Marshall (1991).

7.3 Scan Statistics for Disease Cluster Detection

Besides the Knox test discussed in the previous section, another popular method for detecting disease clusters is based on the *scan statistic* that was originally suggested for detecting clusters in a univariate point process (Loader, 1991; Naus, 1965). It was generalized for detecting disease clusters in a spatial or spatio-temporal point process by Kulldorff (1997), Kulldorff and Hjalmars (1999), Kulldorff (2001), Tango (2010) and many other authors. Its basic idea for detecting disease clusters in the space domain is briefly introduced below.

Let G be the whole space of interest, and Z be a possible disease cluster. See Figure 7.2 for a demonstration, where the small dots denote the locations of the observed disease cases in G. Assume that an individual located in Z has the probability of p_1 to have the disease in concern, and an individual located outside Z has the probability of p_0 to have the disease. Then, the hypotheses of interest are

$$H_0 : p_1 = p_0 \quad \text{versus} \quad H_1 : p_1 > p_0. \tag{7.2}$$

Thus, H_0 implies no disease cluster in G, and H_1 implies that Z is a disease cluster.

To test the hypotheses in (7.2), let us consider a circular region A. Define n_A to be the number of observed disease cases in A, and N_A to be the total number of people in A. Then, under H_0, the expected number of disease cases in A would be $\mu_{0,A} = p_0 N_A$, and under H_1, the expected number of disease cases in A would be $\mu_{1,A} = p_0 N_{A \bigcap Z^c} + p_1 N_{A \bigcap Z}$.

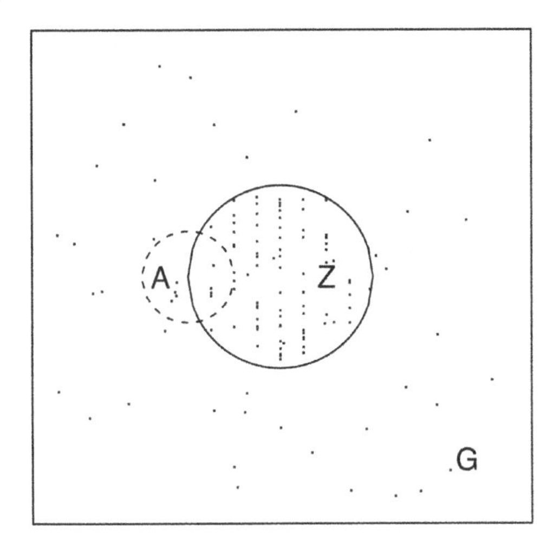

FIGURE 7.2
Demonstration of the scan statistic, where the rectangle G denotes the whole space of interest, the solid circle Z denotes a possible disease cluster, the dashed circle A denotes a circular region considered by the scan statistic, and the small dots denote the observed disease cases in G.

Next, let us further assume that the observed number of disease cases in A follows a Poisson distribution. Namely, $n_A \sim Poisson(\mu_{0,A})$ under H_0, and $n_A \sim Poisson(\mu_{1,A})$ under H_1. By using the likelihood ratio testing framework (cf., Subsection 2.4.3), Kulldorff (1997) and Kulldorff (2001) showed that the likelihood ratio test statistic for testing the hypotheses in (7.2) was

$$\Lambda = \max_{A \in \mathcal{A}} \left\{ \left[\frac{n_A}{\mu_{0,A}} \right]^{n_A} \left[\frac{n_G - n_A}{n_G - \mu_{0,A}} \right]^{n_G - n_A} \right\}, \tag{7.3}$$

where $\mathcal{A}$ was a pre-specified set of all possible regions to scan, and n_G denoted the total number of disease cases in the whole space G. In Expression (7.3), for a specific region A, if $n_A \leq \mu_{0,A}$, then the quantity in the curly braces needs to be replaced by 1. With this modification, Λ defined in (7.3) is the scan statistic, and the hypothesis test based on Λ is the scan test.

From (7.3), it can be seen that the scan statistic Λ is obtained by scanning all possible regions in $\mathcal{A}$. In the literature, there are several different strategies to specify the collection $\mathcal{A}$ of the scanned regions for the maximization procedure (7.3), which include all legitimate circular regions within G, all circular regions with a given radius centered at the grid points of a fixed grid and more. Besides circular regions, some people consider using elliptic regions (e.g., Kulldorff et al., 2006) or other more flexible regions (e.g., Lin et al., 2016; Tango and Takahashi, 2005).

The p-value of the scan test with the test statistic defined in (7.3) can be estimated by a numerical algorithm, such as the (modified) permutation test similar to the ones discussed in Section 3.2, the Gumbel-based p-value approximation (Abrams et al., 2010), and the p-value approximation using the extreme value distributions (Jung and Park, 2015). It can also be estimated by the versatile bootstrap procedure discussed in Subsection 2.4.4. After the p-value is estimated, the estimated p-value can be compared with a pre-specified significance level α. We conclude that there is a significant disease cluster if the estimated p-value is smaller than or equal to α, and the region A in $\mathcal{A}$ that reaches the maximum in (7.3) is the first detected disease cluster. After this region is excluded from $\mathcal{A}$, the above testing procedure can be repeated to detect the second disease cluster. This process can continue until no significant disease clusters are detected.

Although the scan test discussed above is constructed based on the assumption that the observed number n_A of disease cases in A follows a Poisson distribution, it can also be developed based on the assumption that n_A has the $Binomial(N_A, p_0)$ distribution under H_0, and the $Binomial(N_A, p_1)$ distribution under H_1 when $A \subset Z$. See some related discussions in Kulldorff (1997).

The scan test described above is for analyzing spatial data only. Actually, it can be discussed similarly for analyzing spatio-temporal data by considering regions in the 3-dimensional space $[0, T] \times G$, where $[0, T]$ denotes the time period in which disease cases are observed. See Hohl et al. (2020) and Rao et al. (2017) for some specific examples to detect spatio-temporal disease clusters.

The scan test can be implemented using the software *SaTScan* that can be downloaded from the webpage https://www.satscan.org. This method and some of its modified versions can also be accomplished using the *R* packages **rflexscan** and **smerc**. To demonstrate the application of the *R* package **smerc**, let us consider a case study in the example below, which was also discused in Waller and Gotway (2005).

Example 7.3 *Waller and Gotway (2005) presented a dataset that contained numbers of leukemia cases of 281 regions in New York during 1978–1982. To perform a scan test using the R package* **smerc**, *the longitude and latitude of the centroid of each region need to be specified in advance, along with the population of the region. If the scan test is based on the Poisson-distribution assumption, its p-value is determined by the modified permutation approach with 1000 randomly chosen permutations, and the Type-I error probability is set to be* $\alpha = 0.05$, *then the R function* **scan.test()** *in the package* **smerc** *detects two disease clusters that are shown in Figure 7.3. The most significant cluster is the one consisting of certain regions in the bottom part of the plot that are connected by dark lines, and the second most significant cluster is the one consisting of eight regions in the central part of the plot that are connected by light lines.*

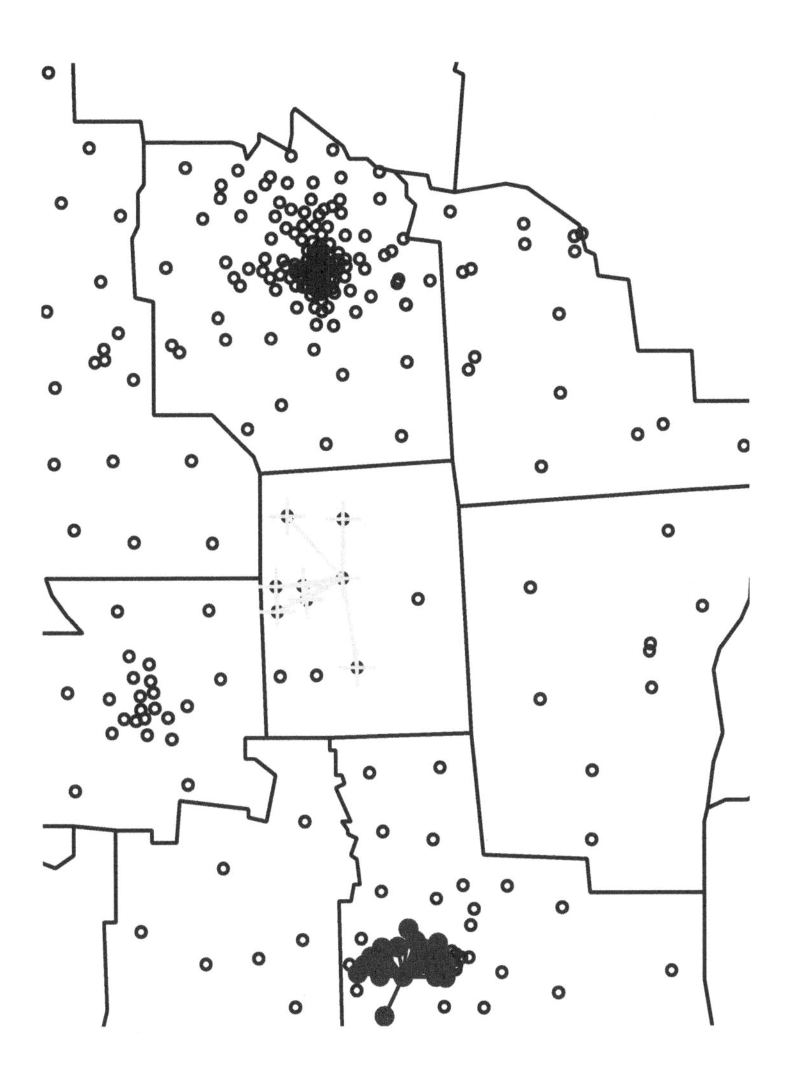

FIGURE 7.3
Leukemia data of 281 regions in New York during 1978–1982. Little circles denote centroids of the regions. Two disease clusters are detected by the scan test described in Example 7.3, where the most significant cluster is the one consisting of certain regions in the bottom part of the plot that are connected by dark lines, and the second most significant cluster is the one consisting of eight regions in the central part of the plot that are connected by light lines.

7.4 Generalized Linear Modeling for Disease Cluster Detection

For the scan test discussed in the previous section, Jung (2009) and Zhang and Lin (2009) generalized it by using a generalized linear model (GLM) described below. Assume that there are a total of I entities in the observed spatial data, where the entities could represent the spatial locations of individual people or sub-areas of the whole space of interest G. For the ith entity, the associated outcome is denoted as Y_i, for $i = 1, 2, \ldots, I$. For instance, the state of Florida has 67 counties. If the observed case numbers of COVID-19 are organized at the county level, then $I = 67$ and $\{Y_i, i = 1, 2, \ldots, I\}$ are the observed case numbers of COVID-19 of the 67 individual counties. To investigate whether a specific region A is a disease cluster, we can consider the following GLM:

$$g(\mu_i) = \alpha + \theta_A d_{i,A} + \boldsymbol{\beta}'\boldsymbol{x}_i, \qquad \text{for } i = 1, 2, \ldots, I, \tag{7.4}$$

where $\mu_i = \mathrm{E}(Y_i)$, $g(\cdot)$ is a pre-specified link function, $d_{i,A}$ is an indicator that equals 1 if the ith entity belongs to A and 0 otherwise, $\boldsymbol{x}_i$ is a vector of q covariates for the ith entity, and α, θ_A and $\boldsymbol{\beta}$ are the related coefficients. In the GLM literature (e.g., McCullagh and Nelder, 1992), the link function $g(\cdot)$ is usually chosen to be the logarithm function $g(u) = \log(u)$ if the outcomes are counts, the logit function $g(u) = \log[u/(1-u)]$ if the outcomes are binary, and the identity function $g(u) = u$ if the outcomes are continuous that can take any values in an interval.

To perform the scan test discussed in the previous section, we can first ignore the covariates in Model (7.4) and then consider the following hypotheses:

$$H_0 : \theta_A = 0, \qquad \text{versus} \qquad H_1 : \theta_A > 0.$$

Let LLR_A denote the log-likelihood ratio test statistic for the above hypotheses (cf., Subsection 2.4.3). Then, Jung (2009) verified that the scan test statistic (cf., (7.3)) was equivalent to $\max_A LLR_A$ in cases when the spatial outcomes take either binary or count values. The equivalence was also confirmed by Zhang and Lin (2009) in cases when the outcomes take count values. The p-value of the test with the test statistic $\max_A LLR_A$ can be estimated in a similar way to that of the test (7.3) discussed in Section 7.3.

From the above discussion, it can be seen that the GLM approach (7.4) is more general than the original scan test discussed in Section 7.3 in that the former can easily accommodate potential impact of certain covariates on the outcomes while the latter is difficult to achieve that. In practice, disease incidence rates are often associated with some covariates. For instance, incidence rates of an infectious disease like flu are usually associated with air temperature, humidity, and other weather or environmental conditions. The GLM approach can explore such association and the association between the detected disease clusters and the related covariates easily. But, it would be difficult for the original scan test discussed in Section 7.3 to explore such associations. In addition, there have been many existing methods and tools developed in the GLM literature for model estimation, hypothesis testing and other purposes. By using the connection discussed above between the scan test and the GLM approach, these existing GLM methods and tools can also be used for detecting disease clusters.

The GLM model (7.4) has been generalized to several different generalized mixed-effects models in the literature for detecting disease clusters (e.g., Gómez-Rubio et al., 2019; Kleinman et al., 2004). For instance, the *R* package **DClusterm** considered several generalizations of Model (7.4), including the following generalized mixed-effects model:

$$g(\mu_i|b_i) = \alpha + \theta_A d_{i,A} + \boldsymbol{\beta}'\boldsymbol{x}_i + b_i, \tag{7.5}$$

where $b_i \sim N(0, \sigma_b^2)$, for all i, is the random-effects term for describing the variation among different entities, and other quantities in (7.5) are the same as those in Model (7.4). By the way, the package **DClusterm** can also be used for analyzing spatio-temporal data.

7.5 Some Discussions

In this chapter, we have introduced some basic retrospective methods developed for disease cluster detection, including the Knox test, the scan test, and the related methods based on the GLM modeling. Our discussion on the scan test and the related GLM modeling approach has focused on analyzing spatial data for simplicity, and it is quite straightforward to generalize these methods for analyzing spatio-temporal data, as mentioned in Section 7.3.

As pointed out at the beginning of this chapter in Section 7.1, the disease surveillance problem is a sequential process monitoring problem, where the related sequential process is usually spatial in the sense that the observed disease incidence data are often collected at multiple spatial locations at each observation time point. To handle a sequential process monitoring problem properly, a sequential decision-making procedure needs to be developed as discussed in Chapters 3–5, and its performance is usually measured by ARL_0 and ARL_1 (cf., Subsection 3.1.2 for their definitions), in which the correctness and timeliness of the signal from the sequential decision-making procedure have both been taken into account. As a comparison, the methods introduced in this chapter are for detecting disease clusters in a given time interval. They are not sequential in nature. Some researchers have used these methods for disease surveillance by applying them to the observed disease incidence data in different time intervals (Kulldorff, 2001; Takahashi et al., 2008). However, such disease surveillance approaches are *ad hoc* in nature, and their performance is difficult to measure properly.

The methods for detecting disease clusters discussed in this chapter are developed based on various model assumptions. For instance, the scan test discussed in Section 7.3 assumes that the number of disease cases in a given region has a binomial or Poisson distribution, and all these methods assume that observed data at different times and locations are independent of each other. However, because of the complexity of the observed spatio-temporal disease incidence data, including the spatio-temporal data correlation that is often hard to describe by a parametric model, it has been confirmed in the literature that such assumptions are rarely valid in practice (Yang and Qiu, 2020; Zhang et al., 2015). Thus, proper model diagnoses become critically important before these methods can be used in an application. Otherwise, the results could be unreliable and/or misleading.

Both the Knox and scan methods involve intensive computation, especially in cases when they are used for analyzing spatio-temporal data. For instance, the Knox test discussed in Section 7.2 considers all $n(n-1)/2$ pairs of n disease cases observed in a given time interval and a spatial region Ω, where n is often a large number in practice. The scan test statistic Λ defined in (7.3) is computed by a maximization procedure that involves scanning of a large number of regions in $\mathcal{A}$. Such computing-intensive methods may not be appropriate for handling certain sequential process monitoring problems, including the disease surveillance problem when a large number of disease cases are involved, because the heavy computing burden would make it hard for them to decide whether there is a disease outbreak at the current observation time immediately after a new batch of data is collected.

7.6 Exercises

7.1 In Sections 2.6 and 2.7, many longitudinal data modeling and spatio-temporal data modeling methods are discussed. Are these methods all retrospective?

7.2 The Knox test discussed in Section 7.2 is designed for detecting space-time interaction in an observed disease incidence dataset. For given values of d_x and d_t, does a relatively large value of N_{d_x,d_t} always imply a large chance of a disease cluster in a space-time region? If the answer is negative, please provide an example in which the value of N_{d_x,d_t} is relatively large, but there are no obvious disease clusters.

7.3 Consider the Knox test statistic N_{d_x,d_t} defined in (7.1).

(i) Confirm that N_{d_x,d_t} denotes the number of disease pairs that the Euclidean distance between two case locations in a pair is less than or equal to d_x and the disease occurrence times of the related two cases is within d_t as well.

(ii) Why is $\widehat{\mu}_{N_{d_x,d_t}} = N_{d_x}N_{d_t}/N$ a good estimator of $\mathrm{E}(N_{d_x,d_t})$? What assumptions have been made to have this conclusion.

7.4 The permutation test discussed in Section 7.2 for computing the p-value of the Knox test is constructed by permuting the observation times of the observed disease cases. The permutation test can also be constructed by permuting the observation locations. Are the two ways to construct the permutation test equivalent? Can we permute observation times and locations together? Explain your answers to these questions.

7.5 An alternative numerical approach to compute the p-value of the Knox test is to use the bootstrap method introduced in Subsection 2.4.4. Discuss in detail how to use the bootstrap method to compute the p-value of the Knox test.

7.6 Use the *R* package **surveillance** to reproduce the results in Example 7.2.

7.7 Derive Expression (7.3) by using the definition of the likelihood ratio test discussed in Subsection 2.4.3.

7.8 Use the *R* package **smerc** to reproduce the results in Example 7.3.

7.9 For the GLM model (7.4),

(i) explain the meaning of all quantities in the model.

(ii) if the term $\boldsymbol{\beta}'\boldsymbol{x}_i$ is ignored in the model, provide an intuitive explanation why the resulting test for testing whether θ_A is 0 or positive would be equivalent to the scan test discussed in Section 7.3.

(iii) when the term $\boldsymbol{\beta}'\boldsymbol{x}_i$ is included in the model, explain the difference between the test for testing whether θ_A is 0 or positive and the scan test discussed in Section 7.3.

7.10 Discuss the major differences between Models (7.4) and (7.5), and the possible impact on the test for testing whether θ_A is 0 or positive by including the random-effects term b_i in Model (7.5).

8

Disease Surveillance by Nonparametric Spatio-Temporal Data Monitoring

8.1 Introduction

Disease surveillance is mainly for detecting *disease outbreaks* that refer to the occurrence of disease cases in excess of what would normally be expected. In recent years, we experienced the outbreaks of COVID-19, Zika, Ebola, SARS, H1N5, H7N9, MERS-CoV, chikungunya and many other damaging infectious diseases. Our society is under a constant threat of bioterrorist attacks and pandemic influenza. It is therefore important to effectively monitor the occurrence of infectious diseases constantly and detect their outbreaks as quickly as possible. Early detection of infectious disease outbreaks can help governments and individuals to take appropriate disease control and prevention measures in a timely manner so that the disease epidemic can be controlled at an early stage and thus their damage can be minimized. In this chapter, we will introduce some recent statistical methodologies developed for disease surveillance.

As discussed in Section 1.2, *disease prevalence* and *disease incidence* are two commonly used measures of disease frequency. The former reflects the total number of existing disease cases while the latter measures the number of newly confirmed disease cases. In disease surveillance, disease incidence is often a preferred measure of disease frequency because it is more helpful for us to understand the disease etiology. To compare the disease incidence numbers of two regions in a given time period, population sizes of the regions should be taken into account. Otherwise, we can have the conclusion like "a region with one million people and 200 newly confirmed disease cases has a more serious disease outbreak than a region with 1000 people and 100 newly confirmed disease cases", which is obviously unreasonable since the rate of newly confirmed disease cases in the first region is 1 out of 5000 people which is much lower than the rate of 1 out of 10 people in the second region. To accommodate the population size of a region, the *disease incidence rate* is often more reasonable to use, which is defined to be the disease incidence in a region divided by the population size of the region within a given time internal.

Disease incidence data used in disease surveillance are often collected at multiple spatial locations at a sequence of time points. Thus, they are

DOI: 10.1201/9781003138150-8

usually spatio-temporal data, although the number of observation times keeps increasing in disease surveillance, instead of fixed in cases considered in most retrospective spatio-temporal data modeling approaches (cf., Section 2.7). In the literature, there have been many existing discussions about disease surveillance. Some basic retrospective methods for solving the disease surveillance problem have been described in Chapter 7. As discussed in Sections 7.1 and 7.5, these methods are generally ineffective for disease surveillance because of their retrospective nature and their inability to accommodate the complex structure of a typical disease incidence dataset. To demonstrate the data complexity in disease surveillance applications, let us consider an example below.

Example 8.1 *Influenza-like illness (ILI) is a respiratory infection caused by a variety of influenza viruses. A suspect ILI case is defined as the severe respiratory illness with fever (> 100° F), cough, sore throat, and difficulty in breathing. It is estimated that 15–40% of the population develop illness from influenza each year in the US. About 36,000 people per year die from influenza infection, and about 114,000 people per year have to be admitted to hospital due to influenza infection (Fiore et al., 2010). A traditional method to estimate the incidence rate of ILI is to carry out repeated seroprevalence surveys. But, such surveys are resource-intensive and slow. Thus, they are infeasible for early detection of disease outbreaks. To overcome that difficulty, the Florida Department of Health (FDOH) has developed an Electronic Surveillance System for the Early Notification of Community-based Epidemics at Florida (ESSENCE-FL), which is a syndromic surveillance system for collecting* **near real-time** *pre-diagnostic data from participating hospitals and urgent care centers in Florida. Currently, the system collects data from acute care visits to 229 emergency departments and 35 urgent care centers distributed in all counties of Florida, and the collected data are updated in a daily basis. Figure 8.1 presents the observed incidence rates of ILI for all 67 counties of Florida on 06/01/2012 (a summer time) and 12/01/2012 (a winter time). From the two plots, we can see that the ILI incidence rates in the winter were generally higher than those in the summer, and the ILI epidemic in some counties (e.g., the Liberty county in the northwestern Florida) was quite serious in the winter of 2012.*

Disease incidence data, such as those shown in Example 8.1, often have complicated structures. For instance, the distribution of disease incidence rate within a given region and a given time interval cannot usually be approximated well by a Poisson, negative binomial, or normal distribution (Yang and Qiu, 2020; Zhang et al., 2015), because of the facts that many confounding risk factors could affect the disease incidence rate in practice, these risk factors may not be easy to measure, and sometimes it is even difficult for us to notice their existence. In addition, disease incidence rates often have complex spatio-temporal patterns like spatial clustering (e.g., some neighboring counties in the northwestern part of Florida seem to have relatively high disease incidence rates in the lower panel of Figure 8.1), seasonality (the incidence rates of ILI

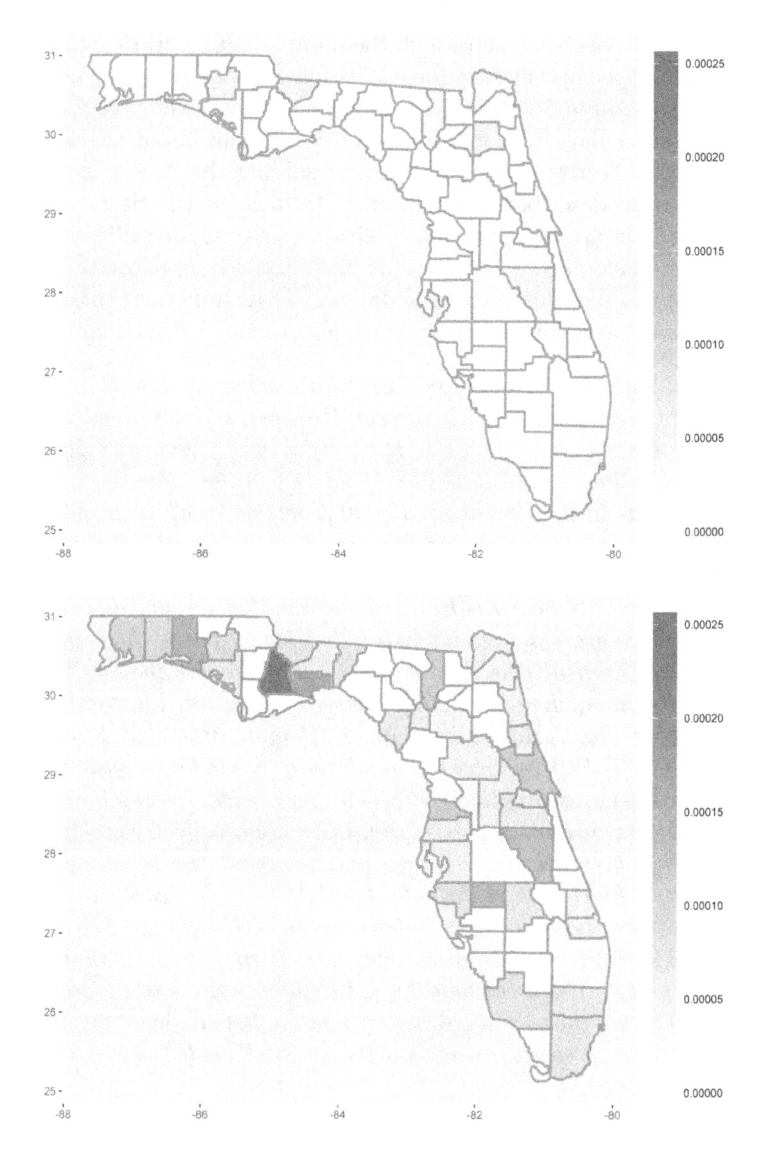

FIGURE 8.1
Observed ILI incidence rates in Florida on 06/01/2012 (left) and 12/01/2012 (right). Darker colors denote larger values.

are generally lower in the summer and higher in the winter as shown in Figure 8.1), and day-of-week variation (cf., Zhao et al., 2011), which cannot usually be described well by a parametric statistical model. Furthermore, the observed disease incidence rates at different time points and spatial locations are usually correlated: the closer the distance between two observation times and/or locations, the stronger the correlation. Such spatio-temporal data correlation is often difficult to describe by a parametric spatio-temporal model either. Thus, the disease surveillance methods discussed in Chapter 7 cannot generally accommodate such complex data structures well because their various model assumptions would be invalid in many disease surveillance applications.

In the disease reporting systems like ESSENCE-FL, some conventional process monitoring tools, such as the cumulative sum (CUSUM) and the exponentially weighted moving average (EWMA) charts, are usually included for routine disease surveillance purposes (cf., Chen et al., 2009; Kite-Powell et al., 2010). These charts, however, require the assumptions that the observed spatio-temporal data are independent at different observation locations and times, and follow a parametric (e.g., normal) distribution when no disease outbreaks are present. See Chapter 3 for a detailed discussion about these conventional control charts. In practice, however, their assumptions are rarely valid, as explained in the previous paragraph. In the statistical process control (SPC) literature, it has been well demonstrated that results from the conventional control charts would be unreliable or even misleading in cases when their required model assumptions are violated (e.g., Capizzi, 2015; Chakraborti et al., 2015; Hackl and Ledolter, 1991; Qiu, 2018a; Qiu and Hawkins, 2001). That explains why these methods did not play an important role in our recent effort in fighting against the infectious diseases like COVID-19 and Ebola.

To accommodate flexible data structure, some new SPC methods have been developed recently. See discussions in Sections 3.3 and 3.4 for a description about some recent SPC methods designed for monitoring processes with correlated data and for cases when a parametric form is unavailable to describe the process distribution. To accommodate the dynamic nature (i.e., the process distribution changes over time) of certain processes, some dynamic screening systems (DySS) have been developed recently, which have been described in detail in Chapters 4–6 in the context of disease screening. Most of these recent SPC methods, however, are designed mainly for monitoring univariate or multivariate non-spatial sequential processes, and they cannot handle spatial processes with complex spatial data structures.

To better model and monitor spatio-temporal data, some nonparametric approaches have been developed recently (Qiu and Yang, 2023; Yang and Qiu, 2018, 2019, 2020, 2022). Because of their generality, besides disease surveillance, they should also be useful for other spatio-temporal data monitoring problems, such as air quality surveillance in environmental research and sea-level pressure monitoring in oceanography. These methods will be introduced in this chapter. More specifically, some nonparametric spatio-temporal data modeling approaches suggested by Yang and Qiu (2018), Yang and Qiu (2019) and Yang and Qiu (2022) will be discussed in Section 8.2. Based on these spatio-temporal data modeling approaches, Yang and Qiu (2020) suggested a disease surveillance method, which will be described in Section 8.3. In practice, disease outbreaks often start in some small clustered regions. A nonparametric disease surveillance method that takes into account this spatial feature was developed recently by Qiu and Yang (2023), which will be discussed in Section 8.4. Incidence rates of an infectious disease like influenza are often associated with some covariates, such as the air temperature, humidity, and other weather and/or environmental conditions. To make use of such covariate information for effective disease surveillance, Qiu and Yang (2021) suggested a new method recently, which will be discussed in Section 8.5. Finally, some concluding remarks will be given in Section 8.6. An *R* package to implement the related methods discussed in this chapter will be introduced in the next chapter.

8.2 Nonparametric Spatio-Temporal Data Modeling

In this section, some recent nonparametric methods for modeling spatio-temporal data collected in a region during a given time interval are described. These methods are retrospective, and will be used for prospective disease surveillance discussed in later sections. Our discussion is organized in four parts. First, a nonparametric spatio-temporal regression model is presented in Subsection 8.2.1 for describing an observed spatio-temporal dataset. Then, a procedure for estimating the nonparametric mean function of the model when the possible spatio-temporal data correlation is ignored is discussed in Subsection 8.2.2. A procedure for estimating the nonparametric variance and covariance functions of the model is discussed in Subsection 8.2.3. Finally, a procedure for estimating the nonparametric mean function of the model with the possible spatio-temporal data correlation accommodated is discussed in Subsection 8.2.4. The methods described in this section were originally suggested in papers Yang and Qiu (2018), Yang and Qiu (2019) and Yang and Qiu (2022). Some technical details about these methods can be found there.

8.2.1 A Nonparametric Spatio-Temporal Regression Model

Assume that a response variable y (e.g., disease incidence rate) is observed at n time points $\{t_i, i = 1, 2, \ldots, n\}$ in the time interval $[0, T]$. At the ith time point t_i, it is observed at m_i spatial locations $\{\boldsymbol{s}_{ij}, j = 1, 2, \ldots, m_i\}$ in a spatial region $\Omega \subset R^2$, for $i = 1, 2, \ldots, n$. For the observed disease incidence rates in different regions in the disease surveillance problem, the observation locations $\{\boldsymbol{s}_{ij}, j = 1, 2, \ldots, m_i\}$ could be the centroids of the regions and they do not change over time in such cases. They are allowed to change over time in the current model to accommodate some scenarios in practice, such as the one when some regions do not have observed data at some specific time points.

The observed spatio-temporal data are assumed to follow the nonparametric spatio-temporal regression (NSTR) model

$$y(t_i, \boldsymbol{s}_{ij}) = \mu(t_i, \boldsymbol{s}_{ij}) + \varepsilon(t_i, \boldsymbol{s}_{ij}), \quad \text{for } j = 1, 2, \ldots, m_i, i = 1, 2, \ldots, n, \tag{8.1}$$

where $y(t_i, \boldsymbol{s}_{ij})$ is the observation of y at time t_i and location $\boldsymbol{s}_{ij}$, $\mu(t_i, \boldsymbol{s}_{ij})$ is its mean, and $\varepsilon(t_i, \boldsymbol{s}_{ij})$ is the zero-mean random error. In the NSTR model (8.1), the covariance structure of the spatio-temporal data can be described by the covariance function

$$V(t, t'; \boldsymbol{s}, \boldsymbol{s}') = \text{Cov}\left[y(t, \boldsymbol{s}), y(t', \boldsymbol{s}')\right], \quad \text{for any } (t, \boldsymbol{s}), (t', \boldsymbol{s}') \in [0, T] \times \Omega. \tag{8.2}$$

When $(t, \boldsymbol{s}) = (t', \boldsymbol{s}')$, $V(t, t; \boldsymbol{s}, \boldsymbol{s})$ is just the variance function of $y(t, \boldsymbol{s})$, denoted as $\sigma^2(t, \boldsymbol{s})$.

It should be pointed out that the NSTR model (8.1) is quite flexible. It does not impose any parametric forms on the mean function $\mu(t, \boldsymbol{s})$, the variance and covariance functions $\sigma^2(t, \boldsymbol{s})$ and $V(t, t'; \boldsymbol{s}, \boldsymbol{s}')$, and the distribution of the response variable $y(t, \boldsymbol{s})$. It even allows the number of observations (i.e., m_i) and the observation locations (i.e., $\{\boldsymbol{s}_{ij}, j = 1, 2, \ldots, m_i\}$) to be different at different observation times. The major model assumptions required by the data modeling approaches described below are that the mean, variance, and covariance functions are all continuous functions of their respective arguments, which should be reasonable in most disease surveillance applications.

8.2.2 Estimation of the Mean Function When the Spatio-Temporal Data Correlation is Ignored

For estimating the mean function $\mu(t, \boldsymbol{s})$ in the NSTR model (8.1), Yang and Qiu (2018) suggested using the local linear kernel (LLK) smoothing procedure (cf., Subsection 2.5.5), after the possible spatio-temporal correlation in the observed data is ignored. More specifically, let

$$\boldsymbol{Y} = (y(t_1, \boldsymbol{s}_{11}), \ldots, y(t_1, \boldsymbol{s}_{1m_1}), \ldots, y(t_n, \boldsymbol{s}_{n1}), \ldots, y(t_n, \boldsymbol{s}_{nm_n}))'$$

be the long vector of all observations. Then, for a given $(t, \boldsymbol{s}) \in [0, T] \times \Omega$, $\mu(t, \boldsymbol{s})$ can be estimated by the following LLK smoothing procedure:

$$\min_{\boldsymbol{\beta} \in R^4} (\boldsymbol{Y} - \boldsymbol{X}\boldsymbol{\beta})' \widehat{\Sigma}_K^{-1} (\boldsymbol{Y} - \boldsymbol{X}\boldsymbol{\beta}), \tag{8.3}$$

where $\boldsymbol{X} = (X_{11}, \ldots, X_{1m_1}, \ldots, X_{n1}, \ldots, X_{nm_n})'$ is the design matrix with $X_{ij} = (1, t_i - t, (\boldsymbol{s}_{ij} - \boldsymbol{s})')'$, for $j = 1, 2, \ldots, m_i$ and $i = 1, 2, \ldots, n$, $\boldsymbol{\beta} = (\beta_0, \beta_1, \beta_2, \beta_3)'$ is the coefficient vector,

$$\begin{aligned}
\widehat{\Sigma}_K &= D_K^{-1/2} \widehat{\Sigma}_{\mathbf{Y}} D_K^{-1/2}, \\
D_K &= \text{diag}\{w_0(1,1), \ldots, w_0(1, m_1), \ldots, w_0(n, 1), \ldots, w_0(n, m_n)\}, \\
w_0(i,j) &= K_1((t_i - t)/h_{t,0}) K_2(d_E(\boldsymbol{s}_{ij}, \boldsymbol{s})/h_{s,0}), \quad \text{for each } i, j,
\end{aligned}$$

$h_{t,0}, h_{s,0} > 0$ are two bandwidths, $K_1(\cdot)$ and $K_2(\cdot)$ are two univariate kernel functions, $d_E(\cdot, \cdot)$ denotes the Euclidean distance in R^2, and $\widehat{\Sigma}_{\mathbf{Y}}$ is an estimated covariance matrix of $\boldsymbol{Y}$, which is set to be the identity matrix in this subsection since the possible data correlation is ignored here. It should be pointed out that (8.3) is the multivariate version of the LLK smoothing procedure discussed in Subsection 2.5.5. It is presented concisely in a matrix format. See a related discussion in Subsection 2.4.3 of Qiu (2005). Then, the LLK estimate of $\mu(t, \boldsymbol{s})$ is defined to be the solution of the minimization problem (8.3) to β_0. It can be checked that the LLK estimate has the following expression:

$$\widetilde{\mu}(t, \boldsymbol{s}) = \boldsymbol{e}_1' \left(\boldsymbol{X}' D_K \boldsymbol{X}\right)^{-1} \boldsymbol{X}' D_K \boldsymbol{Y}, \tag{8.4}$$

where $\boldsymbol{e}_1 = (1, 0, 0, 0)'$.

In (8.3), there are two kernel functions $K_1(\cdot)$ and $K_2(\cdot)$ involved. They are usually chosen to have finite supports so that $\widetilde{\mu}(t, \boldsymbol{s})$ in (8.4) is a weighted average of observations in a neighborhood of $(t, \boldsymbol{s})$, where the neighborhood size is controlled by the two bandwidths $h_{t,0}$ and $h_{s,0}$, and the weights are controlled by the two kernel functions. Yang and Qiu (2018) suggested choosing both kernel functions to be the Epanechnikov kernel function because of its good theoretical properties (Epanechnikov, 1969). Namely, we choose $K_1(x) = K_2(x) = 0.75(1 - x^2)I(|x| \leq 1)$. Because $K_2(x)$ is used in a two-dimensional spatial region, its normalizing constant should be chosen differently from 0.75 to become a density kernel; but, the normalizing constant does not need to be specified correctly here because it will be cancelled out when computing the estimate $\widetilde{\mu}(t, \boldsymbol{s})$.

To choose the two bandwidths $h_{t,0}$ and $h_{s,0}$, one commonly used method is the leave-one-out cross-validation (CV) procedure (cf., Subsection 2.5.5). However, when the observed data are correlated, it has been well demonstrated in the literature that the conventional kernel estimators using the regular bandwidth selection procedures, such as the CV procedure, would not perform well, because they cannot separate the data correlation structure from the mean function effectively in such cases (e.g., Altman, 1990; Opsomer et al., 2001). To overcome this limitation, when choosing a bandwidth in the univariate kernel regression setup, Brabanter et al. (2011) suggested using the so-called ϵ-optimal bimodal kernel function defined as

$$K_\epsilon(u) = \frac{4}{4 - 3\epsilon - \epsilon^2} \begin{cases} \frac{3}{4}(1 - u^2)I(|u| \leq 1), & \text{if } |u| \geq \epsilon, \\ \frac{3(1-\epsilon^2)}{4\epsilon}|u|, & \text{if } |u| < \epsilon, \end{cases} \tag{8.5}$$

where $\epsilon \in (0, 1)$ is a small constant.

Yang and Qiu (2018) generalized the above idea for choosing the two bandwidths $h_{t,0}$ and $h_{s,0}$ in the current problem for estimating $\mu(t, \mathbf{s})$. More specifically, let $\widetilde{\mu}_{-(ij)}(t, \mathbf{s})$ be the estimate of $\mu(t, \mathbf{s})$ obtained by (8.4) from all observations except the one at $(t_i, \mathbf{s}_{ij})$, when both $K_1(\cdot)$ and $K_2(\cdot)$ are chosen to be the ϵ-optimal bimodal kernel function defined in (8.5). Then, the modified

CV (MCV) score is defined to be

$$\mathrm{MCV}(h_{t,0}, h_{s,0}) = \frac{1}{n}\sum_{i=1}^{n}\left\{\frac{1}{m_i}\sum_{j=1}^{m_i}\left[y(t_i, \mathbf{s}_{ij}) - \widetilde{\mu}_{-(ij)}(t_i, \mathbf{s}_{ij})\right]^2\right\}. \quad (8.6)$$

The bandwidths $h_{t,0}$ and $h_{s,0}$ are then chosen to be the minimizers of the MCV score $\mathrm{MCV}(h_{t,0}, h_{s,0})$ defined in (8.6). To use $K_\epsilon(u)$ in (8.5), the parameter ϵ should be determined in advance. Based on an intensive numerical study, Brabanter et al. (2011) suggested choosing $\epsilon = 0.1$. This value is also used here since Yang and Qiu (2018) confirmed that $\widetilde{\mu}(t, \boldsymbol{s})$ performed well when $\epsilon = 0.1$.

The mean function estimate $\widetilde{\mu}(t, \boldsymbol{s})$ in (8.4) ignores the possible spatio-temporal data correlation by setting the estimated covariance matrix $\widehat{\Sigma}_{\mathbf{Y}}$ used in (8.3) to be the identity matrix. Similar to the theory of generalized estimating equations (GEE) (Liang and Zeger, 1986), Yang and Qiu (2018) showed that $\widetilde{\mu}(t, \boldsymbol{s})$ was statistically consistent under some regularity conditions. Many simulation results were presented in that paper to evaluate the numerical performance of the mean function estimate $\widetilde{\mu}(t, \boldsymbol{s})$. Some of them are summarized in the example below.

Example 8.2 *In Model (8.1), assume that $\{t_i, i = 1, 2, \ldots, n\}$ are equally spaced in $[0, 1]$. Both the number of observations and observation locations are assumed to be time-invariant. They are denoted as m and $\{\mathbf{s}_j, j = 1, 2, \ldots, m\}$, respectively, for simplicity. The observation locations $\{\mathbf{s}_j, j = 1, 2, \ldots, m\}$ are assumed to be equally spaced in $\Omega = [0, 1] \times [0, 1]$. The true spatio-temporal mean function is chosen to be*

$$\mu(t, \mathbf{s}) = 0.5 + 0.3\sin\left(\frac{\pi}{2} + \pi s_u\right)\sin\left(\frac{\pi}{2} + \pi s_v\right) + 0.15\cos\left(\frac{3\pi}{2} + 2\pi t\right),$$

where $\mathbf{s} = (s_u, s_v)'$. For the spatio-temporal random errors, we first use the R package **neuRosim** *to generate the spatially correlated noise $\{\widetilde{\varepsilon}(\mathbf{s}_j), j = 1, 2, \ldots, m\}$, and then use the AR(1) model to generate the temporally correlated noise $\{\widetilde{\varepsilon}(t_i), i = 1, 2, \ldots, n\}$. Then, the spatio-temporal random errors are defined to be $\{\varepsilon(t_i, \mathbf{s}_j) = \widetilde{\varepsilon}(t_i)\widetilde{\varepsilon}(\mathbf{s}_j), j = 1, 2, \ldots, m, i = 1, 2, \ldots, n\}$. The related parameters are chosen as follows: $n = 100$, $m = 100$, the parameter controlling the temporal correlation level is chosen to be $\rho_t = 0.5, 0.3$, or 0.05, and the parameter controlling the spatial correlation level is chosen to be $\rho_{\mathbf{s}} = 0.5, 0.3$, or 0.05. In each case, the simulation is repeated 100 times. From each simulation, the averaged squared error (ASE) of the estimate $\widetilde{\mu}(t, \mathbf{s})$ for measuring its accuracy in estimating the mean function $\mu(t, \mathbf{s})$ can be computed by*

$$ASE(\widetilde{\mu}(t, \mathbf{s}), \mu(t, \mathbf{s})) = \frac{1}{n}\sum_{i=1}^{n}\left\{\frac{1}{m}\sum_{j=1}^{m}\left[\widetilde{\mu}(t_i, \mathbf{s}_j) - \mu(t_i, \mathbf{s}_j)\right]^2\right\}.$$

Then, the 100 values of ASE computed from the 100 repeated simulations are averaged to estimate the mean ASE (MASE) of the estimate $\widetilde{\mu}(t, \mathbf{s})$.

In this example, besides the LLK estimate $\widetilde{\mu}(t, \boldsymbol{s})$ *in (8.4), we also consider the estimated mean functions by the following three representative spatio-temporal data modeling methods: the log-Gaussian Cox process (LGCP) method and the dynamic spatio-temporal modeling (DSTM) method that were discussed in Section 2.7, and the weighted average smoothing (WAS) method by Kafadar (1996). For the LLK estimate, the two bandwidths* $h_{t,0}$ *and* $h_{s,0}$ *are chosen by minimizing the MCV score* $MCV(h_{t,0}, h_{s,0})$ *defined in (8.6). For the three competing methods, their parameters are chosen to minimize their estimated MSE values, which would be in their advantage, compared to LLK estimate with its bandwidths chosen by the MCV procedure. The estimated MASE values of the four methods based on 100 replicated simulations are presented in Table 8.1. From the table, we can have the following conclusions. First, the LLK estimate outperforms the estimates of all three competing methods in all cases considered with quite large margins. Second, all methods perform the best when the spatio-temporal data correlation is the weakest (i.e., the case when* $(\rho_t, \rho_{\mathbf{s}}) = (0.05, 0.05)$*), which is intuitively reasonable.*

TABLE 8.1
Estimated MASE values of the mean function estimates by the four methods DSTM, LGCP, WAS and LLK in cases when $n = 100$, $m = 100$ and ρ_t and $\rho_{\mathbf{s}}$ change among 0.5, 0.3 and 0.05. All MASE values are in the unit of 10^{-3}. In each row, the smallest MASE value is in bold.

$(\rho_t, \rho_{\mathbf{s}})$	DSTM	LGCP	WAS	LLK
(0.5,0.5)	5.95	7.07	4.85	**1.73**
(0.5,0.3)	5.26	6.90	3.84	**0.92**
(0.5,0.05)	4.71	6.69	1.12	**0.33**
(0.3,0.5)	5.34	7.11	4.87	**0.69**
(0.3,0.3)	4.54	6.91	3.85	**0.37**
(0.3,0.05)	3.91	6.72	1.12	**0.26**
(0.05,0.5)	4.75	7.15	4.89	**0.34**
(0.05,0.3)	3.86	6.95	3.86	**0.26**
(0.05,0.05)	3.18	6.75	1.13	**0.19**

8.2.3 Estimation of the Variance and Covariance Functions

Although the mean function estimate $\widetilde{\mu}(t, \boldsymbol{s})$ defined in (8.4) is statistically consistent under some regularity conditions, its efficiency could be improved if the possible spatio-temporal correlation in the observed data can be accommodated. To this end, we need to estimate the variance and covariance functions $\sigma^2(t, \boldsymbol{s})$ and $V(t, t'; \boldsymbol{s}, \boldsymbol{s}')$ properly. In the literature, there has been some discussion about estimation of the covariance structure of spatio-temporal data (Choi et al., 2013; Cressie and Huang, 1999; Genton, 2007; Gneiting, 2002). However, most existing methods assume that the covariance structure is separable and/or stationary in space and time. The separability assumption can simplify computation greatly, but it may not be valid in many applications, because of the complicated space-time interaction. In addition, it can be observed in many real spatio-temporal datasets that the sample covariances change significantly over both space and time, indicating that the stationarity assumption may not be appropriate in such cases. To model nonstationary covariance structure, Hsu et al. (2012) suggested a method based on the assumptions that the related covariance function had a complex parametric form, the nonstationarity is in the spatial domain only, and the possible nonstationarity in the time domain can be ignored. Shand and Li (2017) proposed a different method for modeling nonstationary covariance structure, by which a nonstationary process was assumed to be a projection of a stationary process in a higher-dimensional space. This method can model the nonstationarity in both space and time; but, estimation of the extra dimensions depends on the choice of the parametric covariance model. To overcome these limitations of the existing methods, Yang and Qiu (2019) suggested a nonparametric approach to estimate the variance and covariance functions based on the local constant kernel smoothing procedure, which is described below.

Assume that the observed spatio-temporal data $\{y(t_i, \boldsymbol{s}_{ij}), j = 1, 2, \ldots, m_i, i = 1, 2, \ldots, n\}$ follow the NSTR model (8.1), and the mean function estimate $\widetilde{\mu}(t, \boldsymbol{s})$ has been obtained by (8.4). Then, we can define the residuals as follows:

$$\widetilde{\varepsilon}(t_i, \boldsymbol{s}_{ij}) = y(t_i, \boldsymbol{s}_{ij}) - \widetilde{\mu}(t_i, \boldsymbol{s}_{ij}), \qquad \text{for } j = 1, 2, \ldots, m_i, i = 1, 2, \ldots, n.$$

Based on these residuals, Yang and Qiu (2019) suggested estimating the variance function $\sigma^2(t, \boldsymbol{s})$ by the following local constant kernel estimate:

$$\widehat{\sigma}^2(t, \boldsymbol{s}) = \frac{\sum_{i=1}^{n} \sum_{j=1}^{m_i} \widetilde{\varepsilon}^2(t_i, \boldsymbol{s}_{ij}) w_1(i, j)}{\sum_{i=1}^{n} \sum_{j=1}^{m_i} w_1(i, j)}, \quad \text{for } (t, \boldsymbol{s}) \in [0, T] \times \Omega, \tag{8.7}$$

where

$$w_1(i, j) = K_1\left((t_i - t)/h_{t,1}\right) K_2\left(d_E(\mathbf{s}_{ij}, \mathbf{s})/h_{s,1}\right),$$

and $h_{t,1}, h_{s,1} > 0$ were two bandwidths. From Expression (8.7), it can be seen that $\widehat{\sigma}^2(t, \boldsymbol{s})$ is defined to be a weighted average of $\{\widetilde{\varepsilon}^2(t_i, \boldsymbol{s}_{ij})\}$ in a neighborhood of $(t, \boldsymbol{s})$, and the neighborhood size is controlled by the bandwidths $h_{t,1}$ and $h_{s,1}$. Intuitively, if $\widetilde{\mu}(t, \boldsymbol{s})$ is a good estimate of the mean function $\mu(t, \boldsymbol{s})$, then each residual $\widetilde{\varepsilon}(t_i, \boldsymbol{s}_{ij})$ would have the asymptotic mean of 0 and the asymptotic variance of $\sigma^2(t_i, \boldsymbol{s}_{ij})$, for each i and j. Thus, the weighted average of the residual squares in a neighborhood of $(t, \boldsymbol{s})$ should be close to $\sigma^2(t, \boldsymbol{s})$.

Similar to the variance estimate defined in (8.7), the covariance function $V(t, t'; \boldsymbol{s}, \boldsymbol{s}')$, for $(t, \boldsymbol{s}) \neq (t', \boldsymbol{s}')$, can be estimated by

$$\widehat{V}(t, t'; \boldsymbol{s}, \boldsymbol{s}') = \frac{\sum_{i,j} \sum_{(k,l) \neq (i,j)} \widetilde{\varepsilon}(t_i, \boldsymbol{s}_{ij}) \widetilde{\varepsilon}(t_k, \boldsymbol{s}_{kl}) w_2(i, j, k, l)}{\sum_{i,j} \sum_{(k,l) \neq (i,j)} w_2(i, j, k, l)}, \tag{8.8}$$

where

$$\begin{aligned} w_2(i,j,k,l) &= K_1\left((t_i-t)/h_{t,1}\right)K_1\left((t_k-t')/h_{t,1}\right)\times \\ & \quad K_2\left(d_E(\boldsymbol{s}_{ij},\boldsymbol{s})/h_{s,1}\right)K_2\left(d_E(\boldsymbol{s}_{kl},\boldsymbol{s}')/h_{s,1}\right). \end{aligned}$$

In (8.8), $\widehat{V}(t,t';\boldsymbol{s},\boldsymbol{s}')$ is defined to be a weighted sample covariance computed from pairs of the residuals in the neighborhoods of $(t,\boldsymbol{s})$ and $(t',\boldsymbol{s}')$, respectively, and the weights are determined by the kernel functions. Under some regularity conditions, Yang and Qiu (2019) showed that both $\widehat{\sigma}^2(t,\boldsymbol{s})$ and $\widehat{V}(t,t';\boldsymbol{s},\boldsymbol{s}')$ were statistically consistent.

In (8.7) and (8.8), the two kernel functions $K_1(\cdot)$ and $K_2(\cdot)$ can be chosen to be the same as those in (8.3). The two bandwidths $(h_{t,1},h_{s,1})$ could be chosen differently from the bandwidths $(h_{t,0},h_{s,0})$ used in computing the mean function estimate $\widetilde{\mu}(t,\boldsymbol{s})$ in (8.4). For selection of $(h_{t,1},h_{s,1})$, Yang and Qiu (2019) suggested a method based on spatio-temporal prediction, which is described below. First, let us define the cross-validated mean squared prediction error (CV-MSPE) by

$$\text{CV-MSPE}(h_{t,1},h_{s,1}) = \frac{1}{n}\sum_{i=1}^{n}\left\{\frac{1}{m_i}\sum_{j=1}^{m_i}\left[y(t_i,\boldsymbol{s}_{ij})-\widehat{y}_{-(ij)}(t_i,\boldsymbol{s}_{ij})\right]^2\right\}, \tag{8.9}$$

where the predicted values $\{\widehat{y}_{-(ij)}(t_i,\boldsymbol{s}_{ij}), j=1,2,\ldots,m_i, i=1,2,\ldots,n\}$ are obtained by the simple kriging method (Cressie and Wikle, 2011), described below. For each $1\le j\le m_i$ and $1\le i\le n$, let $\widehat{V}_{-(ij)}(t,t';\boldsymbol{s},\boldsymbol{s}')$ be the estimated covariance function by Formula (8.8) when the (i,j)-th residual $\widetilde{\varepsilon}(t_i,\boldsymbol{s}_{ij})$ is excluded, $\boldsymbol{\varepsilon}_{-(ij)}$ be the vector with elements $\{\varepsilon(t_k,\boldsymbol{s}_{kl}), l=1,2,\ldots,m_k, k=1,2,\ldots,n, (k,l)\neq(i,j)\}$, $\mathbf{V}_{ij,-(ij)}$ be the covariance between $\varepsilon(t_i,\boldsymbol{s}_{ij})$ and $\boldsymbol{\varepsilon}_{-(ij)}$, and $\mathbf{V}_{-(ij),-(ij)}$ be the covariance matrix of $\boldsymbol{\varepsilon}_{-(ij)}$. Then, the predicted value $\widehat{y}_{-(ij)}(t_i,\boldsymbol{s}_{ij})$, for $j=1,2,\ldots,m_i$ and $i=1,2,\ldots,n$, is defined to be

$$\widehat{y}_{-(ij)}(t_i,\boldsymbol{s}_{ij}) = \widetilde{\mu}(t_i,\boldsymbol{s}_{ij}) + \widehat{\mathbf{V}}'_{ij,-(ij)}\widehat{\mathbf{V}}^{-1}_{-(ij),-(ij)}\widetilde{\boldsymbol{\varepsilon}}_{-(ij)},$$

where $\widehat{\mathbf{V}}_{ij,-(ij)}$ and $\widehat{\mathbf{V}}_{-(ij),-(ij)}$ are the estimates of $\mathbf{V}_{ij,-(ij)}$ and $\mathbf{V}_{-(ij),-(ij)}$, respectively, computed from $\widehat{V}_{-(ij)}(t,t';\boldsymbol{s},\boldsymbol{s}')$, and $\widetilde{\boldsymbol{\varepsilon}}_{-(ij)}$ is a long vector of the residuals $\{\widetilde{\varepsilon}(t_k,\boldsymbol{s}_{kl}), l=1,2,\ldots,m_k, k=1,2,\ldots,n, (k,l)\neq(i,j)\}$ arranged in the same order as that in $\boldsymbol{\varepsilon}_{-(ij)}$. Then, the bandwidths $(h_{t,1},h_{s,1})$ can be selected by minimizing CV-MSPE$(h_{t,1},h_{s,1})$ defined in (8.9).

Let $\boldsymbol{\varepsilon}$ be a long vector with the elements $\{\varepsilon(t_i,\boldsymbol{s}_{ij}), j=1,2,\ldots,m_i, i=1,2,\ldots,n\}$, $\mathbf{V}$ be its covariance matrix, and $\widehat{\mathbf{V}}$ be the estimate of $\mathbf{V}$ obtained from the estimated variance and convariance functions defined in (8.7) and (8.8). Then, $\widehat{\mathbf{V}}$ may not be a positive semidefinite matrix; thus, it may not be a legitimate covariance matrix. In the literature, there are some existing modification procedures to modify a symmetric matrix to be positive semidefinite (e.g., Hall et al., 1994; Higham, 1988). Yang and Qiu (2019) suggested using the one by Higham (1988), described briefly below. Let $\|\cdot\|_F$ be the Frobenius matrix norm, defined to be the square root of the sum of squares of a matrix's all elements, and $\mathcal{P}$ be the set of all symmetric positive semidefinite matrices with the same dimensions as those of $\widehat{\mathbf{V}}$. Then, we consider the projection of $\widehat{\mathbf{V}}$ onto $\mathcal{P}$, which is the solution of the following minimization problem:

$$\widetilde{\mathbf{V}} = \arg\min_{\mathbf{P}\in\mathcal{P}} \|\mathbf{P} - \widehat{\mathbf{V}}\|_F.$$

Then, the modified covariance matrix is $\widetilde{\mathbf{V}}$, which can be obtained by the *R* function **nearPD()** in the package **Matrix**.

Example 8.3 *Yang and Qiu (2019) presented the following simulation example to evaluate the numerical performance of the estimated variance and covariance functions defined in (8.7) and (8.8). First, in the NSTR model (8.1), the true mean function is set to be*

$$\mu(t, \boldsymbol{s}) = 1.5 + e^{-(s_u^2+s_v^2)} + \cos(2\pi t), \quad \textit{for } t \in [0,1], \boldsymbol{s} \in [0,1]\times[0,1],$$

where $\boldsymbol{s} = (s_u, s_v)'$. *The observation times* $\{t_i = i/n, i = 1, 2, \ldots, n\}$ *are equally spaced in* $[0,1]$, *the number of observations at each observation time is the same to be* m, *and the observation locations* $\{\boldsymbol{s}_j, j = 1, 2, \ldots, m\}$ *do not change over time and are equally spaced in* $[0,1]\times[0,1]$. *For the spatio-temporal data correlation, the following three cases are considered:*

Case 1 *The random errors* $\{\varepsilon(t_i, \boldsymbol{s}_j), i = 1, 2, \ldots, n, j = 1, 2, \ldots, m\}$ *are generated from a non-stationary spatio-temporal model, as discussed in Hsu et al. (2012). More specifically, it is assumed that*

$$\varepsilon(t_i, \boldsymbol{s}_j) = W(t_i, \boldsymbol{s}_j) + \sum_{l=1}^{q} \xi_l(t_i)\psi_l(\boldsymbol{s}_j), \quad \textit{for } i = 1, 2, \ldots, n, j = 1, 2, \ldots, m,$$

where $W(t_i, \boldsymbol{s}_j)$ *is a zero-mean stationary spatio-temporal process,* $\{\psi_l(\boldsymbol{s}), l = 1, 2, \ldots, q\}$ *are* q *pre-specified basis functions, and* $\{\xi_l(t_i), i = 1, 2, \ldots, n\}$, *for* $l = 1, 2, \ldots, q$, *are mutually independent zero-mean stationary time series that are independent of* $W(t_i, \boldsymbol{s}_j)$. *The quantities* $W(t_i, \boldsymbol{s}_j)$, $\{\psi_l(\boldsymbol{s}_j), l = 1, 2, \ldots, q\}$ *and* $\{\xi_l(t_i), l = 1, 2, \ldots, q\}$ *are generated as discussed in Hsu et al. (2012), for each* i *and* j.

Case 2 *Let* $\boldsymbol{\varepsilon}(t_i) = (\varepsilon(t_i, \boldsymbol{s}_1), \varepsilon(t_i, \boldsymbol{s}_2), \ldots, \varepsilon(t_i, \boldsymbol{s}_m))'$. *Then,* $\boldsymbol{\varepsilon}(t_i)$ *is generated from the following vector AR(1) model:*

$$\boldsymbol{\varepsilon}(t_i) = \phi\boldsymbol{\varepsilon}(t_{i-1}) + (1-\phi^2)^{1/2}\boldsymbol{\eta}(t_i),$$

where ϕ *is a coefficient, and* $\{\boldsymbol{\eta}(t_i) = (\eta(t_i, \boldsymbol{s}_1), \eta(t_i, \boldsymbol{s}_2), \ldots, \eta(t_i, \boldsymbol{s}_m))', i = 1, 2, \ldots, n\}$ *are temporally independent spatial processes. For each* i *and* j,

$\eta(t_i, \boldsymbol{s}_j)$ is assumed to have the $N(0,1)$ distribution. At each observation time t_i, the spatial correlation among the elements of $\boldsymbol{\eta}(t_i)$ is described by $Cov(\eta(t_i, \boldsymbol{s}_j), \eta(t_i, \boldsymbol{s}_l)) = \rho(d_E(\boldsymbol{s}_j, \boldsymbol{s}_l))$, for any j and l. In such cases, it can be checked that the covariance between $\varepsilon(t_i, \boldsymbol{s}_j)$ and $\varepsilon(t_k, \boldsymbol{s}_l)$ is

$$V(t_i, t_k; \boldsymbol{s}_j, \boldsymbol{s}_l) = \phi^{|k-i|}\rho(d_E(\boldsymbol{s}_j, \boldsymbol{s}_l)).$$

In the simulation example, we choose $\rho(d) = \exp(-d^2)$, and $\phi = 0.8$.

Case 3 *The random error vector $\boldsymbol{\varepsilon}(t_i)$ is generated from the following vector AR(2) model:*

$$\boldsymbol{\varepsilon}(t_i) = \phi_1\boldsymbol{\varepsilon}(t_{i-1}) + \phi_2\boldsymbol{\varepsilon}(t_{i-2}) + \boldsymbol{\eta}(t_i),$$

where ϕ_1 and ϕ_2 are two coefficients, and $\boldsymbol{\eta}(t_i)$ is the same as the one in the vector AR(1) model considered in Case 2, except that its spatial correlation is determined by a correlation function $\rho(\boldsymbol{s}, \boldsymbol{s}')$, for any $\boldsymbol{s}, \boldsymbol{s}' \in [0,1]\times[0,1]$. In such cases, it can be checked that the covariance between $\varepsilon(t_i, \boldsymbol{s}_j)$ and $\varepsilon(t_k, \boldsymbol{s}_l)$ is

$$V(t_i, t_k; \boldsymbol{s}_j, \boldsymbol{s}_l) = c_{|k-i|}\rho(\boldsymbol{s}_j, \boldsymbol{s}_l),$$

where

$$\begin{aligned} c_0 &= \frac{1-\phi_2}{(1+\phi_2)\left[(1-\phi_2)^2 - \phi_1^2\right]}, \\ c_1 &= \frac{\phi_1}{1-\phi_2}c_0, \\ c_d &= \phi_1 c_{d-1} + \phi_2 c_{d-2}, \text{ for } d > 1. \end{aligned}$$

In the simulation example, we choose $(\phi_1, \phi_2) = (0.5, 0.3)$, and $\rho(\boldsymbol{s}, \boldsymbol{s}') = \exp\{-[(s_u - s_u') + (s_v - s_v')]\}$, where $\boldsymbol{s} = (s_u, s_v)'$ and $\boldsymbol{s}' = (s_u', s_v')'$.

Besides the nonparametric variance estimation method discussed in this subsection, denoted as NP, the following two representative alternative methods are also considered: the group LASSO (GL) method by Hsu et al. (2012) and the B-spline (BS) method by Choi et al. (2013). In the method NP, the bandwidths are chosen by the MSPE procedure (8.9). In the method GL, its parameters are chosen by the CV procedure, as discussed in Hsu et al. (2012). In the method BS, its parameters are chosen to be the recommended values given in Choi et al. (2013). The temporal correlation is assumed to be exponentially decayed in both GL and BS. As a comparison, NP does not require this assumption. To make the comparison fair among different methods, the following truncated mean average squared error (TMASE) is used to measure the performance of the estimated covariance function:

$$TMASE(\vartheta) = \frac{\sum_{i,k=1}^{n}\sum_{j,l=1}^{m}\left[V(t_i, t_k; \boldsymbol{s}_j, \boldsymbol{s}_l) - \widehat{V}(t_i, t_k; \boldsymbol{s}_j, \boldsymbol{s}_l)\right]^2 I(k-i \le \vartheta)}{m^2\sum_{i=1}^{n}\sum_{k=i}^{n} I(k-i \le \vartheta)},$$

where ϑ is a positive integer for truncation. The results based on 100 replicated simulations when $(m, n) = (64, 200)$ and ϑ changes from 5 to 150 are presented in in Figure 8.1. From the plots in the figure, it can be seen that i) NP is much better than the other two methods when ϑ is relatively small in all cases, except in Case 1 where GL is slightly better because all its assumptions are satisfied in that case, and ii) when ϑ gets larger, performance of the three methods tends to be similar. It should be pointed out that both GL and BS are based on the assumptions that the temporal data correlation is stationary and decays monotonically, which are satisfied in this example. But, the method NP does not require these assumptions, which puts it at a disadvantage place in this comparison.

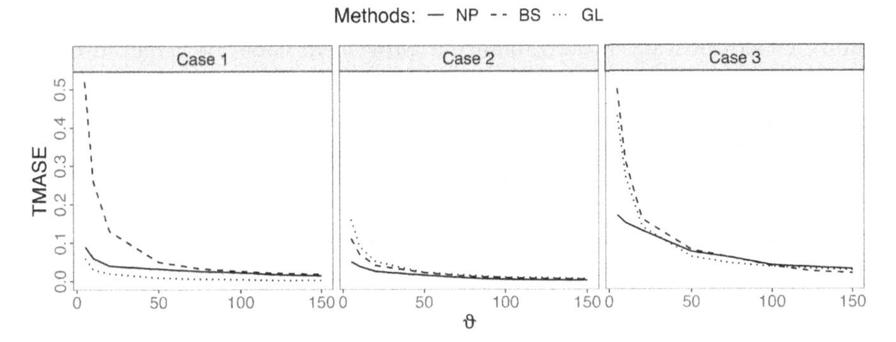

FIGURE 8.2
Calculated TAMSE values of the three variance function estimation methods NP (solid lines), BS (dashed lines) and GL (dotted lines) in three cases when $(m, n) = (64, 200)$ and ϑ changes from 5 to 150.

8.2.4 Estimation of the Mean Function with the Spatio-Temporal Data Correlation Accommodated

After the variance and covariance functions $\sigma^2(t, \boldsymbol{s})$ and $V(t, t'; \boldsymbol{s}, \boldsymbol{s}')$ are estimated by (8.7) and (8.8), the covariance matrix $\Sigma_{\mathbf{Y}}$ of the observed data $\mathbf{Y}$ mentioned below Expression (8.3) can be computed from $\widehat{\sigma}^2(t, \boldsymbol{s})$ and $\widehat{V}(t, t'; \boldsymbol{s}, \boldsymbol{s}')$. The estimated covariance matrix is denoted as $\widehat{\Sigma}_{\mathbf{Y}}$. Then, to accommodate the spatio-temporal data correlation, the estimate of the mean function $\mu(t, \boldsymbol{s})$ can still be computed by (8.4) after D_K there is replaced by $\widehat{\Sigma}_K^{-1} = D_K^{1/2} \widehat{\Sigma}_{\mathbf{Y}}^{-1} D_K^{1/2}$, where D_K is defined immediately after (8.3). Namely, the estimate of $\mu(t, \boldsymbol{s})$ is defined to be

$$\widehat{\mu}(t, \boldsymbol{s}) = \boldsymbol{e}_1' \left(\boldsymbol{X}' \widehat{\Sigma}_K^{-1} \boldsymbol{X} \right)^{-1} \boldsymbol{X}' \widehat{\Sigma}_K^{-1} \mathbf{Y}. \tag{8.10}$$

By comparing (8.10) with (8.4), their major difference is that $\widehat{\Sigma}_{\mathbf{Y}}$ is set to be the identity matrix (i.e., the data correlation in $\mathbf{Y}$ is ignored) in (8.4) while the data correlation in $\mathbf{Y}$ is considered in (8.10) by computing $\widehat{\Sigma}_{\mathbf{Y}}$ from $\widehat{\sigma}^2(t, \boldsymbol{s})$ and $\widehat{V}(t, t'; \boldsymbol{s}, \boldsymbol{s}')$. In (8.10), the bandwidths used in the related LLK smoothing procedure could be chosen to be different from $(h_{t,0}, h_{s,0})$ used in obtaining the estimate $\widetilde{\mu}(t, \boldsymbol{s})$ in (8.4). The new bandwidths used in (8.10) are denoted as $(h_{t,2}, h_{s,2})$.

From (8.4), (8.7), (8.8) and (8.10), it is natural to consider the following iterative procedure: after the mean function $\mu(t, \boldsymbol{s})$ is estimated by (8.10), the estimates of the variance and covariance functions defined in (8.7) and (8.8) can be further updated by replacing the initial mean estimate $\widetilde{\mu}(t, \boldsymbol{s})$ with the mean estimate $\widehat{\mu}(t, \boldsymbol{s})$ in (8.10) when defining the residuals $\{\widetilde{\varepsilon}(t_i, \boldsymbol{s}_{ij})\}$; then, the mean estimate in (8.10) can be further updated by using the updated estimates of the variance and covariance functions and so forth. However, by some theoretical justifications and numerical studies, Yang and Qiu (2022) found that no substantial performance improvement could be achieved by using such an iterative procedure, and the computational burden of the iterative procedure would be heavy. For these reasons, Yang and Qiu (2022) suggested using $\widehat{\mu}(t, \boldsymbol{s})$ in (8.10) as the final estimate of $\mu(t, \boldsymbol{s})$, and proved that it was a statistically consistent estimator under some regularity conditions.

To determine the bandwidths $(h_{t,2}, h_{s,2})$ used in obtaining the final estimate $\widehat{\mu}(t, \boldsymbol{s})$ in (8.10), Yang and Qiu (2022) suggested the following procedure. First, it can be noticed that the mean of the residual mean squares (RMS) of $\widehat{\mu}(t, \boldsymbol{s})$ is

$$\begin{aligned} E(\text{RMS}) =& E\left\{\frac{1}{n}\sum_{i=1}^{n}\left[\frac{1}{m_i}\sum_{j=1}^{m_i}(y(t_i, \boldsymbol{s}_{ij}) - \widehat{\mu}(t_i, \boldsymbol{s}_{ij}))^2\right]\right\} \\ =& \frac{1}{n}\sum_{i=1}^{n}\frac{1}{m_i}\sum_{j=1}^{m_i}\sigma^2(t_i, \boldsymbol{s}_{ij}) + \frac{1}{n}\sum_{i=1}^{n}\frac{1}{m_i}\sum_{j=1}^{m_i}E\left[\mu(t_i, \boldsymbol{s}_{ij}) - \widehat{\mu}(t_i, \boldsymbol{s}_{ij})\right]^2 - \\ & \frac{2}{n}\sum_{i=1}^{n}\frac{1}{m_i}\sum_{j=1}^{m_i}\boldsymbol{e}_1'\left(X'\widehat{\Sigma}_K^{-1}X\right)^{-1}X'\widehat{\Sigma}_K^{-1}\Sigma_{\mathbf{Y}}(\zeta_{ij}), \end{aligned} \tag{8.11}$$

where $\Sigma_{\mathbf{Y}}(\zeta_{ij})$ is the ζ_{ij}th column of the covariance matrix $\Sigma_{\mathbf{Y}}$, and $\zeta_{ij} = \sum_{k=1}^{i-1} m_k + j$. In (8.11), the first term on the right-hand-side of the last equation is not related to $(h_{t,2}, h_{s,2})$, the second term is the mean square error (MSE) of $\widehat{\mu}(t, \boldsymbol{s})$ that measures its performance, and the third term is due to data correlation. In the proposed bandwidth selection procedure, it is suggested to estimate the third term and then choose the bandwidths by minimizing the sum of the RMS and the estimated third term (Note: this sum should be a good estimate of the sum of the first two terms on the right-hand-side of the last equation of (8.11)). More specifically, we first define a bias-corrected estimate of the MSE (BCE-MSE) of $\widehat{\mu}(t, \boldsymbol{s})$ (Note: the first term on the right-hand-side of the last equation of (8.11) has been ignored) to be

$$\begin{aligned}\text{BCE-MSE}(h_{t,2}, h_{s,2}) =& \frac{1}{n}\sum_{i=1}^{n}\left\{\frac{1}{m_i}\sum_{j=1}^{m_i}\left(y(t_i, \boldsymbol{s}_{ij}) - \widehat{\mu}(t_i, \boldsymbol{s}_{ij})\right)^2\right\} + \\ & \frac{2}{n}\sum_{i=1}^{n}\frac{1}{m_i}\sum_{j=1}^{m_i}\boldsymbol{e}_1'\left(X'\widehat{\Sigma}_K^{-1}X\right)^{-1}X'\widehat{\Sigma}_K^{-1}\widehat{\Sigma}_{\mathbf{Y}}(\zeta_{ij}),\end{aligned} \quad (8.12)$$

where $\widehat{\Sigma}_{\mathbf{Y}}(\zeta_{ij})$ is the ζ_{ij}th column of $\widehat{\Sigma}_{\mathbf{Y}}$. Then, $(h_{t,2}, h_{s,2})$ can be chosen by minimizing the quantity BCE-MSE$(h_{t,2}, h_{s,2})$ in (8.12).

Example 8.4 *Yang and Qiu (2022) presented the following simulation example to evaluate the numerical performance of the estimated mean function defined in (8.10). For simplicity, it is assumed that the observation times are* $\{t_i = i/n, i = 1, 2, \ldots, n\}$, *the observation locations at each observation time are equally spaced in* $\Omega = [0,1] \times [0,1]$ *and they do not change over time, and the number of observation locations is* m *at each observation time. In such cases, the observation locations are denoted as* $\{\boldsymbol{s}_j, j = 1, 2, \ldots, m\}$. *In the NSTR model (8.1), it is further assumed that* $(m, n) = (36, 50)$ *or* $(100, 100)$, *and the mean function* $\mu(t, \boldsymbol{s})$ *is chosen to be*

$$\mu(t, \boldsymbol{s}) = 2 + \sin(\pi s_u)\sin(\pi s_v) + \sin(2\pi t),$$

where $\boldsymbol{s} = (s_u, s_v)'$. *Let* $\boldsymbol{\varepsilon}(t_i) = (\varepsilon(t_i, \boldsymbol{s}_1), \varepsilon(t_i, \boldsymbol{s}_2), \ldots, \varepsilon(t_i, \boldsymbol{s}_m))'$. *Then,* $\boldsymbol{\varepsilon}(i)$ *is assumed to be generated from the following vector AR(1) model:*

$$\boldsymbol{\varepsilon}(t_i) = \phi_t\boldsymbol{\varepsilon}(t_{i-1}) + (1 - \phi_t^2)^{1/2}\boldsymbol{\eta}(t_i),$$

where $-1 < \phi_t < 1$ *is a constant controlling the temporal correlation in the observed data, and* $\{\boldsymbol{\eta}(t_i) = (\eta(t_i, \boldsymbol{s}_1), \eta(t_i, \boldsymbol{s}_2), \ldots, \eta(t_i, \boldsymbol{s}_m))', i = 1, 2, \ldots, n\}$ *are temporally independent spatial processes. For each* i *and* j, $\eta(t_i, \boldsymbol{s}_j)$ *is generated from the normal distribution* $N(0, \sigma^2)$. *At each observation time* t_i, *the spatial covariance among the elements of* $\boldsymbol{\eta}(t_i)$ *is described by* $Cov(\eta(t_i, \boldsymbol{s}_j), \eta(t_i, \boldsymbol{s}_l)) = \sigma^2\rho(d_E(\boldsymbol{s}_j, \boldsymbol{s}_l))$, *for any* j *and* l, *where* $\rho(d) = \exp(-\phi_s d)$, *and* $\phi_s > 0$ *is a constant controlling the spatial correlation. In such cases, it can be checked that the covariance between* $\varepsilon(t_i, \boldsymbol{s}_j)$ *and* $\varepsilon(t_k, \boldsymbol{s}_l)$ *is*

$$V(t_i, t_k; \boldsymbol{s}_j, \boldsymbol{s}_l) = \sigma^2\phi_t^{n|t_i - t_k|}\rho(d_E(\boldsymbol{s}_j, \boldsymbol{s}_l)),$$

for any $t_i, t_k \in [0,1]$ *and* $\boldsymbol{s}_j, \boldsymbol{s}_l \in [0,1] \times [0,1]$. *In the simulation, we set* $\sigma = 0.5$, $\phi_t =$ *0.3, 0.6 or 0.9, and* $\phi_s =$ *1, 3 or 5.*

Besides the mean estimate defined in (8.10), we also consider the methods DSTM, LGCP, WAS and LLK discussed in Example 8.2. Because the LLK mean estimate (cf., (8.4)) and the mean estimate defined in (8.10) can be regarded as the steps 1 and 2 in the iterative mean function estimation procedure described in the paragraph below Equation (8.10), they are denoted as

Step1 and Step2, respectively. Then, the estimated MASE values of the mean function estimates by all the related methods based on 100 repeated simulations are presented in Table 8.2. From the table, it can be seen that i) the two methods Step1 and Step2 have a better overall performance than the methods DSTM, LGCP and WAS, ii) Step2 outperforms Step1 in all cases considered, and iii) the performance of Step1 and Step2 improves when the sample size (m, n) *increases from* $(36, 50)$ *to* $(100, 100)$. *The last conclusion is consistent with the theorical consistency results given in Yang and Qiu (2022). The conclusion ii) says that the update from Step1 to Step2 by accommodating the estimated variance and covariance functions is helpful for estimating the mean function* $\mu(t, \boldsymbol{s})$. *The conclusion i) confirms the benefits to use the nonparametric spatio-temporal modeling methods Step1 and Step2, in which the complex spatio-temporal data structure has been accommodated by using flexible models. As a comparison, both the methods DSTM and LGCP require some restrictive model assumptions, and the method WAS ignores the spatio-temporal data correlation completely.*

TABLE 8.2
Estimated MASE values of the mean function estimates by the five spatio-temporal mean function estimation methods DSTM, LGCP, WAS, Step1 and Step2 when $(m, n) = (36, 50)$ or (100,100), and the spatio-temporal data correlation changes from relatively weak to relatively strong cases. In each row, the smallest MASE value is in bold.

(m, n)	(ϕ_t, ϕ_s)	DSTM	LGCP	WAS	Step1	Step2
	(0.3,1)	0.218	0.235	0.237	0.050	**0.048**
	(0.3,3)	0.175	0.231	0.215	0.044	**0.042**
	(0.3,5)	0.152	0.228	0.200	0.037	**0.036**
	(0.6,1)	0.238	0.241	0.239	0.086	**0.077**
(36,50)	(0.6,3)	0.202	0.230	0.216	0.076	**0.064**
	(0.6,5)	0.185	0.221	0.201	0.068	**0.054**
	(0.9,1)	0.246	0.255	0.238	0.184	**0.166**
	(0.9,3)	0.237	0.243	0.217	0.156	**0.130**
	(0.9,5)	0.230	0.237	0.201	0.135	**0.109**
	(0.3,1)	0.225	0.233	0.231	0.034	**0.030**
	(0.3,3)	0.192	0.225	0.202	0.029	**0.026**
	(0.3,5)	0.168	0.208	0.179	0.024	**0.022**
	(0.6,1)	0.233	0.239	0.231	0.064	**0.047**
(100,100)	(0.6,3)	0.211	0.224	0.202	0.054	**0.039**
	(0.6,5)	0.194	0.203	0.179	0.046	**0.033**
	(0.9,1)	0.251	0.244	0.238	0.161	**0.129**
	(0.9,3)	0.241	0.238	0.206	0.133	**0.102**
	(0.9,5)	0.235	0.231	0.181	0.113	**0.083**

As discussed in the paragraph below Equation (8.10), the mean function $\mu(t, \boldsymbol{s})$ *can be estimated by an iterative procedure with the estimates defined in (8.4) and (8.10) as its first and second steps. Next, we study whether the performance of the mean estimate can be further improved by using more iterations. More specifically, besides Step1 and Step2 considered in Table 8.2, we also consider Step3 and Step4, where Step3 denotes the mean estimate obtained by (8.10) after the estimates of the variance and convariance functions are updated by (8.7) and (8.8) with the initial mean estimate* $\widetilde{\mu}(t, \boldsymbol{s})$ *replaced by the mean estimate* $\widehat{\mu}(t, \boldsymbol{s})$ *of Step2 when defining the residuals, and Step4 denotes the mean estimate after another iteration. To compare an alternative estimate with* $\widehat{\mu}(t, \boldsymbol{s})$ *of Step2, we use the following metric:*

$$DASE = MASE \text{ of an alternative estimate} - MASE \text{ of } \widehat{\mu}(t, \boldsymbol{s}) \text{ of Step2}.$$

So, by this metric, the alternative method would perform better than Step2 if the value of DASE is negative, and Step2 would perform better otherwise. In the setup of Table 8.2 when $(m, n) = (36, 50)$*, the results based on 100 replicated simulations are shown in Figure 8.3 by the box plots. From the plots in the figure, it can be seen that i) Step2 is much better than Step1 (i.e., the first iteration is helpful), and ii) Step3 and Step4 improves Step2 only marginally. Because of the computational burden to use more iterations, this example confirms that it is reasonable to use the estimate* $\widehat{\mu}(t, \boldsymbol{s})$ *of Step2 as the final estimate of* $\mu(t, \boldsymbol{s})$*.*

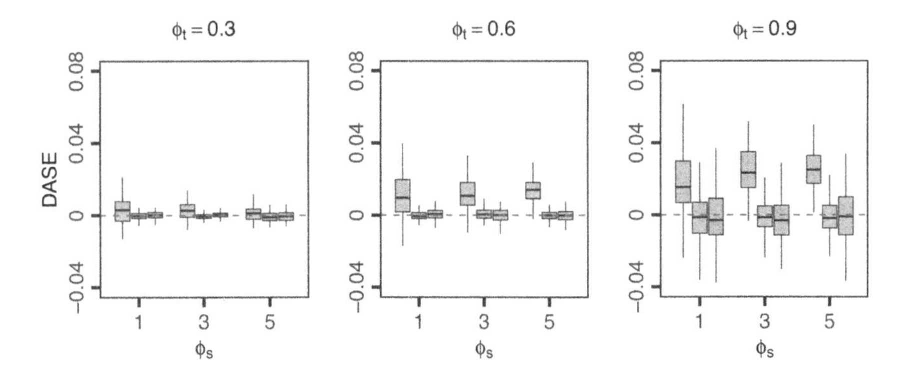

FIGURE 8.3
Boxplots of the DASE values to compare the mean estimates obtained after the first several iterations of the iterative estimation procedure for Model (8.1) in cases when $(m, n) = (36, 50)$, $\phi_s = 1, 3$, or 5, and $\phi_t = 0.3, 0.6$ or 0.9. For a given set of values of (ϕ_t, ϕ_s) in each plot, the three boxes from the left to the right are for comparing Step1, Step3 and Step4 with Step2, respectively, with Step2 as a baseline method.

8.3 Disease Surveillance by Nonparametric Spatio-Temporal Data Modeling

For a given disease, assume that there is a spatio-temporal dataset of its disease incidence rate y available before disease surveillance, which is collected in the time internal $[0, T]$ and a given space Ω when no disease outbreaks are present. This dataset is called an *in-control (IC) dataset*, and its spatio-temporal observations $\{y(t_i, \boldsymbol{s}_{ij}), j = 1, 2, \ldots, m_i, i = 1, 2, \ldots, n\}$ are assumed to follow the NSTR model (8.1). In practice, observed disease incidence data often have seasonality. In such cases, $[0, T]$ should contain at least one complete cycle of seasonality. For simplicity, it is assumed that $[0, T]$ is a whole cycle of seasonality. Then, the mean function $\mu(t, \boldsymbol{s})$, the variance function $\sigma^2(t, \boldsymbol{s})$ and the covariance function $V(t, t'; \boldsymbol{s}, \boldsymbol{s}')$ of the NSTR model (8.1) can be estimated respectively by (8.10), (8.7) and (8.8) from the IC dataset, as discussed in Section 8.2. These estimated functions can be used for describing the estimated *regular spatio-temporal pattern* of the disease incidence rate in cases when no disease outbreaks are present. Then, the estimated regular spatio-temporal pattern can be used for online monitoring of the observed disease incidence rates for disease surveillance, as discussed in Yang and Qiu (2020). The related disease surveillance method developed in Yang and Qiu (2020) is introduced in this section.

Assume that the observed disease incidence rates to monitor are collected at times $\{t_i^*, i \geq 1\}$ and spatial locations $\{\boldsymbol{s}_{ij}^* \in \Omega, j = 1, 2, \ldots, m_i^*, i \geq 1\}$. We use "*" in these notations to distinguish them from those in the IC dataset. When no disease outbreaks are present, the observed disease incidence rates $\{y(t_i^*, \boldsymbol{s}_{ij}^*), j = 1, 2, \ldots, m_i^*, i \geq 1\}$ are assumed to follow the NSTR model (8.1) in the sense that

$$y(t_i^*, \boldsymbol{s}_{ij}^*) = \mu(t_i^*, \boldsymbol{s}_{ij}^*) + \varepsilon(t_i^*, \boldsymbol{s}_{ij}^*), \qquad \text{for } j = 1, 2, \ldots, m_i^*, i \geq 1,$$

where the mean function $\mu(t, \boldsymbol{s})$ has been extended periodically from $[0, T]$ to $[0, \infty)$ with the period T. Namely, $\mu(t_i^*, \boldsymbol{s}_{ij}^*) = \mu(t_i^{**}, \boldsymbol{s}_{ij}^*)$, where $t_i^* = t_i^{**} + \ell T$ for all i, $t_i^{**} \in [0, T]$, and $\ell \geq 1$ is an integer. For instance, if the complete cycle of seasonality in the disease incidence rates is a whole year, which is the case for many infectious diseases, then $T = 1$ (year), and $\mu(t, \boldsymbol{s})$ is assumed to be periodic in different years to reflect the yearly seasonality when no disease outbreaks are present. In some applications, the period T may not be known and thus needs to be estimated from the IC data. In the statistical literature, there have been some discussions on estimation of the period T. See, for instance, Sun et al. (2012) and Vogt and Linton (2014).

As mentioned in Section 8.1, the conventional control charts in the literature are designed for cases when process observations at different observation times are independent and identically distributed when the process under monitoring is IC. In the current disease surveillance problem, however, all these assumptions could be violated. Thus, before online process monitoring, process observations should be decorrelated and standardized properly, as discussed in Li and Qiu (2016) and Li and Qiu (2017). See Section 4.4 for a related description. However, the data decorrelation and standardization procedures discussed in Li and Qiu (2016) and Li and Qiu (2017) cannot be applied to the current problem directly, because the observed data at a given time point is a scalar number or a vector in the problems considered there while they are spatially distributed in the region Ω here. So, data decorrelation and standardization in the current problem would be more challenging. To address this issue, Yang and Qiu (2020) suggested a decorrelation and standardization procedure for handling spatio-temporal data, which is discussed in detail below.

For each i, let

$$\begin{aligned} \boldsymbol{y}(t_i^*) &= \left(y(t_i^*, \boldsymbol{s}_{i1}^*), y(t_i^*, \boldsymbol{s}_{i2}^*), \ldots, y(t_i^*, \boldsymbol{s}_{im_i^*}^*)\right)', \\ \boldsymbol{\mu}(t_i^*) &= \left(\mu(t_i^{**}, \boldsymbol{s}_{i1}^*), \mu(t_i^{**}, \boldsymbol{s}_{i2}^*), \ldots, \mu(t_i^{**}, \boldsymbol{s}_{im_i^*}^*)\right)', \end{aligned}$$

and $\boldsymbol{\varepsilon}(t_i^*) = \boldsymbol{y}(t_i^*) - \boldsymbol{\mu}(t_i^*)$. Assume that t_i^* is the current observation time during online process monitoring, and all historical data at previous time points $t_{i-1}^*, t_{i-2}^*, \ldots, t_1^*$ have been decorrelated and standardized properly. The decorrelated and standardized data at the previous time points are denoted as $\boldsymbol{e}(t_1^*), \boldsymbol{e}(t_2^*), \ldots, \boldsymbol{e}(t_{i-1}^*)$. After the observation $\boldsymbol{y}(t_i^*)$ at the current time point is obtained, we want to decorrelate it with all previous observations, which can be accomplished by the algorithm described below. Let the covariance matrix of $\boldsymbol{\varepsilon}_i = (\boldsymbol{\varepsilon}_{i-1}', \boldsymbol{\varepsilon}(t_i^*)')'$ be denoted as

$$\boldsymbol{\Sigma}_{ii} = \begin{pmatrix} \boldsymbol{\Sigma}_{i-1,i-1} & \boldsymbol{V}_{i-1,i} \\ \boldsymbol{V}_{i-1,i}' & \boldsymbol{V}_{ii} \end{pmatrix},$$

where $\boldsymbol{\varepsilon}_1 = \boldsymbol{\varepsilon}(t_1^*)$, $\boldsymbol{\Sigma}_{i-1,i-1} = \mathrm{Cov}(\boldsymbol{\varepsilon}_{i-1})$, $\boldsymbol{V}_{i-1,i} = \mathrm{Cov}(\boldsymbol{\varepsilon}_{i-1}, \boldsymbol{\varepsilon}(t_i^*))$ and $\boldsymbol{V}_{ii} = \mathrm{Cov}(\boldsymbol{\varepsilon}(t_i^*))$. By the Cholesky decomposition of $\boldsymbol{\Sigma}_{ii}$, we have $\boldsymbol{\Phi}_i \boldsymbol{\Sigma}_{ii} \boldsymbol{\Phi}_i' = \boldsymbol{D}_i$, where

$$\boldsymbol{\Phi}_i = \begin{pmatrix} \boldsymbol{\Phi}_{i-1} & \boldsymbol{0} \\ -\boldsymbol{V}_{i-1,i}' \boldsymbol{\Sigma}_{i-1,i-1}^{-1} & \boldsymbol{I}_{m_i^*} \end{pmatrix},$$

$\boldsymbol{D}_i = \mathrm{diag}\{\boldsymbol{V}_{11}, \boldsymbol{V}_{22\cdot 1}, ..., \boldsymbol{V}_{ii\cdot i-1}\}$, and $\boldsymbol{V}_{ii\cdot i-1} = \boldsymbol{V}_{ii} - \boldsymbol{V}_{i-1,i}' \boldsymbol{\Sigma}_{i-1,i-1}^{-1} \boldsymbol{V}_{i-1,i}$ for each i. Then, we define

$$\boldsymbol{e}(t_i^*) = \boldsymbol{V}_{ii\cdot i-1}^{-\frac{1}{2}} \left(\boldsymbol{\varepsilon}(t_i^*) - \boldsymbol{V}_{i-1,i}' \boldsymbol{\Sigma}_{i-1,i-1}^{-1} \boldsymbol{\varepsilon}_{i-1}\right). \tag{8.13}$$

It can be checked that $\mathrm{Cov}(\boldsymbol{e}_i) = \boldsymbol{I}_{m_1^*+m_2^*+\cdots+m_i^*}$, where

$$\boldsymbol{e}_i = (\boldsymbol{e}_{i-1}', \boldsymbol{e}(t_i^*)')' = \boldsymbol{V}_{ii\cdot i-1}^{-\frac{1}{2}} \Phi_i \boldsymbol{\varepsilon}_i.$$

Thus, $\boldsymbol{e}(t_1^*), \boldsymbol{e}(t_2^*), \ldots, \boldsymbol{e}(t_i^*)$ are mutually uncorrelated with covariance matrices $\boldsymbol{I}_{m_1^*}, \boldsymbol{I}_{m_2^*}, \ldots, \boldsymbol{I}_{m_i^*}$, respectively. Namely, they are spatio-temporally uncorrelated. In practice, the quantities $\boldsymbol{\varepsilon}(t_i^*)$, $\boldsymbol{\varepsilon}_{i-1}$, $\boldsymbol{V}_{ii\cdot i-1}$, $\boldsymbol{V}_{i-1,i}$ and $\boldsymbol{\Sigma}_{i-1,i-1}$ on the right-hand-side of (8.13) are all unobservable. But, they can be replaced by their estimates, using the estimated mean, variance, and covariance functions $\widehat{\mu}(t, \boldsymbol{s})$, $\sigma^2(t, \boldsymbol{s})$, and $\widehat{V}(t, \boldsymbol{s}; t', \boldsymbol{s}')$ defined in (8.10), (8.7) and (8.8), respectively. The resulting decorrelated and standardized data are denoted as $\widehat{\boldsymbol{e}}(t_1^*), \widehat{\boldsymbol{e}}(t_2^*), \ldots, \widehat{\boldsymbol{e}}(t_i^*)$. They should be asymptotically uncorrelated with each other, and each has the asymptotic mean $\boldsymbol{0}$ and the asymptotic identity covariance matrix.

In the above sequential data decorrelation and standardization procedure, we need to calculate the inverse matrix $\boldsymbol{\Sigma}_{ii}^{-1}$, for each i. The matrix $\boldsymbol{\Sigma}_{ii}$ has the dimension of $(m_1^* + m_2^* + \cdots + m_i^*) \times (m_1^* + m_2^* + \cdots + m_i^*)$, which is large when i gets large. Thus, computation of its inverse matrix would be computationally intensive. To reduce the computing burden, the following recursive formula should be helpful: for $i > 1$,

$$\boldsymbol{\Sigma}_{ii}^{-1} = \begin{pmatrix} \boldsymbol{\Sigma}_{i-1,i-1}^{-1} + \boldsymbol{\Sigma}_{i-1,i-1}^{-1}\boldsymbol{V}_{i-1,i}\boldsymbol{V}_{ii\cdot i-1}^{-1}\boldsymbol{V}_{i-1,i}'\boldsymbol{\Sigma}_{i-1,i-1}^{-1} & -\boldsymbol{\Sigma}_{i-1,i-1}^{-1}\boldsymbol{V}_{i-1,i}\boldsymbol{V}_{ii\cdot i-1}^{-1} \\ -\boldsymbol{V}_{ii\cdot i-1}^{-1}\boldsymbol{V}_{i-1,i}'\boldsymbol{\Sigma}_{i-1,i-1}^{-1} & \boldsymbol{V}_{ii\cdot i-1}^{-1} \end{pmatrix}.$$

When i increases, besides the computing burden mentioned above for computing the inverse matrix $\boldsymbol{\Sigma}_{ii}^{-1}$, the storage of this matrix would be demanding as well, because its dimension increases with i. The above recursive formula can partially address these challenges. An alternative strategy suggested in Yang and Qiu (2020) is described below. First, we notice that

$$\boldsymbol{e}(t_i^*) = \boldsymbol{V}_{ii\cdot i-1}^{-\frac{1}{2}} \left[\boldsymbol{\varepsilon}(t_i^*) - \sum_{j=1}^{i-1} \boldsymbol{B}_{i,j}\boldsymbol{V}_{jj\cdot j-1}^{-1}\boldsymbol{e}(t_{j-1}^*) \right],$$

where $\boldsymbol{V}_{11\cdot 0} = \boldsymbol{V}_{11}$, and $\boldsymbol{B}_{i,j} = \mathrm{Cov}(\boldsymbol{\varepsilon}(t_i^*), \boldsymbol{e}(t_j^*))$ for each i and j. In practice, it is often reasonable to assume that the correlation between $\boldsymbol{\varepsilon}(t_i^*)$ and $\boldsymbol{\varepsilon}(t_j^*)$ becomes weaker when the two time points t_i^* and t_j^* are farther apart. Thus, it is often reasonable to assume that $\boldsymbol{B}_{i,j} = \boldsymbol{0}$ when $t_i^* - t_j^* > r_{max}$, where $r_{max} > 0$ denotes the time range of serial data correlation. By using this assumption, the computing and data storage demands can be reduced greatly without sacrificing much effectiveness of the online process monitoring procedure.

After data decorrelation and standardization, the original observations $\{\boldsymbol{y}(t_i^*), i \geq 1\}$ have been transformed to the asymptotically uncorrelated ones $\{\widehat{\boldsymbol{e}}(t_i^*), i \geq 1\}$. Assume that t_i^* is the current observation time during online process monitoring and we need to make a decision whether there is a disease outbreak at t_i^* after the observed data $\boldsymbol{y}(t_i^*)$ have been collected. To this end, because $\widehat{\boldsymbol{e}}(t_i^*)$ is a linear combination of the random errors in the NSTR model (8.1) (cf., Equation (8.13)), its distribution would be close to $N_{m_i^*}(\boldsymbol{0}, \boldsymbol{I}_{m_i^* \times m_i^*})$

if $\boldsymbol{y}(t_i^*)$ is correlated with a substantial number of previous spatial observations. Consequently, the distribution of $\widehat{\boldsymbol{e}}(t_i^*)'\widehat{\boldsymbol{e}}(t_i^*)$ would be close to $\chi^2_{m_i^*}$ in such cases. Then, it is natural to use the following CUSUM charting statistic to sequentially detect shifts in the observed disease incidence rates:

$$C_i^+ = \max\left(0, C_{i-1}^+ + \frac{\widehat{\boldsymbol{e}}(t_i^*)'\widehat{\boldsymbol{e}}(t_i^*) - m_i^*}{\sqrt{2m_i^*}} - k\right), \qquad \text{for } i \geq 1, \tag{8.14}$$

where $C_0^+ = 0$, $k > 0$ is an allowance constant, and $[\widehat{\boldsymbol{e}}(t_i^*)'\widehat{\boldsymbol{e}}(t_i^*) - m_i^*]/\sqrt{2m_i^*}$ is the standardized version of $\widehat{\boldsymbol{e}}(t_i^*)'\widehat{\boldsymbol{e}}(t_i^*)$. The chart gives a signal of an upward mean shift in the observed disease incidence rates when

$$C_i^+ > \rho, \tag{8.15}$$

where $\rho > 0$ is a control limit. The charting statistic C_i^+ has made use of all historical data by using the cumulative information in the observed data. It is reset to 0 each time when the cumulative sum $C_{i-1}^+ + [\widehat{\boldsymbol{e}}(t_i^*)'\widehat{\boldsymbol{e}}(t_i^*) - m_i^*]/\sqrt{2m_i^*}$ is smaller than k. This re-starting mechanism makes it have some good theoretical properties (Moustakides, 1986). See a more detailed discussion about the CUSUM chart in Subsection 3.1.3.

As discussed in Subsection 3.1.3, to evaluate the performance of the CUSUM chart (8.14)–(8.15), in the SPC literature, we usually use the IC average run length (ARL), denoted as ARL_0, which is the average number of observation times from the beginning of process monitoring to the signal time when the process under monitoring is IC, and the OC ARL, denoted as ARL_1, which is the average number of observation times from the process shift time to the signal time after the process under monitoring becomes OC. Usually, the ARL_0 value is pre-specified at a given level, and the chart performs better if its ARL_1 value is smaller when detecting a shift of a given size. In disease surveillance, observation times of disease incidence rates are usually equally spaced. In such cases, ARL_0 and ARL_1 should be reasonable metrics to evaluate the performance of control charts. In cases when the observation times are unequally spaced, they would not be good performance metrics any more, as discussed in Subsection 4.2.3. In such cases, the IC and OC average time to signal (ATS) metrics should be used instead.

In the CUSUM chart (8.14)–(8.15), there are two parameters k and ρ to choose. Usually, k is pre-specified, and then ρ is chosen to achieve a given ARL_0 value. It has been well demonstrated in the SPC literature that a large k value is good for detecting large shifts, and a small k value is good for detecting small shifts (cf., Qiu, 2014). Commonly used k values include 0.1, 0.2, 0.5 and 1.0. If the IC distribution of $\widehat{\boldsymbol{e}}(t_i^*)$ is exactly $N_{m_i^*}(\boldsymbol{0}, \boldsymbol{I}_{m_i^* \times m_i^*})$, for each i, then the control limit ρ can be computed easily by Monte Carlo simulations. However, when i is small or when $\boldsymbol{y}(t_i^*)$ is correlated with a small number of previous spatial observations, the true distribution of $\widehat{\boldsymbol{e}}(t_i^*)$ could be substantially different from $N_{m_i^*}(\boldsymbol{0}, \boldsymbol{I}_{m_i^* \times m_i^*})$ in cases when the distribution of the original data is substantially different from a normal distribution. To make the CUSUM chart (8.14)–(8.15) robust to the normality of $\widehat{e}(t_i^*)$, Yang and Qiu (2020) suggested using a block bootstrap procedure (cf., Lahiri, 2003) for determining the control limit ρ from the IC dataset, which is described below.

For the IC dataset $\{y(t_i, \boldsymbol{s}_{ij}), j = 1, 2, \ldots, m_i, i = 1, 2, \ldots, n\}$, let us divide it into two parts:

$$\left\{y(t_i^{(1)}, \boldsymbol{s}_{ij}^{(1)}), j = 1, 2, \ldots, m_i^{(1)}, i = 1, 2, \ldots, n_1\right\}$$

and

$$\left\{y(t_i^{(2)}, \boldsymbol{s}_{ij}^{(2)}), j = 1, 2, \ldots, m_i^{(2)}, i = 1, 2, \ldots, n_2\right\},$$

where $n_1 + n_2 = n$. The first part is used for obtaining the estimates of $\mu(t, \boldsymbol{s})$, $\sigma^2(t, \boldsymbol{s})$ and $V(t, t'; \boldsymbol{s}, \boldsymbol{s}')$, as described in Section 8.2, and the second part is used for determining ρ as follows.

Step 1 Compute the decorrelated and standardized data $\{\widehat{e}(t_i^{(2)}), i = 1, 2, ..., n_2\}$ from the original data $\{y(t_i^{(2)}, \boldsymbol{s}_{ij}^{(2)}), j = 1, 2, \ldots, m_i^{(2)}, i = 1, 2, \ldots, n_2\}$, as discussed above (cf., Equation (8.13)).

Step 2 Randomly select a sequence of integers from $\{1, 2, ..., n_2 - b + 1\}$ with replacement, where b is a pre-specified block size. The selected integers are denoted as $\{i_1, i_2, \ldots\}$. For a given control limit ρ, calculate the run length (RL) by $RL_0(\rho) = \min\{i \geq 1, C_i^+ > \rho\}$, where C_i^+ is calculated by (8.14) after the decorrelated data $\{\widehat{e}(t_i^*), i \geq 1\}$ are replaced by the bootstrap sample

$$\left\{\widehat{e}(t_{i_1}^{(2)}), \widehat{e}(t_{i_1+1}^{(2)}), \ldots, \widehat{e}(t_{i_1+b-1}^{(2)}), \widehat{e}(t_{i_2}^{(2)}), \widehat{e}(t_{i_2+1}^{(2)}), \ldots, \widehat{e}(t_{i_2+b-1}^{(2)}), \ldots\right\}.$$

This process is then repeated for B times, and the average of the B values of $RL_0(\rho)$ is denoted as $ARL_0(\rho)$.

Step 3 Search for the ρ value by the bisection or other alternative numerical procedures (e.g., Capizzi and Masarotto, 2016) such that $ARL_0(\rho)$ equals the pre-specified value of ARL_0.

Example 8.5 *In this example, let us demonstrate the disease surveillance method discussed in this section using the ILI dataset described in Example 8.1. In this dataset, numbers of new cases of ILI in all 67 counties (i.e., $m_i =$ 67 for all i in the NSTR model (8.1)) were collected daily from 2012 to 2015. Then, the ILI incidence rate on a specific day for each county can be calculated as the ratio of the number of ILI patients on that day and the county population size that can be obtained from the webpage of the Florida Office of Economic and Demographic Research (http://edr.state.fl.us/Content/population-demographics/data/). The calculated ILI incidence rates of the four representative counties Collier, Nassau, Pinellas and Santa Rosa during 2012–2015* *are shown in Figure 8.4. From the plots in the figure, it can be seen that the observed disease incidence rates have seasonal patterns with winter peaks and summer troughs, and that it seems reasonable to assume that the pattern of the observed disease incidence rates is periodic from one year to the next.*

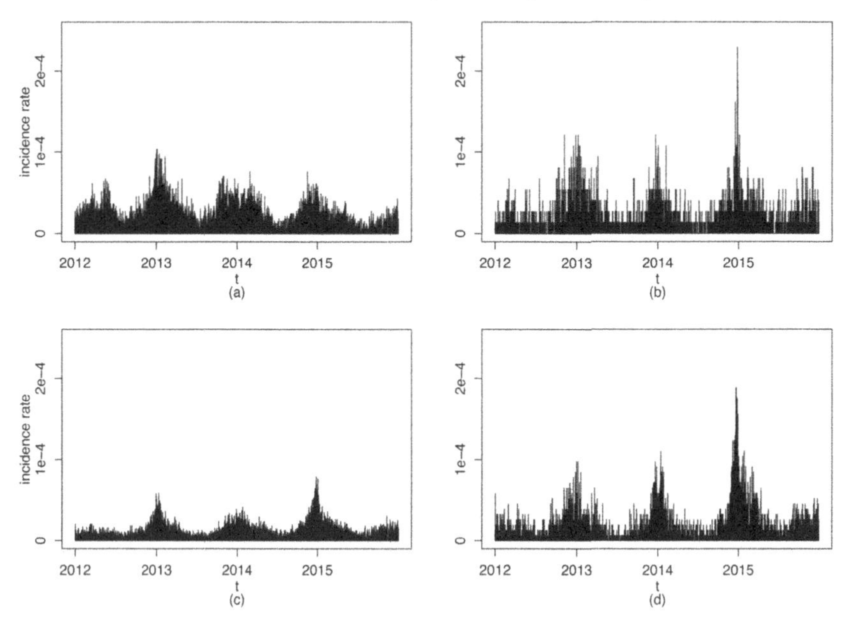

FIGURE 8.4
Observed ILI incidence rates in four representative counties of Florida during 2012–2015: Collier (plot (a)), Nassau (plot (b)), Pinellas (plot (c)) and Santa Rosa (plot (d)).

From Figure 8.4, it seems that there were no major disease outbreaks during the years 2012 and 2013. Therefore, that part of the data is used as the IC data in this example for setting up the CUSUM chart (8.14)–(8.15). For this IC dataset, the Durbin-Watson test for checking the temporal data correlation in the four representative counties Collier, Nassau, Pinellas and Santa Rosa gives the p-values of $2.2 \times 10^{-16}, 0.018, 2.2 \times 10^{-16}$, *and* 2.2×10^{-16}, *respectively, implying significant temporal data correlation in the four counties. The Moran's I test for checking spatial correlation for the data on 06/01/2012 and 12/01/2012 (cf., Figure 8.1) gives the p-values of 0.471 and 0.004, respectively. So, the spatial correlation on 12/01/2012 (a winter time) is significant, although the observed data on 06/01/2012 do not show a significant spatial correlation. The IC data are then divided into two parts, as discussed above. The IC data in the year 2013 are used for estimating the mean, variance and covariance functions of the NSTR model (8.1), and the IC data in the year 2012 are used for determining the control limit* ρ *of the CUSUM chart (8.14)–(8.15) by the block bootstrap procedure with* $B = 10{,}000$ *and* $b = 5$. *In* *the chart, we choose $k = 0.1$ and $ARL_0 = 200$, which are commonly used in the SPC literature. Then, the chart is used to sequentially monitor the observed disease incidence rates, starting on January 1, 2014. This chart is presented in Figure 8.5. From the plot, the chart gives the first signal of disease outbreak on October 16, 2014.*

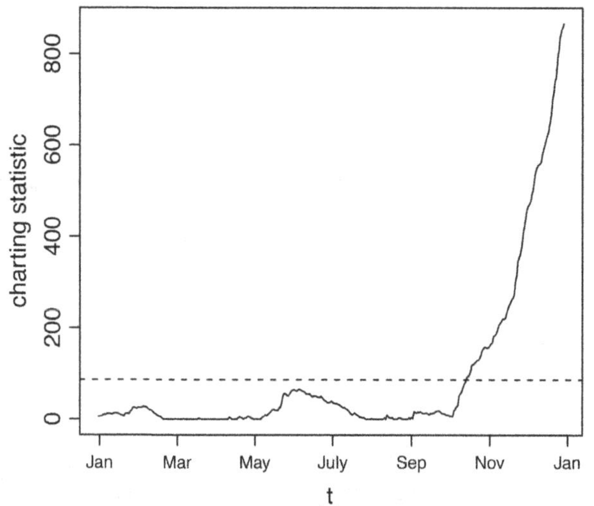

FIGURE 8.5
The CUSUM chart (8.14)–(8.15) for monitoring the observed ILI incidence rates starting from January 1, 2014 in cases when $k = 0.1$ and $ARL_0 = 200$. The dashed horizontal line in the plot denotes its control limit.

To check whether the signal of the CUSUM chart (8.14)–(8.15) is valid, the observed disease incidence rates in the entire Florida state from September 1 to December 31 in the years 2012, 2013 and 2014 are shown in Figure 8.6. From the figure, it can be seen that the observed disease incidence rates are quite similar in the month of September among the three years, and the observed data in 2014 start to deviate upward from those in 2012 and 2013 beginning in October. This plot shows that a real disease outbreak occurs in the first half of October in 2014, and the CUSUM chart (8.14)–(8.15) can detect such a disease outbreak shortly after it occurs.

To further study the validity of the signal by the CUSUM chart (8.14)–(8.15), we present the residuals $\widehat{\boldsymbol{\varepsilon}}(t_i^*) = \boldsymbol{y}(t_i^*) - \widehat{\boldsymbol{\mu}}(t_i^{**})$ on October 16th of the years 2012, 2013, and 2014 in the three maps of Figure 8.7, where $\widehat{\boldsymbol{\mu}}(t_i^{**})$ is the estimated values of $\boldsymbol{\mu}(t_i^{**})$ from the IC data and t_i^{**} is the time in $[0, T]$ that corresponds to t_i^* (cf., the related discussion in the second paragraph of this section). It can be seen that the residual map for the year 2014 has stronger colors, implying that the residual values are larger in that year, compared to those in the years 2012 and 2013. As an example, the Jackson county on the northern border has a strong color in the year 2014, and its color is light in the previous two years. The observed disease incidence rates of this county

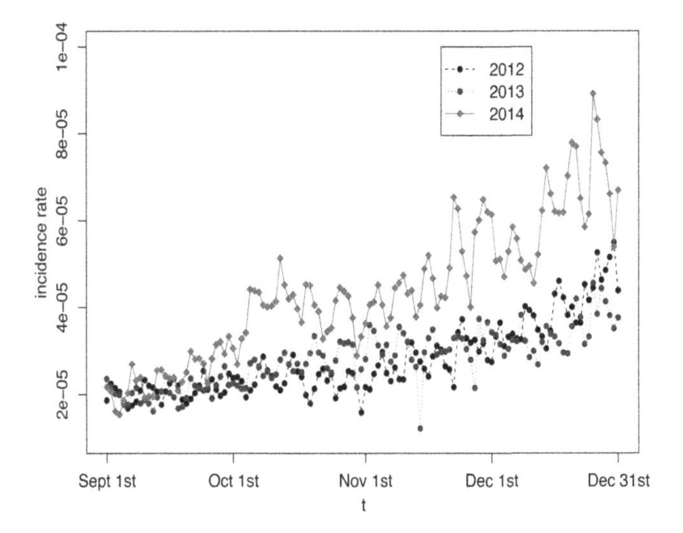

FIGURE 8.6
Observed disease incidence rates of the entire Florida state from September 1 to December 31 in the years 2012, 2013 and 2014.

during the years 2012–2015 are shown in Figure 8.8, where the vertical line denotes the signal time of the CUSUM chart (8.14)–(8.15). It can be seen that the observed disease incidence rates in this county start to increase a bit earlier than the signal time and the CUSUM chart can successfully detect the increasing trend before the major disease outbreak in December 2014.

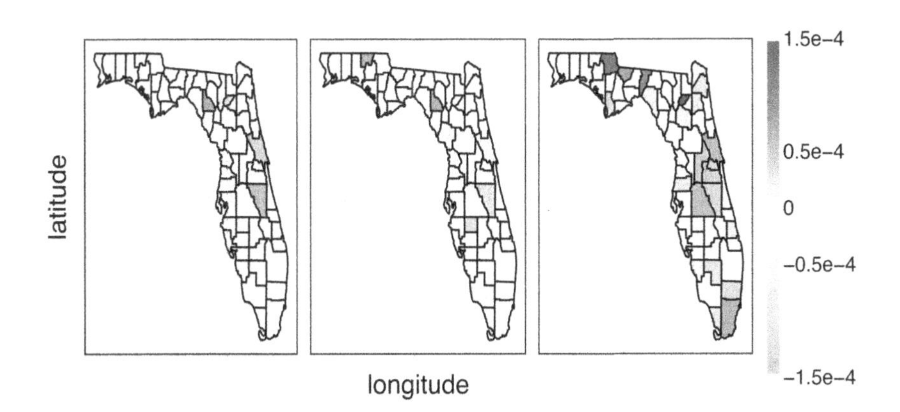

FIGURE 8.7
Maps of the residuals on October 16th of the years 2012 (left), 2013 (middle) and 2014 (right).

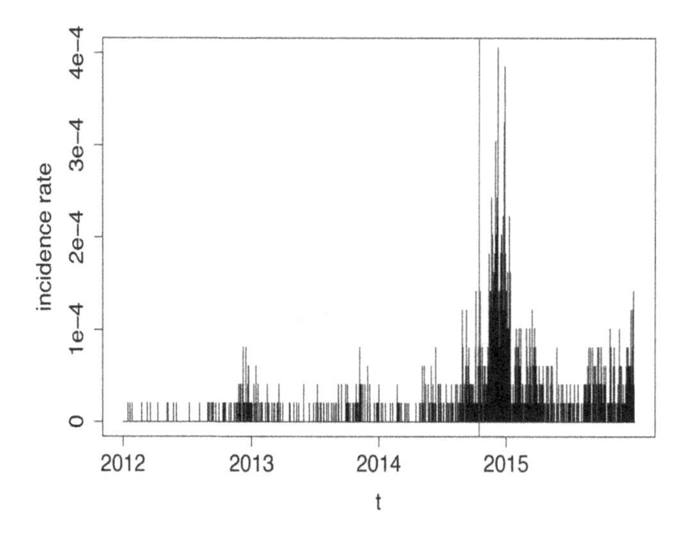

FIGURE 8.8
Observed disease incidence rates of the Jackson county in the years 2012–2015. The vertical line indicates the signal time of the CUSUM chart (8.14)–(8.15).

8.4 Disease Surveillance by Exponentially Weighted Spatial LASSO

In disease surveillance, a disease outbreak often starts in small clustered regions. For instance, outbreaks of infectious diseases like Ebora and COVID-19 usually start in some small communities and then spread to a larger population. For such applications, one intuitive idea is to first find the small regions with possible shifts in the disease incidence rates at each observation time during process monitoring, and then focus on the observed data in these small regions to make a decision about the process status at a given observation time. To this end, variable selection methods like the LASSO and adaptive LASSO procedures (cf., Tibshirani, 1996; Zou, 2006) should be helpful. In the SPC literature, there have been some discussions on process monitoring using such variable selection methods. See, for instance, Wang and Jiang (2009), Zou and Qiu (2009) and Zou et al. (2012a). However, these process monitoring methods are designed mainly for monitoring high-dimensional data or linear profiles. They are not suitable for monitoring spatio-temporal data because the spatio-temporal data structure is not considered by them. Also, these existing methods assume that process observations at different time points are independent, which is rarely valid in applications like disease surveillance. To overcome these limitations, Qiu and Yang (2023) developed a new control chart for spatio-temporal disease surveillance. The new method is based on the following two major ideas. First, to find small regions with possible shifts in the observed disease incidence rates at each observation time, a spatial LASSO procedure is suggested in the space domain, which can accommodate spatial data structure during variable selection. Second, to make use of all historical data for online process monitoring, an exponentially weighted smoothing procedure is suggested in the time domain to combine helpful information in all available spatio-temporal data by the current observation time for effective process monitoring. These two ideas are then combined seamlessly in the space-time domain for disease surveillance. This method is introduced in detail below.

Assume that an IC dataset has been collected before online process monitoring, and

$$\{y(t_i, \boldsymbol{s}_{ij}), j = 1, 2, \ldots, m_i, i = 1, 2, \ldots, n\}$$

are the observations in the IC dataset, where $t_i \in [0, T]$ is the ith observation time, $\boldsymbol{s}_{ij} \in \Omega$ is the jth observation location at time t_i, m_i is the number of spatial locations at t_i, and n is the number of observation times in the IC data. These IC data are assumed to follow the NSTR model (8.1). Then, the mean function $\mu(t, \boldsymbol{s})$, the variance function $\sigma^2(t, \boldsymbol{s})$, and the covariance function $V(t, t'; \boldsymbol{s}, \boldsymbol{s}')$ can be estimated by the methods discussed in Section 8.2 (cf., Expressions (8.10), (8.7) and (8.8)). Their estimates are denoted as $\widehat{\mu}(t, \boldsymbol{s})$, $\widehat{\sigma}^2(t, \boldsymbol{s})$, and $\widehat{V}(t, t'; \boldsymbol{s}, \boldsymbol{s}')$, respectively,

After the NSTR model (8.1) is estimated, the estimated regular spatio-temporal pattern of the observed disease incidence rates can be described by the estimated mean, variance, and covariance functions $\widehat{\mu}(t, \boldsymbol{s})$, $\widehat{\sigma}^2(t, \boldsymbol{s})$, and $\widehat{V}(t, t'; \boldsymbol{s}, \boldsymbol{s}')$, for $t, t' \in [0, T]$ and $\boldsymbol{s}, \boldsymbol{s}' \in \Omega$. Then, the estimated regular spatio-temporal pattern can be used for online process monitoring, after the estimated mean, variance, and covariance functions are extended periodically in the time domain from $[0, T]$ to $[0, \infty)$, as discussed in Section 8.3.

Let $\{y(t_i^*, \boldsymbol{s}_{ij}^*), j = 1, 2, \ldots, m_i^*, i \geq 1\}$ be the spatio-temporal process observations for online monitoring, where $\{t_i^* \in (T, \infty), i \geq 1\}$ are the observation times and $\{\boldsymbol{s}_{ij}^* \in \Omega, j = 1, 2, \ldots, m_i^*, i \geq 1\}$ are the observation locations. These process observations could be spatio-temporally correlated and their IC mean and variance values could vary over both space and time. Therefore, they need to be decorrelated and standardized properly before a control chart can be applied to them for disease surveillance since a conventional control chart is designed for cases when process observations are independent and have an identical IC distribution. To this end, the data decorrelation and standardization procedure described in Section 8.3 can be used. After using this procedure, the original process observations $\{y(t_i^*, \boldsymbol{s}_{ij}^*), j = 1, 2, \ldots, m_i^*, i \geq 1\}$ are transformed to the decorrelated and standardized observations $\{\widehat{e}(t_i^*, \boldsymbol{s}_{ij}^*), j = 1, 2, \ldots, m_i^*, i \geq 1\}$. These decorrelated and standardized observations would be asymptotically uncorrelated with each other, and each has the asymptotic mean 0 and the asymptotic variance 1 when the process under monitoring is IC.

After data decorrelation and standardization, we are ready to monitor the decorrelated and standardized observations $\{\widehat{e}(t_i^*, \boldsymbol{s}_{ij}^*), j = 1, 2, \ldots, m_i^*, i \geq 1\}$. To this end, by the general principles of sequential process monitoring (cf., Qiu, 2014, Chapters 4 and 5), we should use as much available information as possible about the process under monitoring, and give less weights to process observations collected farther away from the current observation time. To accomplish these goals, the following exponentially weighted kernel smoothing (EWKS) procedure can be considered for estimating the mean function of $\widehat{e}(t_i^*, \boldsymbol{s})$, denoted as $\mu_{\widehat{e}}(t_i^*, \boldsymbol{s})$, at the current observation time t_i^* and at a given spatial location $\boldsymbol{s} \in \Omega$:

$$\min_{a \in \mathbb{R}} \sum_{k=1}^{i} \sum_{j=1}^{m_k^*} \left[\widehat{e}(t_k^*, \boldsymbol{s}_{kj}^*) - a\right]^2 K_s\left(\frac{d_E(\boldsymbol{s}_{kj}^*, \boldsymbol{s})}{h}\right)(1-\lambda)^{(t_i^* - t_k^*)}, \tag{8.16}$$

where $K_s(\cdot)$ is a pre-specified kernel function, $h > 0$ is a bandwidth, $d_E(\cdot, \cdot)$ denotes the Euclidean distance, and $\lambda \in (0, 1]$ is a weighting parameter. The solution to a of the minimization procedure (8.16), denoted as $\widetilde{\mu}_{\widehat{e}}(t_i^*, \boldsymbol{s})$, is the local constant kernel estimate of $\mu_{\widehat{e}}(t_i^*, \boldsymbol{s})$ (cf., Subsection 2.5.5). Here, the local constant kernel smoothing procedure, instead of the more popular local linear kernel smoothing procedure, is used because the spatio-temporal trend in the observed data has been mostly removed when computing the decorrelated and standardized observations $\{\widehat{e}(t_i^*, \boldsymbol{s}_{ij}^*), j = 1, 2, \ldots, m_i^*, i \geq 1\}$.

In the minimization procedure (8.16), the kernel function $K_s(\cdot)$ should be chosen to be a decreasing function in $[0, \infty)$ so that process observations collected at places farther away from the given location $\boldsymbol{s}$ would receive less weights in function estimation. Similarly, the exponential weights $(1-\lambda)^{(t_i^* - t_k^*)}$ are used in (8.16) so that process observations collected at times farther away from the current observation time t_i^* would receive less weights. By similar arguments to those in Subsection 2.5.5 (cf., Equation (2.50)), it can be checked that $\widetilde{\mu}_{\widehat{e}}(t_i^*, \boldsymbol{s})$ is a linear combination of all current and previous process observations, with the weights exponentially decaying for older observations.

From the above intuitive explanation, the EWKS procedure (8.16) can be regarded as a combination of the exponentially weighted moving average (EWMA) procedure (cf., Subsection 3.1.4) commonly used in the SPC literature and the local constant kernel smoothing procedure in nonparametric regression (cf., Subsection 2.5.5). The bandwidth h used in (8.16) can be chosen by minimizing the following cross-validation (CV) score (cf., Subsection 2.5.5):

$$CV(h) = \frac{1}{m_i^*} \sum_{j=1}^{m_i^*} \left[\widehat{e}(t_i^*, \boldsymbol{s}_{ij}^*) - \widetilde{\mu}_{\widehat{e}, -(ij)}(t_i^*, \boldsymbol{s}_{ij}^*)\right]^2, \tag{8.17}$$

where $\widetilde{\mu}_{\widehat{e},-(ij)}(t_i^*, \boldsymbol{s}_{ij}^*)$ is the estimate of $\mu_{\widehat{e}}(t_i^*, \boldsymbol{s}_{ij}^*)$ obtained by the EWKS procedure (8.16) after the data point $\widehat{e}(t_i^*, \boldsymbol{s}_{ij}^*)$ is excluded from the estimation. It should be pointed out that although the original process observations are spatio-temporally correlated, the decorrelated and standardized observations $\{\widehat{e}(t_i^*, \boldsymbol{s}_{ij}^*), j = 1, 2, \ldots, m_i^*, i \geq 1\}$ would be asymptotically uncorrelated. Thus, the regular CV procedure should be appropriate to use here, instead of the modified CV procedure (8.6) discussed in Subsection 8.2.2.

Intuitively, when the process under monitoring is IC at t_i^*, the values of $\{|\widetilde{\mu}_{\widehat{e}}(t_i^*, \boldsymbol{s}_{ij}^*)|, j = 1, 2, \ldots, m_i^*\}$ should be all small. Thus, a natural charting statistic for process monitoring would be

$$\widetilde{T}_i = \widetilde{\boldsymbol{\mu}}_{\widehat{e},i}' \widetilde{\Sigma}_{\widetilde{\boldsymbol{\mu}}_{\widehat{e},i}}^{-1} \widetilde{\boldsymbol{\mu}}_{\widehat{e},i},$$

where $\widetilde{\boldsymbol{\mu}}_{\widehat{e},i} = (\widetilde{\mu}_{\widehat{e}}(t_i^*, \boldsymbol{s}_{i1}^*), \widetilde{\mu}_{\widehat{e}}(t_i^*, \boldsymbol{s}_{i2}^*), \ldots, \widetilde{\mu}_{\widehat{e}}(t_i^*, \boldsymbol{s}_{im_i^*}^*))'$ and $\widetilde{\Sigma}_{\widetilde{\boldsymbol{\mu}}_{\widehat{e},i}}$ is the estimated covariance matrix of $\widetilde{\boldsymbol{\mu}}_{\widehat{e},i}$. But, this statistic treats all observation locations $\{\boldsymbol{s}_{ij}^*, j = 1, 2, \ldots, m_i^*\}$ equally. Thus, it would not be effective for many disease surveillance problems in which a disease outbreak starts in small clustered regions in the design space Ω. To overcome this limitation, one idea is to first detect the small regions with possible process shifts at t_i^*, and then construct the charting statistic based on the detected small regions. To this end, the LASSO variable selection procedure (Tibshirani, 1996) can be considered. By considering the fact that spatial locations with possible process shifts are usually clustered in small connected regions, instead of a set of isolated spatial locations scattered in Ω, Qiu and Yang (2023) suggested using a spatial LASSO procedure (e.g., Samarov et al., 2015) that took into account the spatial data structure when detecting small clustered regions with possible process shifts. By combining the spatial LASSO idea with the EWKS procedure (8.16), the following penalized EWKS procedure is considered for estimating $\{\mu_{\widehat{e}}(t_i^*, \boldsymbol{s}_{ij}^*), j = 1, 2, \ldots, m_i^*\}$:

$$\min_{a_1, a_2, \ldots, a_{m_i^*}} \left\{ \sum_{j=1}^{m_i^*} \sum_{k=1}^{i} \sum_{l=1}^{m_k^*} \left[\widehat{e}(t_k^*, \boldsymbol{s}_{kl}^*) - a_j\right]^2 K_s\left(\frac{d_E(\boldsymbol{s}_{kl}^*, \boldsymbol{s}_{ij}^*)}{h}\right) (1-\lambda)^{(t_i^* - t_k^*)} \right.$$
$$\left. + \gamma_1 \sum_{j=1}^{m_i^*} \varpi_{1j} |a_j| + \gamma_2 \sum_{j=1}^{m_i^*} \varpi_{2j} \left| a_j - \frac{\sum_{1 \leq l \leq m_i^*} K_s(d_E(\boldsymbol{s}_{ij}^*, \boldsymbol{s}_{il}^*)/h) a_l}{\sum_{1 \leq l \leq m_i^*} K_s(d_E(\boldsymbol{s}_{ij}^*, \boldsymbol{s}_{il}^*)/h)} \right| \right\}, \tag{8.18}$$

where $\varpi_{1j} = 1/|\widetilde{\mu}_{\widehat{e}}(t_i^*, \boldsymbol{s}_{ij}^*)|$ and

$$\varpi_{2j} = 1 \Bigg/ \left| \widetilde{\mu}_{\widehat{e}}(t_i^*, \boldsymbol{s}_{ij}^*) - \frac{\sum_{1 \leq l \leq m_i^*} K_s(d_E(\boldsymbol{s}_{ij}^*, \boldsymbol{s}_{il}^*)/h) \widetilde{\mu}_{\widehat{e}}(t_i^*, \boldsymbol{s}_{il}^*)}{\sum_{1 \leq l \leq m_i^*} K_s(d_E(\boldsymbol{s}_{ij}^*, \boldsymbol{s}_{il}^*)/h)} \right|$$

are the adaptive LASSO weights (Zou, 2006), and $\gamma_1, \gamma_2 > 0$ are two tuning parameters. In (8.18), the last term is the adaptive spatial LASSO penalty. In this term,

$$\left| a_j - \frac{\sum_{1 \le l \le m_i^*} K_s(d_E(\boldsymbol{s}_{ij}^*, \boldsymbol{s}_{il}^*)/h) a_l}{\sum_{1 \le l \le m_i^*} K_s(d_E(\boldsymbol{s}_{ij}^*, \boldsymbol{s}_{il}^*)/h)} \right|$$

measures the difference between the estimated process mean at the jth location with a weighted average of the estimated process means at neighboring locations at the current observation time t_i^*. Thus, this term penalizes the difference among estimated means at neighboring locations, which is desirable for applications in which process shifts are spatially clustered. By a reparameterization, it can be shown that the minimization problem (8.18) is a generalized LASSO procedure and can be implemented by using the path algorithm suggested by Tibshirani and Taylor (2011). The solutions of the minimization problem to $\{a_1, a_2, \ldots, a_{m_i^*}\}$ are defined as the estimates of $\{\mu_{\widehat{e}}(t_i^*, \boldsymbol{s}_{ij}^*), j = 1, 2, \ldots, m_i^*\}$, denoted as $\{\widehat{\mu}_{\widehat{e}}(t_i^*, \boldsymbol{s}_{ij}^*), j = 1, 2, \ldots, m_i^*\}$.

In the penalized EWKS procedure (8.18), the bandwidth h can still be chosen to be the one determined by the CV procedure (8.17), since the only difference between $\{\widetilde{\mu}_{\widehat{e}}(t_i^*, \boldsymbol{s}_{ij}^*), j = 1, 2, \ldots, m_i^*\}$ determined by (8.16) and $\{\widehat{\mu}_{\widehat{e}}(t_i^*, \boldsymbol{s}_{ij}^*), j = 1, 2, \ldots, m_i^*\}$ determined by (8.18) is that the penalized EWKS procedure would enforce those estimates in the latter that are located outside the small clustered regions with process shifts to be shrunk to zero. Because the overall impact of the shrinkage is quite small for the two sets of estimates, a selected bandwidth that is good for the former should also be reasonably good for the latter. Regarding the two tuning parameters γ_1 and γ_2, they can be chosen by the following Bayesian information criterion (BIC) (Schwarz, 1978):

$$\begin{aligned} BIC(\gamma_1, \gamma_2) \quad = \quad & \log\left(\sum_{j=1}^{m_i^*} \left[\widehat{e}(t_i^*, \boldsymbol{s}_{ij}^*) - \widehat{\mu}_{\widehat{e}}(t_i^*, \boldsymbol{s}_{ij}^*) \right]^2 \right) + \qquad (8.19) \\ & \log(m_i^*) \sum_{j=1}^{m_i^*} I\left(\widehat{\mu}_{\widehat{e}}(t_i^*, \boldsymbol{s}_{ij}^*) \neq 0 \right). \end{aligned}$$

Then, γ_1 and γ_2 are chosen by minimizing $BIC(\gamma_1, \gamma_2)$. The BIC procedure (8.19) is used here because of its consistency property in selecting the true model (cf., Yang, 2005).

From the construction of the penalized EWKS procedure (8.18), it can be seen that the estimates $\{\widehat{\mu}_{\widehat{e}}(t_i^*, \boldsymbol{s}_{ij}^*), j = 1, 2, \ldots, m_i^*\}$ have taken into account the previous process observations through its EWKS component (i.e., the first term of the objective function in (8.18)). The procedure (8.18) is an adaptive LASSO procedure and its shrinkage property guarantees that some elements in $\{\widehat{\mu}_{\widehat{e}}(t_i^*, \boldsymbol{s}_{ij}^*), j = 1, 2, \ldots, m_i^*\}$ would be zero and only those at locations with process shifts would be non-zero. So, to detect process shifts, it is natural to consider

$$T_i = \widehat{\boldsymbol{\mu}}_{\widehat{e},i}' \widehat{\Sigma}_{\widehat{\boldsymbol{\mu}}_{\widehat{e},i}}^{-1} \widehat{\boldsymbol{\mu}}_{\widehat{e},i},$$

where $\widehat{\boldsymbol{\mu}}_{\widehat{e},i} = (\widehat{\mu}_{\widehat{e}}(t_i^*, \boldsymbol{s}_{i1}^*), \widehat{\mu}_{\widehat{e}}(t_i^*, \boldsymbol{s}_{i2}^*), \ldots, \widehat{\mu}_{\widehat{e}}(t_i^*, \boldsymbol{s}_{im_i^*}^*))'$, and $\widehat{\Sigma}_{\widehat{\boldsymbol{\mu}}_{\widehat{e},i}}$ is an estimate of the covariance matrix of $\widehat{\boldsymbol{\mu}}_{\widehat{e},i}$. Then, the charting statistic for disease surveillance is the following standardized version of T_i:

$$ST_i = \frac{T_i - \widehat{\mathrm{E}}(T_i)}{\sqrt{\widehat{\mathrm{Var}}(T_i)}}, \quad \text{for } i \geq 1, \tag{8.20}$$

where $\widehat{\mathrm{E}}(T_i)$ and $\widehat{\mathrm{Var}}(T_i)$ are the estimates of the mean and variance of T_i, respectively. The chart gives a signal of process shift at time t_i^* if

$$ST_i > L, \tag{8.21}$$

where $L > 0$ is a control limit. This chart is called the exponentially weighted spatial LASSO (EWSL) chart hereafter.

To use the control chart (8.20)–(8.21), the two parameters λ and L should be specified properly beforehand. Regarding λ, it is similar to the regular weighting parameter used in an EWMA chart. In the SPC literature, it has been well demonstrated that a large value of the weighting parameter is good for detecting relatively large shifts, and a small value is good for detecting relatively small shifts (cf., Qiu, 2014, Chapter 5). Based on our extensive numerical experience, this is also true here if λ is chosen in the range $(0, 0.1]$. It should be pointed out that, in the current penalized EWKS procedure (8.18), if λ is chosen too large, then the estimate $\widehat{\mu}_{\widehat{e}}(t_i^*, \boldsymbol{s}_{ij}^*)$ would have a relatively large variability in estimating $\mu_{\widehat{e}}(t_i^*, \boldsymbol{s}_{ij}^*)$, for all i and j, because only observed data at a few previous observation times will be used in function estimation in such cases. See Qiu et al. (2010) for a related discussion on this issue. Based on these considerations and our numerical experience, we suggest choosing $\lambda \in [0.02, 0.1]$. Once λ is chosen, the control limit L can be selected based on the IC dataset such that a pre-specified ARL_0 value is reached, which can be accomplished by a block bootstrap procedure described below. From this block bootstrap procedure, the estimates $\widehat{\Sigma}_{\widehat{\boldsymbol{\mu}}_{\widehat{e},i}}$, $\widehat{\mathrm{E}}(T_i)$ and $\widehat{\mathrm{Var}}(T_i)$ used in (8.20) can also be obtained.

Block Bootstrap Procedure for Determing the Control Limit L

Step 1 Decorrelate and standardize the IC data by the data decorrelation and standardization procedure discussed in Section 8.3, and obtain the decorrelated and standardized IC observations $\{\widehat{e}(t_i), i = 1, 2, \ldots, n\}$. Then, these decorrelated and standardized observations are used to form $n - b + 1$ overlapping blocks $\{B_k, k = 1, 2, \ldots, n - b + 1\}$, where b is a block size and the kth block is defined to be $B_k = \{\widehat{e}(t_i), i = k, k + 1, \ldots, k + b - 1\}$.

Step 2 Sample with replacement from $\{B_k, k = 1, 2, \ldots, n - b + 1\}$, the selected blocks are placed one after another, and they form the lth bootstrap sample of process observations for online process monitoring, denoted as $\{\widehat{e}_i^{(l)}, i \geq 1\}$. Repeat this block bootstrap sampling procedure for B times and obtain B bootstrap samples.

Step 3 For sequential monitoring of the lth bootstrap sample, compute the values of $\{\widehat{\boldsymbol{\mu}}_{\widehat{e},i}, i \geq 1\}$ by the penalized EWKS procedure (8.18), denoted as $\{\widehat{\boldsymbol{\mu}}_{\widehat{e},i}^{(l)}, i \geq 1\}$, for $l = 1, 2, \ldots, B$. For each i, use the sample covariance of $\{\widehat{\boldsymbol{\mu}}_{\widehat{e},i}^{(l)}, 1 \leq l \leq B\}$ to estimate $\Sigma_{\widehat{\boldsymbol{\mu}}_{\widehat{e},i}}$, and the resulting estimate is used as $\widehat{\Sigma}_{\widehat{\boldsymbol{\mu}}_{\widehat{e},i}}$.

Step 4 For each l and i, compute $T_i^{(l)} = (\widehat{\boldsymbol{\mu}}_{\widehat{e},i}^{(l)})' \widehat{\Sigma}_{\widehat{\boldsymbol{\mu}}_{\widehat{e},i}}^{-1} \widehat{\boldsymbol{\mu}}_{\widehat{e},i}^{(l)}$. Then, $\mathrm{E}(T_i)$ and $\mathrm{Var}(T_i)$ can be estimated by the sample mean and sample variance of $\{T_i^{(l)}, 1 \leq l \leq B\}$, for each i, and denoted as $\widehat{\mathrm{E}}(T_i)$ and $\widehat{\mathrm{Var}}(T_i)$.

Step 5 For each l, the charting statistic values can be computed by (8.20) and denoted as $\{ST_i^{(l)}, i \geq 1\}$. For a given control limit L, record the IC run length to be $\mathrm{RL}_0^{(l)}(L) = \min\{i, ST_i^{(l)} > L\}$. Then, the ARL_0 value is computed to be $\mathrm{ARL}_0(L) = \frac{1}{B}\sum_{l=1}^{B} \mathrm{RL}_0^{(l)}(L)$.

Step 6 Use the bisection or other alternative numerical procedures to search for L such that the computed value of $\mathrm{ARL}_0(L)$ equals the pre-specified value of ARL_0.

It should be pointed out that the IC dataset for estimating the NSTR model (8.1) could be different from the one for determining the control limit L, as discussed in Section 8.3. Based on extensive numerical studies, we find that the EWSL chart (8.20)–(8.21) would have a more reliable IC performance, in the sense that its actual ARL_0 value would be closer to the nominal ARL_0 value, if two different IC datasets are used for these two purposes. In addition, the estimated covariance matrix $\widehat{\Sigma}_{\widehat{\boldsymbol{\mu}}_{\widehat{e},i}}$ obtained from the above block bootstrap procedure may not be positive semidefinite. To modify it to be positive semidefinite, we can use the matrix modification procedure discussed in Subsection 8.2.3 that is based on matrix projection to the space of all positive semidefinite matrices.

Example 8.6 *To evaluate the numerical performance of the EWSL chart (8.20)–(8.21), Qiu and Yang (2023) presented some simulation results in the following setup. First, in the NSTR model (8.1), the IC observation times are* $\{t_i = i/n, i = 1, 2, \ldots, n\}$ *which are equally spaced in* $[0, T] = [0, 1]$, *and the observation locations at each observation time are* $\{\boldsymbol{s}_j, j = 1, 2, \ldots, m\}$ *which are unchanged over time and equally spaced in* $\Omega = [0, 1] \times [0, 1]$, *where* $(n, m) = (300, 64)$. *The mean function is assumed to be*

$$\mu(t, \boldsymbol{s}) = \cos(2\pi t) + \exp\left[-\frac{(s_u - 0.5)^2 + (s_v - 0.5)^2}{2}\right] + 1,$$

where $t \in [0, 1]$ *and* $\boldsymbol{s} \in [0, 1] \times [0, 1]$. *The random errors are generated in one of the following six ways to consider six different cases of spatio-temporal data correlation and distribution.*

Case I *The random errors* $\{\varepsilon(t_i, \boldsymbol{s}_j), i = 1, 2, \ldots, n, j = 1, 2, \ldots, m\}$ *are independent and identically distributed (i.i.d.) with the common distribution being* $N(0, 1)$.

Cases II and III *For each* i, *let* $\boldsymbol{\varepsilon}(t_i) = (\varepsilon(t_i, \boldsymbol{s}_1), \varepsilon(t_i, \boldsymbol{s}_2), \ldots, \varepsilon(t_i, \boldsymbol{s}_m))'$. *Then,* $\boldsymbol{\varepsilon}(t_i)$ *is generated from the vector AR(1) model*

$$\boldsymbol{\varepsilon}(t_i) = \rho_t \boldsymbol{\varepsilon}(t_{i-1}) + (1 - \rho_t^2)^{1/2} \boldsymbol{\eta}(t_i),$$

where $\boldsymbol{\eta}(t_i) = (\eta(t_i, \boldsymbol{s}_1), \eta(t_i, \boldsymbol{s}_2), \ldots, \eta(t_i, \boldsymbol{s}_m))'$ *is a realization of a temporally independent Gaussian spatial process whose spatial correlation is described by the covariance function*

$$Cov(\eta(t_i, \boldsymbol{s}_j), \eta(t_i, \boldsymbol{s}_l)) = \exp\left[-\frac{d_E(\boldsymbol{s}_j, \boldsymbol{s}_l)}{\rho_s}\right], \quad \text{for } 1 \le j, l \le m,$$

and $\rho_t, \rho_s > 0$ *are the two parameters controlling the temporal and spatial data correlation, respectively. In such cases, it can be checked that the covariance between* $y(t_i, \boldsymbol{s}_j)$ *and* $y(t_k, \boldsymbol{s}_l)$ *is*

$$V(t_i, t_k; \boldsymbol{s}_j, \boldsymbol{s}_l) = \rho_t^{|k-i|} \exp\left[-\frac{d_E(\boldsymbol{s}_j, \boldsymbol{s}_l)}{\rho_s}\right], \quad \text{for } 1 \le i, k \le n, 1 \le j, l \le m.$$

To consider cases with different levels of spatio-temporal data correlation, $(\rho_t, \rho_s) = (0.25, 0.1)$ *in Case II and* $(\rho_t, \rho_s) = (0.5, 0.2)$ *in Case III.*

Case IV *The random errors are generated from the vector AR(2) model*

$$\boldsymbol{\varepsilon}(t_i) = 0.5\boldsymbol{\varepsilon}(t_{i-1}) + 0.25\boldsymbol{\varepsilon}(t_{i-2}) + \boldsymbol{\eta}(t_i), \qquad \text{for } i = 1, 2, \ldots, n,$$

where $\boldsymbol{\eta}(t_i)$ *is the same as that considered in Case II, except that its spatial covariance function is*

$$\rho(\boldsymbol{s}, \boldsymbol{s}') = \exp\left\{-10\left[(\boldsymbol{s} - \boldsymbol{s}')'\mathbf{M}(\boldsymbol{s} - \boldsymbol{s}')\right]^{1/2}\right\}, \qquad \text{for } \boldsymbol{s}, \boldsymbol{s}' \in \Omega,$$

where

$$\mathbf{M} = \begin{pmatrix} 1 & 0.5 \\ 0.5 & 1 \end{pmatrix}.$$

The spatial data correlation described by this covariance function is non-stationary.

Case V *The random errors are generated from the vector AR(1) model*

$$\boldsymbol{\varepsilon}(t_i) = 0.25\boldsymbol{\varepsilon}(t_{i-1}) + (1 - 0.25^2)^{1/2} \boldsymbol{\eta}(t_i),$$

where $\boldsymbol{\eta}(t_i) = \boldsymbol{\eta}_1(t_i) + \boldsymbol{\eta}_2(t_i)$, $\{\boldsymbol{\eta}_1(t_i)\}$ *are temporally independent Gaussian spatial processes whose spatial correlation is described by*

$$Cov(\eta_1(t_i, \boldsymbol{s}_j), \eta_1(t_i, \boldsymbol{s}_l)) = \exp[-10 d_E(\boldsymbol{s}_j, \boldsymbol{s}_l)],$$

$\boldsymbol{\eta}_2(t_i) = (\eta_2(t_i, \boldsymbol{s}_1), \eta_2(t_i, \boldsymbol{s}_2), \ldots, \eta_2(t_i, \boldsymbol{s}_m))'$, *and* $\{\eta_2(t_i, \boldsymbol{s}_j)\}$ *are i.i.d. with the standardized* $t(3)$ *distribution.*

Case VI *The random errors are generated from the vector AR(1) model*

$$\varepsilon(t_i) = 0.25\varepsilon(t_{i-1}) + \left(1 - 0.25^2\right)^{1/2} \eta(t_i),$$

where $\eta(t_i) = \eta_1(t_i) + \eta_2(t_i)$, $\{\eta_1(t_i)\}$ *are generated in the same way as that in Case V, and* $\{\eta_2(t_i, s_j)\}$ *are i.i.d. with the standardized* $\chi^2(3)$ *distribution.*

In each of the above six cases, the random errors $\{\varepsilon(t_i, s_j)\}$ *are all standardized to have mean 0 and variance 1. From the above description, it can be seen that Case I is the conventional case without any spatio-temporal data correlation, which is considered by many existing methods. Cases II and III have the AR(1) temporal data correlation and a stationary spatial data correlation, with different levels of spatio-temporal data correlation. Case IV has the AR(2) temporal data correlation and a nonstationary spatial data correlation. Case V is the same as Case II, except that its AR(1) model has an extra error term with the standardized* $t(3)$ *distribution, which is heavy-tailed. Case VI is the same as Case V, except that the extra error term has the standardized* $\chi^2(3)$ *distribution which is skewed.*

After the process under monitoring becomes OC, the process observations are assumed to follow the OC model

$$y(t, s) = \mu(t, s) + \delta(t, s) + \varepsilon(t, s), \qquad \text{for } (t, s) \in [0, 1] \times \Omega,$$

where $\delta(t, s)$ *is the shift function. The following three types of shift functions are considered, and each type has four different shift magnitudes:*

Type (i) $\delta(t, s) = 0.25\nu I(s \in \Delta)$, *for* $\nu = 1, 2, 3, 4$;

Type (ii) $\delta(t, s) = (0.25 + 0.5\nu t)I(s \in \Delta)$, *for* $\nu = 1, 2, 3, 4$;

Type (iii) $\delta(t, s) = [0.25 + 0.5t + 0.1\nu d_E(s, s_0)]I(s \in \Delta)$, *for* $\nu = 1, 2, 3, 4$,

where $s_0 = (0.5, 0.5)'$, *and* $\Delta = \{s, d_E(s, s_0) \leq d\} \subset \Omega$ *is the circular spatial region with process mean shifts. Without further specification, d is chosen to be 0.2. From the above expressions of the shifts, it can be seen that Type (i) shifts keep unchanged across both space and time, Type (ii) shifts can change over time but not space and Type (iii) shifts can change over both space and time. So, the three types of shift functions represent constant, time-varying and space/time-varying shifts in the small region* Δ, *respectively.*

In the simulation study, besides the EWSL chart (8.20)–(8.21), the following five alternative charts are also considered.

- *Yan et al. (2018) suggested a real-time monitoring method for spatio-temporal processes based on the spatio-temporal smooth sparse decomposition (SSD). This method can accommodate space/time-varying mean structure and it has been shown to be effective for detecting sparse anomalies. However, it is assumed that the random noises at different times and locations are independent and normally distributed. This method is denoted as ST-SSD.*

- *Zhao et al. (2011) proposed a spatio-temporal process monitoring method by using the kernel smoothing (KS) procedure to estimate the IC space/time-varying mean function. In process monitoring, the observed data are first compared with the IC mean function to compute the raw residuals. Then, at each location, the raw residuals are decorrelated by an AR(2) time series model to obtain the model-based residuals. Finally, this method gives a signal of process shift if a model-based residual exceeds a threshold value c, where c is chosen by a parametric bootstrap procedure under the assumption that the observations at different locations are independent and the model-based residuals follow a normal distribution. This method is denoted as ST-KS.*

- *Yang and Qiu (2020) proposed a CUSUM chart for online monitoring of spatio-temporal data, denoted as ST-CUSUM, which has been described in detail in Section 8.3. This method does not impose any parametric assumptions on the spatio-temporal data variation, spatio-temporal data correlation, or data distribution. So, this method should be reliable to use in many applications. However, it may not be effective for detecting spatially clustered shifts that start in some small regions, since it treats all observation locations equally in its chart construction.*

- *Zou and Qiu (2009) suggested a LASSO-based EWMA chart, denoted as LEWMA, for monitoring multivariate processes. It has been shown to be effective for detecting shifts that occur in a small number of quality variables. In this numerical study, observation locations do not change over time. So, this method can be used here if observations at each spatial location are considered to be observations of a quality variable. However, this method cannot accommodate IC temporal data variation and/or temporal data correlation since it assumes that the IC process observations at different time points are independent and the IC process distribution does not change over time. To make the comparison fair, we have applied this chart to the decorrelated and standardized data* $\{\widehat{e}(t_i^*, \boldsymbol{s}_j), j = 1, 2, \ldots, m, i = 1, 2, \ldots\}$ *here. For simplicity in notation, the resulting chart is still denoted as LEWMA. Obviously, this chart is not designed for monitoring spatial data, and thus may not be effective for detecting spatially clustered shifts.*

- *Finally, we consider a modified version of the EWSL chart, described below. First, let us construct an EWMA chart as follows:*

$$\xi(t_i^*, \boldsymbol{s}_j) = \lambda \widehat{e}(t_i^*, \boldsymbol{s}_j) + (1 - \lambda)\xi(t_{i-1}^*, \boldsymbol{s}_j),$$

where $\xi(t_0^*, \boldsymbol{s}_j) = 0$ *and* $\lambda > 0$ *is a weighting parameter. Then, the mean vector* $\boldsymbol{\mu}_{\widehat{e},i} = (\mu_{\widehat{e}}(t_i^*, \boldsymbol{s}_1), \ldots, \mu_{\widehat{e}}(t_i^*, \boldsymbol{s}_m))'$ *is estimated by the following adaptive spatial LASSO (ASL) procedure:*

$$\min_{a_1, a_2, \ldots, a_m} \left\{ \sum_{j=1}^m \left(\xi(t_i^*, \boldsymbol{s}_j) - a_j\right)^2 + \gamma_1 \sum_{j=1}^m \varpi_{1j}|a_j| + \right.$$
$$\left. \gamma_2 \sum_{j=1}^m \varpi_{2j} \left| a_j - \frac{\sum_{l=1}^m K_s(d_E(\boldsymbol{s}_j, \boldsymbol{s}_l)/h) a_l}{\sum_{l=1}^m K_s(d_E(\boldsymbol{s}_j, \boldsymbol{s}_l)/h)} \right| \right\},$$

where ϖ_{1j} and ϖ_{2j} are the adaptive weights defined to be the same as those in (8.18), and γ_1 and γ_2 are two tuning parameters chosen by the BIC criterion (8.19). Other components of the modified chart are the same as those of EWSL. So, the major difference between this modified method and EWSL is that the EWMA procedure in the time domain and the ASL procedure in the space domain are separated in the modified method, while these two components are mixed in EWSL. To use the modified method, denoted as ASL, spatial locations are required to be unchanged over time.

We first compare the IC performance of the six control charts described above. In the charts LEWMA, ASL and EWSL, the weighting parameter λ is chosen to be 0.02, 0.05 or 0.1. The allowance constant ϕ in the ST-CUSUM chart is chosen to be 0.1, 0.3 or 0.5. For all the charts, the nominal ARL_0 value is fixed 200. The control limits of the charts ST-CUSUM, LEWMA, ASL and EWSL are determined by the block bootstrap procedures with the bootstrap sample size $B = 1000$ and the block size $b = 5$. The threshold value c in the ST-KS method is determined by the parametric bootstrap procedure, as discussed in Zhao et al. (2011). The control limit of the chart ST-SSD is determined by the simulation-based procedure discussed in Yan et al. (2018). For a given chart, its actual ARL value is estimated based on 1000 replicated simulations of online monitoring. Because such an ARL value depends on the IC datasets used for estimating the IC model and/or for determining the control limit, which are random, the entire simulation described above, from generation of the IC datasets, estimation of the IC model, determination of the control limit, to estimation of the actual ARL value, is repeated for 100 times. Then, the average of the 100 estimated ARL values is used as the final estimate of the true ARL value. The estimated actual ARL_0 values of the six charts are presented in Table 8.3. From the table, it can be seen that (i) the four charts EWSL, ASL, LEWMA and ST-CUSUM have a satisfactory IC performance in most cases considered, since their calculated ARL_0 values are close to the nominal level of 200, (ii) the two charts ST-KS and ST-SSD have a worse IC performance, compared to the charts EWSL, ASL, LEWMA and ST-CUSUM, in Cases II-VI when there is spatio-temporal data correlation, and (iii) by comparing the results in Cases I-III, the IC performance of all six charts becomes worse from Case I to Case III when the data correlation gets stronger, although the impact of the data correlation on the four charts EWSL, ASL, LEWMA and ST-CUSUM seems quite small.

We then study the OC performance of the six control charts in Cases I-VI for detecting the three types of shifts described earlier. In each case, let d $= 0.2$ and the nominal ARL_0 level be 200. The other setups are the same as those in Table 8.3. To make the comparison fair, the control limit or the threshold value of each chart has been adjusted so that its actual ARL_0 value equals the nominal level of 200. Also, procedure parameters in each chart (e.g., λ in LEWMA, ASL and EWSL) are chosen such that the ARL_1 value reaches the minimum for detecting a given shift. Namely, the optimal ARL_1 values of different charts are compared here, because it has been pointed out in the

TABLE 8.3
Estimated ARL_0 values of the six control charts in different cases when the nominal ARL_0 value is 200. In the table, each λ value is used for all three charts LEWMA, ASL and EWSL.

Case	ST-SSD	ST-KS	ϕ	ST-CUSUM	λ	LEWMA	ASL	EWSL
			0.1	191	0.02	195	204	198
I	197	193	0.3	191	0.05	194	198	199
			0.5	195	0.10	196	200	200
			0.1	186	0.02	186	194	195
II	171	182	0.3	188	0.05	195	197	197
			0.5	192	0.10	195	198	199
			0.1	185	0.02	186	191	190
III	150	169	0.3	186	0.05	189	192	193
			0.5	190	0.10	191	196	195
			0.1	187	0.02	190	192	193
IV	164	182	0.3	189	0.05	193	195	196
			0.5	193	0.10	196	198	198
			0.1	182	0.02	183	191	192
V	144	165	0.3	183	0.05	188	194	193
			0.5	188	0.10	191	195	195
			0.1	177	0.02	179	190	191
VI	138	156	0.3	181	0.05	183	192	192
			0.5	184	0.10	189	193	194

literature that the OC performance of different charts with pre-specified parameter values may not be comparable (e.g., Qiu et al., 2020a). The optimal ARL_1 values of the six charts are presented in Figure 8.9. From the figure, we can have the following conclusions. (i) The charts ST-CUSUM, LEWMA, ASL and EWSL perform better than the charts ST-SSD and ST-KS in most cases considered, which is reasonable because some assumptions in ST-SSD and ST-KS are violated here. (ii) LEWMA has a better performance than ST-CUSUSM, which confirms the benefit to build a LASSO-based variable selection procedure into a control chart. (iii) the charts ASL and EWSL perform better than LEWMA in this example, which confirms that the spatial information used in ASL and EWSL is helpful for spatio-temporal process monitoring. (iv) The chart EWSL has the best performance in all cases considered. Thus, compared to ASL in which the EWMA procedure in the time domain and the adaptive spatial LASSO procedure in the space domain are separated, EWSL with the two procedures mixed in the space-time domain would be more effective in detecting spatially clustered process shifts that start in small collected regions.

In the previous example, the parameter d that controls the size of the shift region Δ is fixed at 0.2. Next, we consider cases when d changes its value

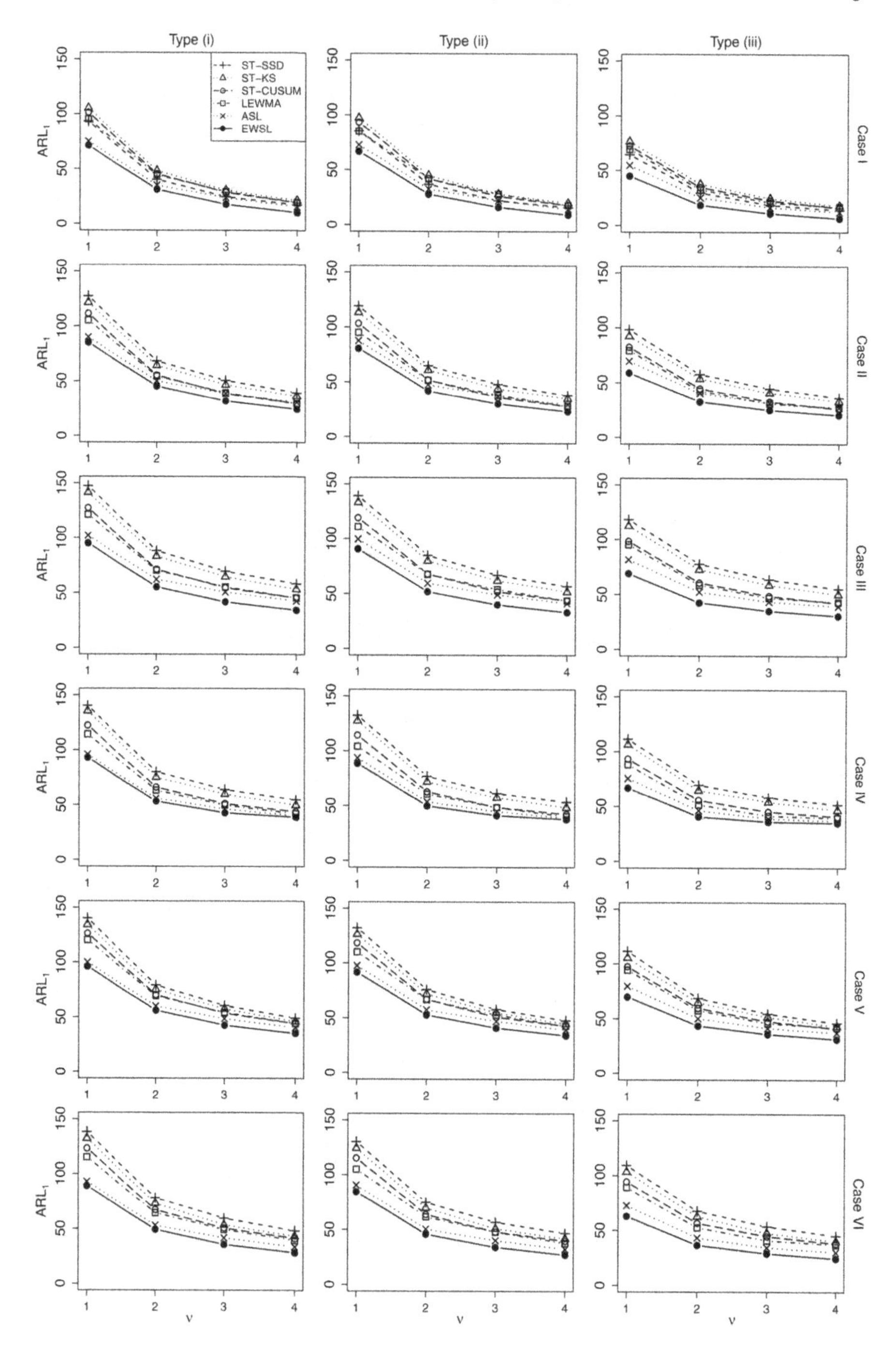

FIGURE 8.9
Calculated optimal ARL_1 values of the six charts for detecting the shifts of Types (i)–(iii) in Cases I–VI when the nominal ARL_0 level of each chart is fixed at 200 and $d = 0.2$.

among 0.1, 0.3, 0.4 or 0.5, and other setups are the same as those in Figure 8.9. The optimal ARL$_1$ *values of the six charts for detecting the shifts of Type (iii) in Case II are shown in Figure 8.10. From the figure, we can see that EWSL still performs the best among the six charts in all cases considered. Results for detecting the other two types of shifts have similar patterns, and thus are omitted here.*

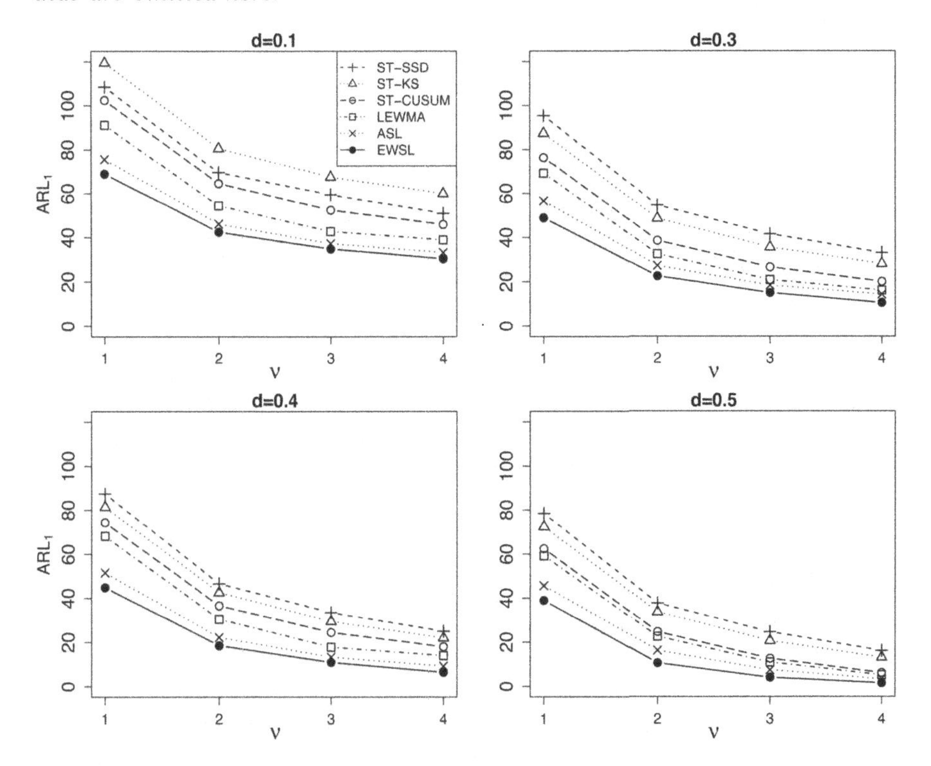

FIGURE 8.10
Calculated optimal ARL_1 values of the six charts for detecting the shifts of Type (iii) in Case II when the nominal ARL_0 level of each chart is fixed at 200 and $d = 0.1$, 0.3, 0.4 or 0.5.

8.5 Disease Surveillance by Using Covariate Information

The disease surveillance methods discussed in the previous sections concentrate on the observed disease incidence rates only without considering the impact of any covariates. In practice, however, disease incidence rates are often associated with some covariates, including the air temperature, humidity, and other weather or environmental conditions if infectious diseases like flu are concerned. Recently, Yang and Qiu (2021) suggested an EWMA chart for monitoring univariate sequential processes, which can take into account helpful information in covariates. A major feature of that method is that the covariate information is used in choosing the weighting parameter of the EWMA chart: it is chosen large when the observed data of the covariates show that the likelihood for the covariates to have a shift is large, and small otherwise. Because of this feature, the resulting EWMA chart can react to a future shift in the related process performance variable under monitoring quickly when such a shift is associated with the covariates. On the other hand, because the covariate information is used in choosing the weighting parameter only and the EWMA charting statistic is a weighted average of observations of the related process performance variable, the chart would be sensitive to shifts in the process performance variable only and insensitive to shifts in the covariates if such shifts do not result in shifts in the process performance variable. These properties should be especially relevant to disease surveillance since disease incidence data are often associated with weather and/or environmental conditions and some other covariates. Thus, on one hand, such covariate information should be used in disease surveillance to make the related disease surveillance methods more effective. On the other hand, the disease surveillance methods should be robust to shifts in the covariates that would not result in disease outbreaks.

The method suggested in Yang and Qiu (2021), however, cannot be applied to the disease surveillance problem directly for the following reasons. First, this method is designed for monitoring univariate processes only, while the disease surveillance problem discussed here is for monitoring spatial processes that often have complicated spatio-temporal data structure, as discussed in the previous sections. Second, this method is for handling the conventional process monitoring problem in which the IC process distribution is assumed to be unchanged over time. In the disease surveillance problem, however, distribution of the observed disease incidence rates often changes over time even in cases when no disease outbreaks are present, representing seasonality and other temporal variation. In other words, the disease incidence process is usually dynamic in nature. To address these challenges, Qiu and Yang (2021) developed a disease surveillance method based on the idea of the method discussed in Yang and Qiu (2021). The new method has all the favorable properties of the method in Yang and Qiu (2021) mentioned above, while it can accommodate the complicated structure of the observed spatio-temporal disease incidence data. This method is described below in two subsections.

8.5.1 Estimation of the Regular Spatio-Temporal Pattern

IC spatio-temporal model and its estimation. The method by Qiu and Yang (2021) requires that an IC dataset is available for estimating the regular spatio-temporal pattern of the disease incidence rates. To this end, let

$\{y(t_i, \boldsymbol{s}_{ij}), j = 1, 2, \ldots, m_i, i = 1, 2, \ldots, n\}$ be the observed disease incidence rates in the IC data, where $t_i \in [0, T]$ is the ith observation time, $\boldsymbol{s}_{ij} \in \Omega$ is the jth observation location at time t_i, m_i is the number of observation locations at t_i, and n is the number of observation times. These observed IC disease incidence rates are assumed to follow the model

$$\begin{aligned} y(t_i, \boldsymbol{s}_{ij}) &= \mu(t_i, \boldsymbol{s}_{ij}) + \mathbf{X}_1'(t_i)\boldsymbol{\beta}_1 + \mathbf{X}_2'(t_i, \boldsymbol{s}_{ij})\boldsymbol{\beta}_2 + \varepsilon(t_i, \boldsymbol{s}_{ij}), \quad (8.22) \\ & \quad \text{for } j = 1, 2, \ldots, m_i, i = 1, 2, \ldots, n, \end{aligned}$$

where $\mathbf{X}_1(t)$ is a vector of p_1 time-dependent covariates, $\mathbf{X}_2(t, \boldsymbol{s})$ is a vector of p_2 space/time-dependent covariates, $\boldsymbol{\beta}_1$ and $\boldsymbol{\beta}_2$ are their regression coefficients, $\mu(t, \boldsymbol{s})$ is the mean of $y(t, \boldsymbol{s})$ after the part explained by $\mathbf{X}_1(t)$ and $\mathbf{X}_2(t, \boldsymbol{s})$ being excluded, and $\varepsilon(t, \boldsymbol{s})$ is a zero-mean random error, for any $(t, \boldsymbol{s}) \in [0, T] \times \Omega$. The covariance function of $y(t, \boldsymbol{s})$ is denoted as

$$V_y(t, t'; \boldsymbol{s}, \boldsymbol{s}') = \text{Cov}\left[y(t, \boldsymbol{s}), y(t', \boldsymbol{s}')\right], \quad \text{for any } (t, \boldsymbol{s}), (t', \boldsymbol{s}') \in [0, T] \times \Omega.$$

For convenience, $V_y(t, t; \boldsymbol{s}, \boldsymbol{s})$ is also denoted as $\sigma_y^2(t, \boldsymbol{s})$, for any $(t, \boldsymbol{s}) \in [0, T] \times \Omega$. In model (8.22), no parametric forms are imposed on $\mu(t, \boldsymbol{s})$, $V_y(t, t'; \boldsymbol{s}, \boldsymbol{s}')$ and the distribution of $\varepsilon(t, \boldsymbol{s})$. Thus, it is flexible. In practice, besides time-dependent and space/time-dependent covariates, there could be covariates that do not depend on time (e.g., geographic features that depend on space only), but are associated with the disease incidence rates. Such covariates, however, would not provide any information about the temporal variation of the disease incidence rates. Thus, they are not included explicitly in model (8.22) since they would not be helpful for sequential spatial process monitoring discussed later.

Model (8.22) can be regarded as a semiparametric model, in which $\mu(t, \boldsymbol{s})$ is the nonparametric part and $\mathbf{X}_1'(t)\boldsymbol{\beta}_1 + \mathbf{X}_2'(t, \boldsymbol{s})\boldsymbol{\beta}_2$ is the parametric part. To estimate a semiparametric model, it is natural to consider an iterative estimation procedure (e.g., Speckman, 1988), in which the nonparametric and parametric parts can be estimated iteratively. To this end, let us first assume that $\boldsymbol{\beta} = (\boldsymbol{\beta}_1', \boldsymbol{\beta}_2')' = \mathbf{0}$ in model (8.22). Then, the resulting model becomes the NSTR model (8.1) considered in Section 8.2, and $\mu(t, \boldsymbol{s})$ can be estimated by $\widehat{\mu}(t, \boldsymbol{s})$ defined in (8.10). The entire iterative estimation procedure is described below.

Iterative Algorithm for Estimating Model (8.22)

Initialization Set $\boldsymbol{\beta} = \mathbf{0}$ in Model (8.22) and obtain an initial estimate of $\mu(t, \boldsymbol{s})$ by (8.10), denoted as $\widehat{\mu}^{(0)}(t, \boldsymbol{s})$.

Iteration In the kth iteration, for $k \geq 1$, implement the following two steps:

a) Compute the least squares estimate of $\boldsymbol{\beta}$, denoted as $\widehat{\boldsymbol{\beta}}^{(k)}$, from the linear model $Z^{(k-1)}(t, \boldsymbol{s}) = \mathbf{X}_1'(t)\boldsymbol{\beta}_1 + \mathbf{X}_2'(t, \boldsymbol{s})\boldsymbol{\beta}_2 + \varepsilon(t, \boldsymbol{s})$, where $Z^{(k-1)}(t, \boldsymbol{s}) = y(t, \boldsymbol{s}) - \widehat{\mu}^{(k-1)}(t, \boldsymbol{s})$, and $\widehat{\mu}^{(k-1)}(t, \boldsymbol{s})$ is the estimate of $\mu(t, \boldsymbol{s})$ obtained at the $(k-1)$-th iteration.

b) Update the estimate of $\mu(t, \boldsymbol{s})$ by replacing $\mathbf{Y}$ in (8.10) by $\mathbf{Y}^{(k)} = (y^{(k)}(t_1, \boldsymbol{s}_{11}), \ldots, y^{(k)}(t_n, \boldsymbol{s}_{nm_n}))'$, where $y^{(k)}(t_i, \boldsymbol{s}_{ij}) = y(t_i, \boldsymbol{s}_{ij}) - \mathbf{X}_1'(t_i)\widehat{\boldsymbol{\beta}}_1^{(k)} - \mathbf{X}_2'(t_i, \boldsymbol{s}_{ij})\widehat{\boldsymbol{\beta}}_2^{(k)}$, for $j = 1, 2, \ldots, m_i$ and $i = 1, 2, \ldots, n$. The updated estimate is denoted as $\widehat{\mu}^{(k)}(t, \boldsymbol{s})$.

Exit The iterative algorithm stops when $\|\widehat{\boldsymbol{\beta}}^{(k)} - \widehat{\boldsymbol{\beta}}^{(k-1)}\|_1 / \|\widehat{\boldsymbol{\beta}}^{(k-1)}\|_1 \leq \varsigma$, where $\varsigma > 0$ is a pre-specified small number and $\|\boldsymbol{a}\|_1$ denotes the summation of the absolute values of all elements in the vector $\boldsymbol{a}$. Then, $\widehat{\boldsymbol{\beta}}^{(k)}$ and $\widehat{\mu}^{(k)}(t, \boldsymbol{s})$ are the final estimates of $\boldsymbol{\beta}$ and $\mu(t, \boldsymbol{s})$, respectively. These final estimates are denoted as $\widehat{\boldsymbol{\beta}}$ and $\widehat{\mu}(t, \boldsymbol{s})$.

The variance and covariance functions $\sigma_y^2(t, \boldsymbol{s})$ and $V_y(t, t'; \boldsymbol{s}, \boldsymbol{s}')$ can be estimated by (8.7) and (8.8), respectively, after $\{\widetilde{\varepsilon}(t_i, \boldsymbol{s}_{ij}), j = 1, 2, \ldots, m_i, i = 1, 2, \ldots, n\}$ are replaced by $\{\widehat{\varepsilon}(t_i, \boldsymbol{s}_{ij}), j = 1, 2, \ldots, m_i, i = 1, 2, \ldots, n\}$, where

$$
\begin{aligned}
\widehat{\varepsilon}(t_i, \boldsymbol{s}_{ij}) &= y(t_i, \boldsymbol{s}_{ij}) - \widehat{\mu}_y(t_i, \boldsymbol{s}_{ij}), \\
\widehat{\mu}_y(t_i, \boldsymbol{s}_{ij}) &= \widehat{\mu}(t_i, \boldsymbol{s}_{ij}) + \widehat{\mu}_z(t_i, \boldsymbol{s}_{ij}),
\end{aligned}
$$

and $\widehat{\mu}_z(t, \boldsymbol{s})$ is the estimated mean function of $\widehat{z}(t, \boldsymbol{s}) = \mathbf{X}_1'(t)\widehat{\boldsymbol{\beta}}_1 + \mathbf{X}_2'(t, \boldsymbol{s})\widehat{\boldsymbol{\beta}}_2$ obtained by (8.10) which will be discussed in detail below. The related estimates are denotes as $\widehat{\sigma}_y^2(t, \boldsymbol{s})$ and $\widehat{V}_y(t, t'; \boldsymbol{s}, \boldsymbol{s}')$. Then, the estimated regular spatio-temporal pattern of the disease incidence rates is described by $\widehat{\mu}_y(t, \boldsymbol{s})$, $\widehat{\sigma}_y^2(t, \boldsymbol{s})$ and $\widehat{V}_y(t, t'; \boldsymbol{s}, \boldsymbol{s}')$.

It should be pointed out that the estimates $\widehat{\sigma}_y^2(t, \boldsymbol{s})$ and $\widehat{V}_y(t, t'; \boldsymbol{s}, \boldsymbol{s}')$ may not be positive semidefinite to become legitimate variance and covariance functions. So, the modification procedure discussed in Subsection 8.2.3 is also relevant here. Also, the bandwidths used in estimating $\mu(t, \boldsymbol{s})$ can be selected in a similar way to that discussed in Subsection 8.2.3.

Estimation of the IC covariate effect. From Model (8.22), the covariates $\mathbf{X}_1(t)$ and $\mathbf{X}_2(t, \boldsymbol{s})$ affect the disease incidence rate $y(t, \boldsymbol{s})$ through $z(t, \boldsymbol{s}) = \mathbf{X}_1'(t)\boldsymbol{\beta}_1 + \mathbf{X}_2'(t, \boldsymbol{s})\boldsymbol{\beta}_2$. Let $\widehat{z}(t, \boldsymbol{s}) = \mathbf{X}_1'(t)\widehat{\boldsymbol{\beta}}_1 + \mathbf{X}_2'(t, \boldsymbol{s})\widehat{\boldsymbol{\beta}}_2$, where $\widehat{\boldsymbol{\beta}} = (\widehat{\boldsymbol{\beta}}_1', \widehat{\boldsymbol{\beta}}_2')'$ is obtained from the iterative algorithm described above. Then, $\widehat{z}(t, \boldsymbol{s})$ should be a reasonable estimate of $z(t, \boldsymbol{s})$. For any $(t, \boldsymbol{s}), (t', \boldsymbol{s}') \in [0, T] \times \Omega$, define

$$
\mu_z(t, \boldsymbol{s}) = \mathrm{E}\left[\widehat{z}(t, \boldsymbol{s})\right], \quad V_z(t, t'; \boldsymbol{s}, \boldsymbol{s}') = \mathrm{Cov}\left[\widehat{z}(t, \boldsymbol{s}), \widehat{z}(t', \boldsymbol{s}')\right]
$$

to be the mean and covariance functions of $\widehat{z}(t, \boldsymbol{s})$. For simplicity, let $\sigma_z^2(t, \boldsymbol{s}) = V_z(t, t; \boldsymbol{s}, \boldsymbol{s})$. Next, we discuss how to estimate $\mu_z(t, \boldsymbol{s})$, $\sigma_z^2(t, \boldsymbol{s})$ and $V_z(t, t'; \boldsymbol{s}, \boldsymbol{s}')$ from the data $\{\widehat{z}(t_i, \boldsymbol{s}_{ij}), j = 1, 2, \ldots, m_i, i = 1, 2, \ldots, n\}$.

The mean function $\mu_z(t, \boldsymbol{s})$ can be estimated by the LLK estimate obtained by (8.10), denoted as $\widehat{\mu}_z(t, \boldsymbol{s})$, after $\mathbf{Y}$ is replaced by

$$
\widehat{\mathbf{Z}} = (\widehat{z}(t_1, \boldsymbol{s}_{11}), \ldots, \widehat{z}(t_1, \boldsymbol{s}_{1m_1}), \ldots, \widehat{z}(t_n, \boldsymbol{s}_{n1}), \ldots, \widehat{z}(t_n, \boldsymbol{s}_{nm_n}))'.
$$

The bandwidths used here could be different from those used for estimating

$\mu(t, \boldsymbol{s})$. But, they can still be chosen by the MCV procedure (8.6) or the BCE-MSE procedure (8.12), after all the related quantities changed properly from those computed from $\{y(t_i, \boldsymbol{s}_{ij}), j = 1, 2, \ldots, m_i, i = 1, 2, \ldots, n\}$ to the corresponding ones computed from $\{\widehat{z}(t_i, \boldsymbol{s}_{ij}), j = 1, 2, \ldots, m_i, i = 1, 2, \ldots, n\}$. The variance and covariance functions $\sigma_z^2(t, \boldsymbol{s})$ and $V_z(t, t'; \boldsymbol{s}, \boldsymbol{s}')$ can be estimated in the same way as that for estimating $\sigma_y^2(t, \boldsymbol{s})$ and $V_y(t, t'; \boldsymbol{s}, \boldsymbol{s}')$, except that the quantities $\{\widehat{\varepsilon}_y(t_i, \boldsymbol{s}_{ij}), j = 1, 2, \ldots, m_i, i = 1, 2, \ldots, n\}$ should be replaced by $\{\widehat{\varepsilon}_z(t_i, \boldsymbol{s}_{ij}) = \widehat{z}(t_i, \boldsymbol{s}_{ij}) - \widehat{\mu}_z(t_i, \boldsymbol{s}_{ij}), j = 1, 2, \ldots, m_i, i = 1, 2, \ldots, n\}$.

8.5.2 Spatio-Temporal Disease Surveillance by Using Covariate Information

Construct a control chart for disease surveillance. After the regular spatio-temporal pattern of the disease incidence rates is estimated from an IC dataset, we are ready to construct a method for disease surveillance. A main feature of the method is that it can make use of helpful covariate information when detecting disease outbreaks, while its signal of disease outbreak can only be triggered by unusual spatio-temporal pattern of the observed disease incidence rates, instead of the pattern of the covariates. To be more specific, assume that the disease incidence rates to monitor are observed at times $\{t_i^* \in (T, \infty), i \geq 1\}$. At the ith time t_i^*, for $i \geq 1$, they are observed at spatial locations $\{\boldsymbol{s}_{ij}^* \in \Omega, j = 1, 2, \ldots, m_i^*\}$. These spatio-temporal observations are denoted as

$$\left\{y(t_i^*, \boldsymbol{s}_{ij}^*), j = 1, 2, \ldots, m_i^*, i \geq 1\right\}.$$

The related observations of the time-dependent and space/time-dependent covariates are denoted as

$$\left\{\mathbf{X}_1(t_i^*), j = 1, 2, \ldots, m_i^*, i \geq 1\right\}, \quad \left\{\mathbf{X}_2(t_i^*, \boldsymbol{s}_{ij}^*), j = 1, 2, \ldots, m_i^*, i \geq 1\right\},$$

respectively. As in Section 8.3, "*" is used in the notations here to distinguish them from those in the IC dataset.

To detect disease outbreaks, let us first consider the following standardized residuals:

$$\widehat{e}_y(t_i^*, \boldsymbol{s}_{ij}^*) = \frac{y(t_i^*, \boldsymbol{s}_{ij}^*) - \widehat{\mu}_y(t_i^*, \boldsymbol{s}_{ij}^*)}{\widehat{\sigma}_y(t_i^*, \boldsymbol{s}_{ij}^*)}, \quad \text{for } j = 1, 2, \ldots, m_i^*, \ i \geq 1, \tag{8.23}$$

where $\widehat{\mu}_y(t_i^*, \boldsymbol{s}_{ij}^*)$ and $\widehat{\sigma}_y(t_i^*, \boldsymbol{s}_{ij}^*)$ are obtained from the IC data (cf., Subsection 8.5.1), after they are extended periodically in the time domain from $[0, T]$ to $[0, \infty)$ with the period of T, as discussed in the second paragraph of Section 8.3. For instance, if $t_i^* = t_i^{**} + \ell T$, where $t_i^{**} \in [0, T]$ and $\ell \geq 1$ is an integer, then we define $\widehat{\mu}_y(t_i^*, \boldsymbol{s}_{ij}^*) = \widehat{\mu}_y(t_i^{**}, \boldsymbol{s}_{ij}^*)$, for all i and j. In Expression (8.23), the observed spatio-temporal pattern of the disease incidence rates has been compared to the estimated regular spatio-temporal pattern described by $\widehat{\mu}_y(t_i^*, \boldsymbol{s}_{ij}^*)$ and $\widehat{\sigma}_y(t_i^*, \boldsymbol{s}_{ij}^*)$. So, the quantities $\{\widehat{e}_y(t_i^*, \boldsymbol{s}_{ij}^*), j = 1, 2, \ldots, m_i^*, i \geq 1\}$ can be used for detecting disease outbreaks: the larger their values, the more likely a disease outbreak.

From Model (8.22), the covariates $\mathbf{X}_1(t)$ and $\mathbf{X}_2(t, \boldsymbol{s})$ affect the disease incidence rate $y(t, \boldsymbol{s})$ through $z(t, \boldsymbol{s}) = \mathbf{X}_1'(t)\boldsymbol{\beta}_1 + \mathbf{X}_2'(t, \boldsymbol{s})\boldsymbol{\beta}_2$. A shift in $z(t, \boldsymbol{s})$ could result in a shift in $y(t, \boldsymbol{s})$. Similar to (8.23), the following standardized residuals could be useful for detecting a shift in the observed values of $z(t, \boldsymbol{s})$:

$$\widehat{e}_z(t_i^*, \boldsymbol{s}_{ij}^*) = \frac{\widehat{z}(t_i^*, \boldsymbol{s}_{ij}^*) - \widehat{\mu}_z(t_i^*, \boldsymbol{s}_{ij}^*)}{\widehat{\sigma}_z(t_i^*, \boldsymbol{s}_{ij}^*)}, \quad \text{for } j = 1, \ldots, m_i^*, \quad i \geq 1, \tag{8.24}$$

where $\widehat{z}(t_i^*, \boldsymbol{s}_{ij}^*) = \mathbf{X}_1'(t_i^*)\widehat{\boldsymbol{\beta}}_1 + \mathbf{X}_2'(t_i^*, \boldsymbol{s}_{ij}^*)\widehat{\boldsymbol{\beta}}_2$, $\widehat{\mu}_z(t_i^*, \boldsymbol{s}_{ij}^*)$ and $\widehat{\sigma}_z(t_i^*, \boldsymbol{s}_{ij}^*)$ are computed from the IC data (cf., Subsection 8.5.1) after they are extended periodically in the time domain from $[0, T]$ to $[0, \infty)$ with the period of T. Next, the standardized residuals at different observation locations are combined at each observation time, so that a univariate control chart can be used for detecting shifts in $z(t, \boldsymbol{s})$. To this end, because of the spatial data correlation among $\{\widehat{e}_z(t_i^*, \boldsymbol{s}_{ij}^*), j = 1, 2, \ldots, m_i^*\}$ defined in (8.24), we first decorrelate them by defining

$$\widetilde{\mathbf{e}}_z(t_i^*) = \widehat{\mathcal{C}}_z(t_i^*)^{-1/2}\widehat{\mathbf{e}}_z(t_i^*),$$

where $\widehat{\mathbf{e}}_z(t_i^*) = (\widehat{e}_z(t_i^*, \boldsymbol{s}_{i1}^*), \widehat{e}_z(t_i^*, \boldsymbol{s}_{i2}^*), \ldots, \widehat{e}_z(t_i^*, \boldsymbol{s}_{im_i^*}^*))'$, and $\widehat{\mathcal{C}}_z(t_i^*)$ is the estimated correlation matrix of $\widehat{\mathbf{e}}_z(t_i^*)$ computed from the covariance function $\widehat{V}_z(t_i^*, t_i^*; \boldsymbol{s}, \boldsymbol{s}')$, for $\boldsymbol{s}, \boldsymbol{s}' \in \Omega$. It can be checked that the elements of $\widetilde{\mathbf{e}}_z(t_i^*)$, denoted as $\{\widetilde{e}_z(t_i^*, \boldsymbol{s}_{ij}^*), j = 1, 2, \ldots, m_i^*\}$, are asymptotically uncorrelated with each other and each element has the asymptotic mean 0 and the asymptotic variance 1 when there is no disease outbreak at the time t_i^*. Then, the following EWMA charting statistic can be considered:

$$E_{z,i} = \lambda \check{e}_z(t_i^*) + (1 - \lambda)E_{z,i-1}, \quad \text{for } i \geq 1, \tag{8.25}$$

where $E_{z,0} = 0$, $\lambda \in (0, 1]$ is a weighting parameter, and $\check{e}_z(t_i^*) = \sum_{j=1}^{m_i^*} \widetilde{e}_z(t_i^*, \boldsymbol{s}_{ij}^*)/\sqrt{m_i^*}$, for each i. If there is an upward mean shift in $z(t, \boldsymbol{s})$ at or before the time t_i^*, then the value of $E_{z,i}$ would be relatively large because of the shift (cf., Subsection 3.1.4). Therefore, the EWMA charting statistic $E_{z,i}$ provides a measure of the likelihood of an upward mean shift in $z(t, \boldsymbol{s})$.

In the current spatio-temporal disease surveillance problem, our ultimate goal is to detect shifts in the disease incidence rate $y(t, \boldsymbol{s})$, which may or may not be caused by shifts in $z(t, \boldsymbol{s})$. In addition, shifts in $z(t, \boldsymbol{s})$ alone would not be our major concern in the disease surveillance problem, although any helpful information in $z(t, \boldsymbol{s})$ should be used in disease surveillance. By these considerations and the idea in Yang and Qiu (2021) to use covariate information for online monitoring of the observed process observations, Qiu and Yang (2021) suggested using the following EWMA charting statistic for disease surveillance: for $i \geq 1$,

$$E_{y,i} = \mathrm{W}(E_{z,i}; \lambda, \kappa)\, \check{e}_y(t_i^*) + [1 - \mathrm{W}(E_{z,i}; \lambda, \kappa)]\, E_{y,i-1}, \tag{8.26}$$

where $E_{y,0} = 0$, and $\mathrm{W}(E_{z,i}; \lambda, \kappa) \in (0,1]$ was a weighting parameter for $\breve{e}_y(t_i^*)$ that depended on the covariate charting statistic $E_{z,i}$ and two parameters $\lambda \in (0,1]$ and $\kappa > 0$. In (8.26), the quantity $\breve{e}_y(t_i^*)$ is defined similarly to $\breve{e}_z(t_i^*)$, as

$$\breve{e}_y(t_i^*) = \frac{1}{\sqrt{m_i^*}} \sum_{j=1}^{m_i^*} \widetilde{e}_y(t_i^*, \boldsymbol{s}_{ij}^*),$$

where

$$\begin{aligned} \widetilde{\mathbf{e}}_y(t_i^*) &= \left(\widetilde{e}_y(t_i^*, \boldsymbol{s}_{i1}^*), \widetilde{e}_y(t_i^*, \boldsymbol{s}_{i2}^*), \ldots, \widetilde{e}_y(t_i^*, \boldsymbol{s}_{im_i^*}^*)\right)' \\ &= \widehat{\mathcal{C}}_y(t_i^*)^{-1/2} \widehat{\mathbf{e}}_y(t_i^*), \\ \widehat{\mathbf{e}}_y(t_i^*) &= \left(\widehat{e}_y(t_i^*, \boldsymbol{s}_{i1}^*), \widehat{e}_y(t_i^*, \boldsymbol{s}_{i2}^*), \ldots, \widehat{e}_y(t_i^*, \boldsymbol{s}_{im_i^*}^*)\right)', \end{aligned}$$

and $\widehat{\mathcal{C}}_y(t_i^*)$ is the estimated correlation matrix of $\widehat{\mathbf{e}}_y(t_i^*)$ obtained from the covariance function estimate $\widehat{V}_y(t_i^*, t_i^*; \boldsymbol{s}, \boldsymbol{s}')$, for any $\boldsymbol{s}, \boldsymbol{s}' \in \Omega$. Then, the chart gives a signal of disease outbreak at time t_i^* if

$$E_{y,i} > L, \tag{8.27}$$

where $L > 0$ is a control limit.

From its construction, it can be seen that the EWMA charting statistic $E_{y,i}$ in (8.26) is a weighted average of the observed disease incidence rates. Thus, only shifts in the disease incidence rates can trigger a signal of the chart. The covariate information is used in the weighting parameter $\mathrm{W}(E_{z,i}; \lambda, \kappa)$ only, which will be chosen to be an increasing function of $E_{z,i}$. So, when $E_{z,i}$ is larger, or when there is more evidence of a shift in the combination $z(t, \boldsymbol{s})$ of the time-dependent covariates, the weight $\mathrm{W}(E_{z,i}; \lambda, \kappa)$ will be chosen larger so that the current and several most recent observations of the disease incidence rate will receive more weights. In such cases, the possible shift in the disease incidence rates that is associated with the covariates can be detected more effectively. Because the covariate information has been used in the weighting parameter only, a shift in $z(t, \boldsymbol{s})$ would not trigger a signal from the chart (8.26)–(8.27) if that shift does not result in a shift in the disease incidence rates. Thus, the chart (8.26)–(8.27) can accomplish the research goals stated at the beginning of this section.

Determination of the weighting function $\mathbf{W}(u; \lambda, \kappa)$ and the control limit L. To use the EWMA chart (8.26)–(8.27), we need to properly specify the weighting function $\mathrm{W}(u; \lambda, \kappa)$ (as a function of u) in advance. As mentioned earlier, this function should be chosen to be an increasing function of u. Since it is a weight used in an EWMA chart, its value should be in the interval $(0,1]$. By taking into account all these considerations, Qiu and Yang (2021) suggested using the following weighting function:

$$\mathrm{W}(u; \lambda, \kappa) = \begin{cases} \min\{1, \lambda + (u/\kappa - 1)\}, & \text{if } u > \kappa, \\ \lambda, & \text{otherwise.} \end{cases} \tag{8.28}$$

This function is shown in Figure 8.11. From the figure and Expression (8.28), it can be seen that $\mathrm{W}(u;\lambda,\kappa)$ is a linear function of u with a lower bound of $\lambda > 0$ and an upper bound of 1. The lower bound λ is reached when $u \leq \kappa$. So, by using this weighting function in the EWMA chart (8.26)–(8.27), when $E_{z,i} \leq \kappa$, $\mathrm{W}(u;\lambda,\kappa)$ becomes the regular weighting parameter λ. The parameter κ is similar to a control limit for the EWMA charting statistic $E_{z,i}$. So, when $E_{z,i} \leq \kappa$, it is unlikely that there is an upward mean shift in $z(t,\boldsymbol{s})$ by the time t_i^*. In such cases, it is reasonable to use the regular weighting parameter λ in (8.26). When $E_{z,i} > \kappa$, it is likely that an upward mean shift in $z(t,\boldsymbol{s})$ has occurred at or before the time t_i^*. In such cases, the weight $\mathrm{W}(E_{z,i};\lambda,\kappa)$ defined in (8.28) will be larger than λ, implying that the observed disease incidence rates at t_i^* and a few previous time points will receive more weights, which is intuitively reasonable, as explained before.

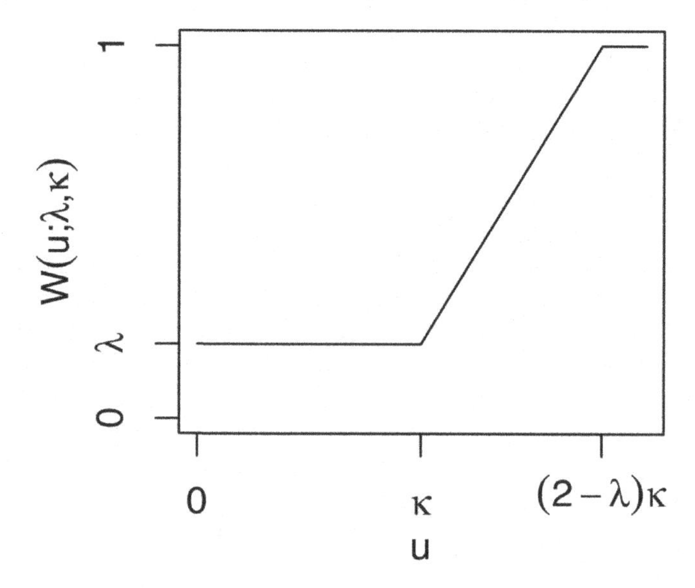

FIGURE 8.11
The weighting function $\mathrm{W}(u;\lambda,\kappa)$ defined in (8.28).

In the weighting function $\mathrm{W}(u;\lambda,\kappa)$ defined in (8.28), there are two parameters λ and κ involved. As explained above, λ is a regular weighting parameter used in an EWMA chart. It can be chosen to be the same as the one used in defining the EWMA charting statistic $E_{z,i}$ in (8.25). Regarding κ, it can be selected similarly to a control limit of an EWMA chart. Let the IC ARL value of the EWMA chart with the charting statistic $E_{z,i}$ be $\mathrm{ARL}_{0,z}$. Then, κ can be chosen from an IC dataset $\{(\mathbf{X}_1(t_i'),\mathbf{X}_2(t_i',\boldsymbol{s}_{ij}'),y(t_i',\boldsymbol{s}_{ij}')), j = 1,2,\ldots,m_i', i = 1,2,\ldots,n'\}$ by a block bootstrap procedure consisting of the following five steps, where the IC data used here could be different from the one used for estimating the IC model (8.22).

1) The standardized residuals $\{\breve{e}_z(t_i'), i = 1, 2, \ldots, n'\}$ are first computed as discussed above, and then $n' - b + 1$ blocks $\{Q_k, k = 1, 2, \ldots, n' - b + 1\}$ can be constructed from these standardized residuals, where $Q_k = \{\breve{e}_z(t_i'), i = k, k+1, \ldots, k+b-1\}$, and b is a block size.

2) A sequence of blocks can be randomly selected with replacement from $\{Q_k, k = 1, 2, \ldots, n' - b + 1\}$, and the selected blocks are placed one after another to form a bootstrap sample, denoted as $\{\breve{e}_{z,i}^{(l)}, i \geq 1\}$.

3) For $i \geq 1$, we calculate the EWMA charting statistic values from the bootstrap sample, defined as $E_{z,i}^{(l)} = \lambda \breve{e}_{z,i}^{(l)} + (1 - \lambda) E_{z,i-1}^{(l)}$, and record the IC run length as $\mathrm{RL}_0^{(l)}(\kappa) = \min\{i, E_{z,i}^{(l)} > \kappa\}$, for a given value of κ.

4) The second and third steps are then repeated for B times, and the average of the B values of $\mathrm{RL}_0^{(l)}(\kappa)$ is used for approximating $\mathrm{ARL}_0(\kappa)$ which is the ARL_0 value of the chart when κ is used as its control limit.

5) The bisection or an alternative numerical search algorithm is used to search for a value of κ such that $\mathrm{ARL}_0(\kappa)$ equals a pre-specified value of $\mathrm{ARL}_{0,z}$.

For the EWMA chart (8.26)–(8.27), its control limit L can be determined in the same way by the above block bootstrap procedure, once its IC ARL value, denoted as $\mathrm{ARL}_{0,y}$, is given and the weighting function $\mathrm{W}(u; \lambda, \kappa)$ is determined. So, to use the EWMA chart (8.26)–(8.27), the following three parameters need to be pre-specified: λ, $\mathrm{ARL}_{0,z}$ and $\mathrm{ARL}_{0,y}$. Based on a large simulation study, the following conclusions were made in Qiu and Yang (2021) regarding the selection of λ and $\mathrm{ARL}_{0,z}$. First, the general conclusion about the impact of λ on the performance of an EWMA chart is still true here that a smaller λ is good for detecting a smaller shift and a larger λ is good for detecting a larger shift (cf., Qiu, 2014, Chapter 5). Second, selection of $\mathrm{ARL}_{0,z}$ depends on whether a future shift is related to a shift in covariates: if the answer is "yes", then $\mathrm{ARL}_{0,z}$ should be chosen relatively small. Otherwise, it should be chosen large. In practice, we may not have such prior information. In such cases, Qiu and Yang (2021) suggested choosing $\mathrm{ARL}_{0,z} = \mathrm{ARL}_{0,y}$. The corresponding results when $\mathrm{ARL}_{0,z} = \mathrm{ARL}_{0,y}$ may not be the best, but they would be reasonably good. Regarding the block size b in the above block bootstrap procedure, Qiu and Yang (2021) suggested choosing it in the interval $[10, 15]$.

A modified version of the chart (8.26)–(8.27). It should be pointed out that the chart (8.26)–(8.27) may not be effective for detecting an upward mean shift in the disease incidence rate $y(t, \boldsymbol{s})$ in cases when $y(t, \boldsymbol{s})$ actually has downward shifts at some spatial locations. The reason is that the decorrelated and standardized residuals $\{\widetilde{e}_y(t_i^*, \boldsymbol{s}_{ij}^*), j = 1, 2, \ldots, m_i^*\}$ have been averaged across different spatial locations to obtain $\breve{e}_y(t_i^*)$ at the current observation time t_i^* when computing the charting statistic $E_{y,i}$. So, positive and negative residuals at different spatial locations would be cancelled out, making the resulting chart ineffective in such cases. To overcome this limitation, the following modified version of the chart (8.26)–(8.27) was suggested in Qiu and Yang (2021). Let

$$\begin{aligned}\widehat{e}_{y,+}(t_i^*, \boldsymbol{s}_{ij}^*) &= \max(\widehat{e}_y(t_i^*, \boldsymbol{s}_{ij}^*), 0),\\ \widehat{e}_{z,+}(t_i^*, \boldsymbol{s}_{ij}^*) &= \max(\widehat{e}_z(t_i^*, \boldsymbol{s}_{ij}^*), 0),\end{aligned}$$

for $j = 1, 2, \ldots, m_i^*$ and $i \geq 1$. Then, the means of these quantities would be non-zero, and their standardized values are defined to be

$$\begin{aligned}\widehat{e}_{y,0}(t_i^*, \boldsymbol{s}_{ij}^*) &= \frac{\widehat{e}_{y,+}(t_i^*, \boldsymbol{s}_{ij}^*) - \widehat{\mu}_{y,+}(t_i^*, \boldsymbol{s}_{ij}^*)}{\widehat{\sigma}_{y,+}(t_i^*, \boldsymbol{s}_{ij}^*)},\\ \widehat{e}_{z,0}(t_i^*, \boldsymbol{s}_{ij}^*) &= \frac{\widehat{e}_{z,+}(t_i^*, \boldsymbol{s}_{ij}^*) - \widehat{\mu}_{z,+}(t_i^*, \boldsymbol{s}_{ij}^*)}{\widehat{\sigma}_{z,+}(t_i^*, \boldsymbol{s}_{ij}^*)},\end{aligned} \tag{8.29}$$

where $\widehat{\mu}_{y,+}(t_i^*, \boldsymbol{s}_{ij}^*)$ and $\widehat{\mu}_{z,+}(t_i^*, \boldsymbol{s}_{ij}^*)$ are the estimated means of $\widehat{e}_{y,+}(t_i^*, \boldsymbol{s}_{ij}^*)$ and $\widehat{e}_{z,+}(t_i^*, \boldsymbol{s}_{ij}^*)$, respectively, and $\widehat{\sigma}_{y,+}(t_i^*, \boldsymbol{s}_{ij}^*)$ and $\widehat{\sigma}_{z,+}(t_i^*, \boldsymbol{s}_{ij}^*)$ are their estimated standard deviations. The estimated mean functions $\widehat{\mu}_{y,+}(t, \boldsymbol{s})$ and $\widehat{\mu}_{z,+}(t, \boldsymbol{s})$ can both be obtained by the formula (8.10) after $\{y(t_i, \boldsymbol{s}_{ij}), j = 1, 2, \ldots, m_i, i = 1, 2, \ldots, n\}$ are replaced respectively by $\{\widehat{e}_{y,+}(t_i, \boldsymbol{s}_{ij}), j = 1, 2, \ldots, m_i, i = 1, 2, \ldots, n\}$ and $\{\widehat{e}_{z,+}(t_i, \boldsymbol{s}_{ij}), j = 1, 2, \ldots, m_i, i = 1, 2, \ldots, n\}$. Similarly, the variance and covariance functions $\widehat{\sigma}^2_{y,+}(t, \boldsymbol{s})$, $\widehat{\sigma}^2_{z,+}(t, \boldsymbol{s})$, $\widehat{V}_{y,+}(t, t'; \boldsymbol{s}, \boldsymbol{s}')$ and $\widehat{V}_{z,+}(t, t'; \boldsymbol{s}, \boldsymbol{s}')$ can be obtained by the estimation procedures (8.7) and (8.8) after $\{\widehat{\varepsilon}_y(t_i, \boldsymbol{s}_{ij}), j = 1, 2, \ldots, m_i, i = 1, 2, \ldots, n\}$ are replaced respectively by

$$\{\widehat{\varepsilon}_{y,+}(t_i, \boldsymbol{s}_{ij}) = \widehat{e}_{y,+}(t_i, \boldsymbol{s}_{ij}) - \widehat{\mu}_{y,+}(t_i, \boldsymbol{s}_{ij}), j = 1, 2, \ldots, m_i, i = 1, 2, \ldots, n\}$$

and

$$\{\widehat{\varepsilon}_{z,+}(t_i, \boldsymbol{s}_{ij}) = \widehat{e}_{z,+}(t_i, \boldsymbol{s}_{ij}) - \widehat{\mu}_{z,+}(t_i, \boldsymbol{s}_{ij}), j = 1, 2, \ldots, m_i, i = 1, 2, \ldots, n\}.$$

The bandwidths used in computing $\widehat{\mu}_{y,+}(t, \boldsymbol{s})$ and $\widehat{\mu}_{z,+}(t, \boldsymbol{s})$ can be selected by the MCV procedure (8.6) or the BCE-MSE procedure (8.12), while the bandwidths used for computing $\widehat{\sigma}^2_{y,+}(t, \boldsymbol{s})$, $\widehat{\sigma}^2_{z,+}(t, \boldsymbol{s})$, $\widehat{V}_{y,+}(t, t'; \boldsymbol{s}, \boldsymbol{s}')$ and $\widehat{V}_{z,+}(t, t'; \boldsymbol{s}, \boldsymbol{s}')$ can be chosen by the MSPE procedure (8.9). Then, the modified charting statistic is defined by (8.26), after the quantities $\{\check{e}_y(t_i^*), i \geq 1\}$ computed from $\{\widehat{e}_y(t_i^*, \boldsymbol{s}_{ij}^*), j = 1, 2, \ldots, m_i^*, i \geq 1\}$ are replaced by the corresponding ones computed from $\{\widehat{e}_{y,0}(t_i^*, \boldsymbol{s}_{ij}^*), j = 1, 2, \ldots, m_i^*, i \geq 1\}$.

Example 8.7 *Qiu and Yang (2021) presented the following simulation results to investigate the numerical performance of the disease surveillance method based on the EWMA chart (8.26)–(8.27), denoted as NEW, and its modified version discussed above, denoted as MNEW. The similation setup is described as follows. First, it is assumed that* $[0, T] = [0, 1]$*, the observation times in the IC data are* $\{t_i = i/n, i = 1, 2, \ldots, n\}$*, and the observation locations* $\{\boldsymbol{s}_j, j =$

$1,2,\ldots,m\}$ are unchanged over time and equally spaced in $\Omega=[0,1]\times[0,1]$. Second, the IC model (8.22) is assumed to be

$$y(t,\boldsymbol{s})=\mu(t,\boldsymbol{s})+\beta_1 X_1(t)+\beta_2 X_2(t,\boldsymbol{s})+\varepsilon(t,\boldsymbol{s}),\quad \textit{for}\quad (t,\boldsymbol{s})\in[0,1]\times\Omega,$$

where

$$\begin{aligned} X_1(t) &= \mu_1(t)+\varepsilon_1(t),\\ X_2(t,\boldsymbol{s}) &= \mu_2(t,\boldsymbol{s})+\varepsilon_2(t,\boldsymbol{s}), \end{aligned}$$

and $\varepsilon_1(t)$, $\varepsilon_2(t,\boldsymbol{s})$ and $\varepsilon(t,\boldsymbol{s})$ are mutually independent zero-mean random errors. In the above model, it is assumed that

$$\begin{aligned} \beta_1 &= \beta_2=0.3,\\ \mu_1(t) &= 0.01(t-0.5)^2,\\ \mu_2(t,\boldsymbol{s}) &= 0.01(t-0.5)^2+0.01\left[(s_u-0.5)^2+(s_v-0.5)^2\right],\\ \mu(t,\boldsymbol{s}) &= 0.01\cos(2\pi t)+0.01\exp[-(s_u+s_v)/2]+0.02, \end{aligned}$$

where $\boldsymbol{s}=(s_u,s_v)'$. The random errors $\{\varepsilon(t_i,\boldsymbol{s}_j)\}$, $\{\varepsilon_1(t_i)\}$ and $\{\varepsilon_2(t_i,\boldsymbol{s}_j)\}$ are generated as follows:

- *The quantities $\{\varepsilon_1(t_i)\}$ are generated from the AR(1) model*

  $$\varepsilon_1(t_i)=\rho_t\varepsilon_1(t_{i-1})+(1-\rho_t^2)^{1/2}\eta_1(t_i),$$

  where $|\rho_t|<1$ is a constant and $\{\eta_1(t_i)\}$ are i.i.d. with the common distribution $N(0,0.006^2)$.

- *Let $\boldsymbol{\varepsilon}_2(t_i)=(\varepsilon_2(t_i,\boldsymbol{s}_1),\varepsilon_2(t_i,\boldsymbol{s}_2),\ldots,\varepsilon_2(t_i,\boldsymbol{s}_m))'$. Then, $\boldsymbol{\varepsilon}_2(t_i)$ is generated from the vector AR(1) model*

  $$\boldsymbol{\varepsilon}_2(t_i)=\rho_t\boldsymbol{\varepsilon}_2(t_{i-1})+(1-\rho_t^2)^{1/2}\boldsymbol{\eta}_2(t_i),$$

  where $\boldsymbol{\eta}_2(t_i)=(\eta_2(t_i,\boldsymbol{s}_1),\eta_2(t_i,\boldsymbol{s}_2),\ldots,\eta_2(t_i,\boldsymbol{s}_m))'$ are temporally independent Gaussian spatial processes whose spatial correlation is described by the covariance function

  $$Cov(\eta_2(t_i,\boldsymbol{s}_j),\eta_2(t_i,\boldsymbol{s}_l))=0.006^2\exp\left[-d_E(\boldsymbol{s}_j,\boldsymbol{s}_l)/\rho_s\right],$$

  and $\rho_s>0$ is a constant.

- *Let $\boldsymbol{\varepsilon}(t_i)=(\varepsilon(t_i,\boldsymbol{s}_1),\varepsilon(t_i,\boldsymbol{s}_2),\ldots,\varepsilon(t_i,\boldsymbol{s}_m))'$. Then, $\boldsymbol{\varepsilon}(t_i)$ is generated in the same way as that for $\boldsymbol{\varepsilon}_2(t_i)$, except that its spatial covariance at each time point is assumed to be*

  $$Cov(\eta(t_i,\boldsymbol{s}_j),\eta(t_i,\boldsymbol{s}_l))=0.003^2\exp[-d_E(\boldsymbol{s}_j,\boldsymbol{s}_l)/\rho_s].$$

In the above setup, it can be checked that, for any $1 \leq i, k \leq n$ and $1 \leq j, l \leq m$, the covariance between $y(t_i, \boldsymbol{s}_j)$ and $y(t_k, \boldsymbol{s}_l)$ is

$$\begin{aligned} & V_y(t_i, t_k; \boldsymbol{s}_j, \boldsymbol{s}_l) \\ = & \rho_t^{|k-i|}\left\{0.006^2\beta_1^2 + (0.006^2\beta_2^2 + 0.003^2)\exp\left[-\frac{d_E(\boldsymbol{s}_j, \boldsymbol{s}_l)}{\rho_s}\right]\right\}. \end{aligned}$$

Thus, the parameters ρ_t and ρ_s control the data correlation in the time and space domains, respectively. The larger their values, the stronger the correlation. To consider cases with different spatio-temporal data correlation, (ρ_t, ρ_s) are chosen to be (0.2, 0.1), (0.4, 0.2) or (0.6, 0.3) in this study.

Third, the OC model for the disease incidence rates after a disease outbreak is assumed to be

$$y^{(\delta)}(t, \boldsymbol{s}) = \mu^{(\delta)}(t, \boldsymbol{s}) + z^{(\delta)}(t, \boldsymbol{s}) + \varepsilon(t, \boldsymbol{s}),$$

where

$$\begin{aligned} \mu^{(\delta)}(t, \boldsymbol{s}) &= \mu(t, \boldsymbol{s}) + \sigma_y\delta_\mu(t, \boldsymbol{s}), \\ z^{(\delta)}(t, \boldsymbol{s}) &= z(t, \boldsymbol{s}) + \sigma_y\delta_z(t, \boldsymbol{s}), \end{aligned}$$

$\sigma_y = (0.006^2 \times 2 \times 0.3^2 + 0.003^2)^{1/2} = 0.0039$ is the IC standard deviation of $y(t, \boldsymbol{s})$, $z(t, \boldsymbol{s}) = \beta_1 X_1(t) + \beta_2 X_2(t, \boldsymbol{s})$, $\delta_z(t, \boldsymbol{s})$ and $\delta_\mu(t, \boldsymbol{s})$ describe the shift sizes in $y(t, \boldsymbol{s})$ due to the covariates and other factors that are not included in the model, respectively, and $\mu(t, \boldsymbol{s})$, $X_1(t)$, $X_2(t, \boldsymbol{s})$ and $\varepsilon(t, \boldsymbol{s})$ are the same as those in the IC model. By some simple calculation, it can be checked that the OC mean function of $y(t, \boldsymbol{s})$ in the above setup is

$$\mu_y^{(\delta)}(t, \boldsymbol{s}) = \mu_y(t, \boldsymbol{s}) + \sigma_y[\delta_\mu(t, \boldsymbol{s}) + \delta_z(t, \boldsymbol{s})],$$

where $\mu_y(t, \boldsymbol{s})$ is the IC mean function of $y(t, \boldsymbol{s})$. The following four scenarios are considered about the shift sizes $\delta_\mu(t, \boldsymbol{s})$ and $\delta_z(t, \boldsymbol{s})$: for $\nu = 1, 2, 3, 4$,

(I) $\delta_\mu(t, \boldsymbol{s}) = 0.2\nu\xi_1(t, \boldsymbol{s})$, $\delta_z(t, \boldsymbol{s}) = 0$,

(II) $\delta_\mu(t, \boldsymbol{s}) = 0.04\nu\xi_1(t, \boldsymbol{s})$, $\delta_z(t, \boldsymbol{s}) = 0.16\nu\xi_1(t, \boldsymbol{s})$,

(III) $\delta_\mu(t, \boldsymbol{s}) = 0.2\nu\xi_2(t, \boldsymbol{s})$, $\delta_z(t, \boldsymbol{s}) = 0$, *and*

(IV) $\delta_\mu(t, \boldsymbol{s}) = 0.04\nu\xi_2(t, \boldsymbol{s})$, $\delta_z(t, \boldsymbol{s}) = 0.16\nu\xi_2(t, \boldsymbol{s})$,

where

$$\begin{aligned} \xi_1(t, \boldsymbol{s}) &= 2(t - 0.5)^2 + \exp\left\{-[(s_u - 0.5)^2 + (s_v - 0.5)^2]\right\}, \\ \xi_2(t, \boldsymbol{s}) &= 2(t - 0.5)^2 + \exp\{-[(s_u - 0.5)^2 + (s_v - 0.5)^2]\} \times \\ & \quad sign\{|s_u - 0.5| + |s_v - 0.5| - 0.5\}, \end{aligned}$$

and sign(u) is the sign function that equals 1, 0 and -1 when $u > 0$, $= 0$ and < 0. From the above expressions, it can be seen that $\xi_1(t, \boldsymbol{s})$ is always *positive in* $[0,T] \times \Omega$, *and* $\xi_2(t, \boldsymbol{s})$ *could be negative in regions close to the center (0.5,0.5) of* Ω. *In addition, the shifts of types (I) and (III) are not due to the covariates at all, while those of types (II) and (IV) are due to both covariates and other factors. By comparing the shifts of types (I) and (III), those of type (I) are always positive at all observation times and locations, but those of type (III) could be negative in spatial regions close to the center (0.5,0.5) of* Ω. *Similarly, the shifts of type (II) are always positive, but shifts of type (IV) could be negative for both components* $\delta_\mu(t, \boldsymbol{s})$ *and* $\delta_z(t, \boldsymbol{s})$.

In the simulation study, the regression coefficients (β_1, β_2), *and the mean and covariance functions are estimated from an IC dataset of size* (n, m) *generated from the IC model. The control limits* κ *and L of the charts (8.25) and (8.26)–(8.27) are determined from another IC dataset of the same size by the block bootstrap procedure with the bootstrap sample size* $B = 10{,}000$ *and the block size* $l = 10$. *The actual* ARL_0 *and* ARL_1 *values of the charts are then computed based on 1000 replicated simulations of online process monitoring once the values of* λ, $ARL_{0,z}$ *and* $ARL_{0,y}$ *are pre-specified. Because these actual* ARL_0 *and* ARL_1 *values depend on the randomly generated IC datasets, the entire simulation process, from generation of the IC datasets, estimation of the IC model, determination of the control limits, to computation of the actual* ARL_0 *and* ARL_1 *values of a chart, is repeated for 100 times. The average of the 100* ARL_0 *(or* ARL_1*) values is used as the final estimate of the true* ARL_0 *(or* ARL_1*) value in each case considered.*

Besides the charts NEW and MNEW, the following four alternative methods are also considered in the numerical study.

- *Zhao et al. (2011) suggested a spatio-temporal disease surveillance method, denoted as DODZ, which is described briefly in Example 8.6.*

- *Chen et al. (2016) suggested a distribution-free EWMA chart, denoted as DFEWMA, for monitoring high-dimensional processes under the assumptions that the IC process distribution is unchanged over time and process observations at different time points are independent. In the DFEWMA chart, time-varying control limits are used, and they are obtained by a permutation testing procedure.*

- *In the chart NEW, a regular weighting parameter* λ *is used in (8.26), replacing the covariate-dependent weight* $W(E_{z,i}; \lambda, \kappa)$. *The resulting chart does not use any covariate information. It is denoted as WOC, represeting "without using covariate" information.*

- *In the chart MNEW, a regular weighting parameter* λ *is used. The resulting chart is denoted as MWOC.*

We first study the IC performance of all six methods discussed above. In the charts DFEWMA, WOC, MWOC, NEW and MNEW, the weighting parameter λ *is chosen to be 0.1, 0.2 or 0.3. In the method DODZ, the threshold value c is determined by a parametric bootstrap procedure, as discussed in*

Zhao et al. (2011). In the chart DFEWMA, there is a window size parameter w to choose. We adopt the suggestion by Chen et al. (2016) that w is chosen to be the smallest integer satisfying $(1-\lambda)^w \leq 0.05$. As mentioned above, the control limit of DFEWMA is chosen by a permutation testing procedure suggested by Chen et al. (2016). The control limits of WOC, MWOC, NEW and MNEW are determined by the block bootstrap procedure discussed earlier in this section with $B = 10{,}000$ and $l = 10$. In both NEW and MNEW, $ARL_{0,z}$ is chosen to be the same as $ARL_{0,y}$. Then, in cases when the nominal ARL_0 value of each chart is fixed at 200, $(n,m) = (200,64)$ or $(400,100)$, and $(\rho_t, \rho_s) = (0.2, 0.1)$, $(0.4, 0.2)$ or $(0.6, 0.3)$, the calculated actual ARL_0 values of the six control charts are presented in Table 8.4. From the table, it can be seen that (i) the actual ARL_0 values of DODZ and DFEWMA are quite far away from the nominal ARL_0 value of 200, due to the fact that some of their model assumptions are violated in this example, (ii) the actual ARL_0 values of WOC, MWOC, NEW and MNEW are all close to the nominal ARL_0 value, and thus these four charts all have a reliable IC performance, and (iii) for each chart, its actual ARL_0 values are closer to the nominal ARL_0 value when (n,m) are larger and/or (ρ_t, ρ_s) are smaller, which is intuitively reasonable.

TABLE 8.4
Actual ARL_0 values of six control charts in different cases when their nominal ARL_0 values are all fixed at 200.

(n,m)	(ρ_t,ρ_s)	λ	DODZ	DFEWMA	WOC	MWOC	NEW	MNEW
(200,64)	(0.2,0.1)	0.1	174	112	193	195	192	194
		0.2		127	197	197	196	197
		0.3		140	198	203	198	200
	(0.4,0.2)	0.1	161	97	187	189	185	186
		0.2		108	192	192	191	192
		0.3		114	195	197	192	195
	(0.6,0.3)	0.1	141	86	182	185	181	183
		0.2		94	190	190	189	187
		0.3		104	193	192	192	193
(400,100)	(0.2,0.1)	0.1	189	121	198	197	204	203
		0.2		129	199	202	198	201
		0.3		147	200	201	200	200
	(0.4,0.2)	0.1	174	103	191	191	190	190
		0.2		111	195	192	193	194
		0.3		121	199	202	198	199
	(0.6,0.3)	0.1	158	92	187	189	188	186
		0.2		102	192	191	191	190
		0.3		111	195	196	196	195

Next, we compare the OC performance of all six methods in cases when their nominal ARL_0 values are all fixed at 200, $(n,m) = (200,64)$ or

$(400, 100)$, *and* $(\rho_t, \rho_s) = (0.2, 0.1)$, $(0.4, 0.2)$ *or* $(0.6, 0.3)$. *To make the comparison fair, the control limits of the six charts, especially the charts DODZ and DFEWMA, are all adjusted such that their actual* ARL_0 *values equal to 200. In addition, a weighting parameter* λ *is involved in the charts DFEWMA, WOC, MWOC, NEW and MNEW, and the OC performance of the related charts may not be comparable if they use a same value of* λ *(cf., Qiu, 2008). To overcome this difficulty, their optimal OC performance is considered here, which is obtained by changing the value of* λ *for each method such that its* ARL_1 *value is minimized for detecting a given shift. In the charts NEW and MNEW,* $ARL_{0,z}$ *is chosen to be the same as* $ARL_{0,y}$*, and other setups are the same as those in Table 8.4. Then, the optimal* ARL_1 *values of the six methods are shown in Figures 8.12 and 8.13. From the figures, we can have the following conclusions. (i) The four charts WOC, MWOC, NEW and MNEW perform uniformly better than the remaining two charts DODZ and DFEWMA in all cases considered. (ii) WOC performs slightly better than MWOC, NEW and MNEW for detecting shifts of type (I). (iii) For detecting shifts of type (II), NEW and MNEW are better than WOC and MWOC. (iv) MNEW and MWOC are better than NEW and WOC for detecting shifts of type (III). (v) To detect shifts of type (IV), MNEW performs the best. The conclusion (i) is reasonable because some model assumptions of DODZ and DFEWMA are invalid in this example. All shifts of type (I) are positive and not due to the covariates. So, the conclusion (ii) is reasonable because the chart WOC did not use any covariate information in its construction, it did not consider any modifications for handling negative shifts, and thus the variability of its charting statistic would be smaller than that of the charts MWOC, NEW and MNEW. Since the shifts of type (II) are partially due to covariates and all positive, NEW and MNEW would be better than WOC and MWOC, and NEW would be better than MNEW. This explains why the conclusion (iii) is also reasonable. The remaining two conclusions can be explained in a similar way. From this example, it can be seen that the chart MNEW performs the best or close to the best in all cases considered. Because it is often difficult to know in practice whether a future shift would be related to the covariates and whether it could be negative at some spatial locations, the chart MNEW is recommended in Qiu and Yang (2021).*

8.6 Some Discussions

In this chapter, we have introduced several recent statistical methods for spatio-temporal disease surveillance. These methods are based on nonparametric spatio-temporal regression modeling approaches discussed in Section 8.2 for estimating the regular spatio-temporal pattern of the observed disease incidence rates. These nonparametric modeling approaches do not impose restrictive assumptions on the spatio-temporal mean, variance/covariance,

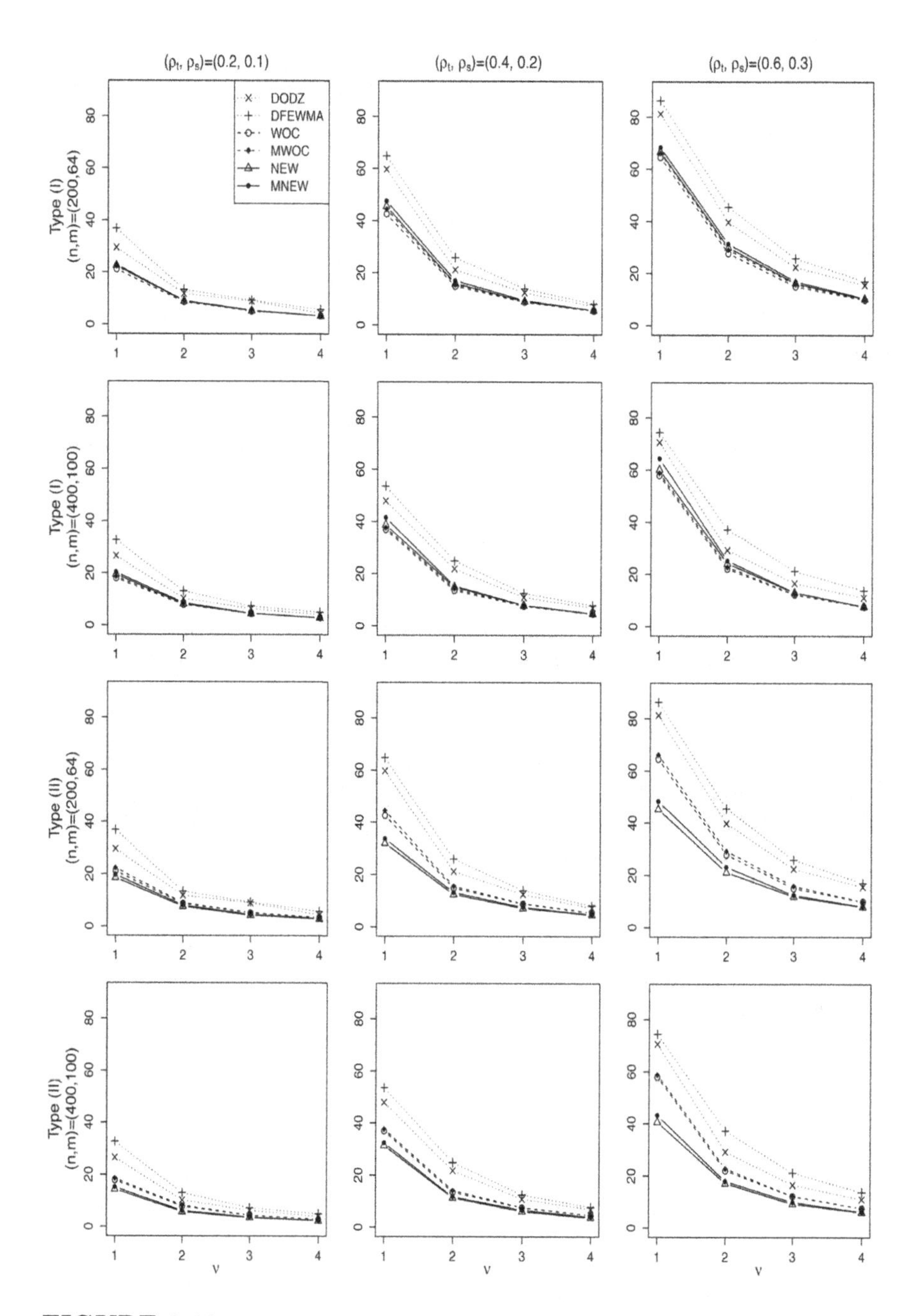

FIGURE 8.12
Optimal ARL_1 values of the six charts DODZ, DFEWMA, WOC, MWOC, NEW and MNEW for detecting shifts of types (I) and (II).

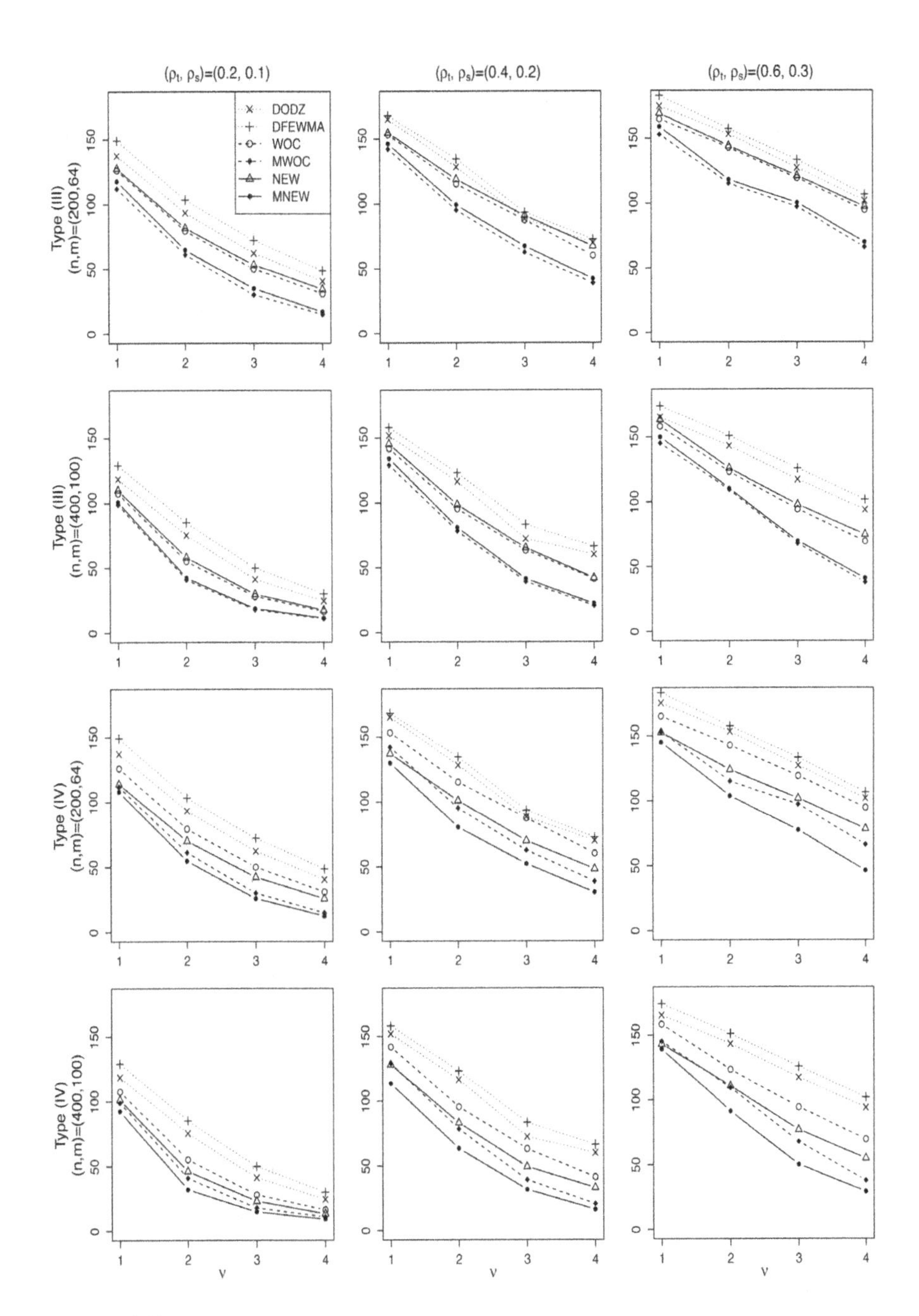

FIGURE 8.13
Optimal ARL_1 values of the six charts DODZ, DFEWMA, WOC, MWOC, NEW and MNEW for detecting shifts of types (III) and (IV).

and data distribution functions. Thus, they are flexible enough to accommodate the complex data structure of the observed disease incidence rates. The resulting disease surveillance methods are also flexible and can accommodate time-varying IC distribution of the disease incidence rates and other complexities of the observed data.

Three specific spatio-temporal disease surveillance methods have been introduced in this chapter. The one discussed in Section 8.3 makes its decision about whether a disease outbreak is present at the current observation time by comparing the observed spatio-temporal pattern of the disease incidence rates with the estimated regular spatio-temporal pattern, after the observed data are properly decorrelated and standardized in advance. This method is effective, compared to the ones based on some conventional multivariate control charts. But, it has not taken into account the special feature of the disease surveillance problem that a disease outbreak often starts in small clustered regions. The disease surveillance method introduced in Section 8.4 has been developed based on this feature. It combines seamlessly a spatial LASSO procedure in the space domain with the exponentially weighted smoothing procedure in the time domain. Numerical results show that it is more effective than the one discussed in Section 8.3 in most cases considered. In practice, disease incidence rates are often associated with some covariates, and the methods discussed in Sections 8.3 and 8.4 have not used any covariate information. Intuitively, proper use of helpful covariate information should be able to improve disease surveillance, which has been confirmed by the method and the related numerical results introduced in Section 8.5.

There are still some issues about the disease surveillance methods introduced in this chapter. For instance, all of them require to have an IC dataset available in advance, from which the regular spatio-temporal pattern of the disease incidence rates can be estimated. In practice, such an IC dataset is only available for some diseases that we have a reasonably good knowledge, such as the influenza and some other respiratory diseases. For some other diseases, especially those relatively new, it is often challenging to know whether disease outbreaks are present or not in a given period of time. It is also challenging to collect a suitable amount of IC data in such cases. This issue is related to the Phase-I SPC problem discussed in Subsection 3.1.1. But, the conventional Phase-I SPC charts cannot be applied to the current problem because they require the assumptions that the IC distribution of the disease incidence rates remains unchanged over time and the observed data are independent at different times and/or locations, which are obviously invalid here. These difficulties might be possible to overcome, using similar methods to those discussed in Sections 8.2 and 8.3 for data decorrelation and standardization, which needs to be confirmed in future research. Another possible method to handle the challenges mentioned above is to use the self-starting control charts introduced in Subsection 3.2.1. The major idea of such charts is to keep expanding the IC data by combining the existing IC data with the new observations collected at the current time point after the spatial process under monitoring is confirmed to be IC. Again, the conventional self-starting control charts cannot be applied to the current problem directly due to their restrictive assumptions, which should be addressed properly. In addition, after a signal is given by the control chart in a disease surveillance method, it is important to know when and where the detected disease outbreak occurs. This is related to the post-signal diagnosis discussed in the SPC literature (cf., Li et al., 2017; Xian et al., 2019), and has not been discussed in this chapter yet.

Regarding the disease surveillance method based on the exponentially weighted spatial LASSO (EWSL) chart discussed in Section 8.4, the EWSL chart is based on the L_1 adaptive spatial LASSO penalty. In the statistical literature, there are some alternative penalized approaches for variable selection, such as the elastic net (Zou and Hastie, 2005) and the smoothly clipped absolute deviation procedure (Fan and Li, 2001). It should be interesting to study these alternative variable selection procedures in the context of spatio-temporal process monitoring and then select a more effective variable selection approach. Furthermore, performance of the EWSL chart depends on the weighting parameter λ. Since this parameter is similar to the weighting parameter in a conventional EWMA chart, it is expected that the optimal selection of λ depends on the shift size that is often unknown in practice. To overcome the difficulty to select a proper value for λ, one strategy is to combine a sequence of potential values of λ to achieve a robust OC performance (e.g., Qiu et al., 2018). Another strategy is to consider an adaptive EWMA chart discussed in Subsection 3.2.2 in which the shift size is estimated sequentially and the value of λ is adjusted accordingly.

For the disease surveillance method using covariate information that is discussed in Section 8.5, there could be a large number of covariates that are all potentially relevant to the disease incidence rates in practice. Intuitively, only those highly important ones should be included in the IC model (8.22), to reduce the variability of the estimated IC model and improve the efficiency of the subsequent process monitoring. Therefore, a reliable and effective variable selection procedure should be helpful when estimating the IC model. In addition, although the semiparametric IC model (8.22) is already quite flexible, it assumes that the relationship between the covariates and the response (i.e., the disease incidence rate) is linear, which may not be appropriate in some applications. This model is possible to be further generalized to a semiparametric model with space/time-varying coefficients or even a completely nonparametric model. However, such possible generalizations are not straightforward and require much future research effort.

8.7 Exercises

8.1 Summarize the major complexities of the spatio-temporal data discussed in Example 8.1 about the observed incidence rates of influenza-like illness (ILI) for all 67 counties of Florida. Explain intuitively why such data would be spatio-temporally correlated.

8.2 In cases when the observed data at different times and/or spatial locations are assumed independent (i.e., $\widehat{\Sigma}_{\mathbf{Y}}$ in (8.3) is the identity matrix), $\widetilde{\mu}(t, \boldsymbol{s})$ in (8.4) is the conventional local linear kernel (LLK) estimate of the mean function $\mu(t, \boldsymbol{s})$. The current formula (8.4) is in a matrix format. Please rewrite this formula using the elements of the related matrices.

8.3 Explain intuitively why the estimates of the variance and covariance functions defined in (8.7) and (8.8) would be good estimates.

8.4 Use the R function **nearPD()** in the package **Matrix** to find the modified covariance matrix of $\widehat{\mathbf{V}}$, where

$$\widehat{\mathbf{V}} = \begin{pmatrix} 1 & 0.5 & 0.5 \\ 0.5 & 1 & 0.5 \\ 0.5 & 0.5 & -0.25 \end{pmatrix}.$$

8.5 In Example 8.3 discussed in Subsection 8.2.3,

(i)Check that in Case 2, $V(t_i, t_k; \boldsymbol{s}_j, \boldsymbol{s}_l) = \phi^{|k-i|}\rho(d_E(\boldsymbol{s}_j, \boldsymbol{s}_l))$.

(ii)Check that in Case 3, $V(t_i, t_k; \boldsymbol{s}_j, \boldsymbol{s}_l) = c_{|k-i|}\rho(\boldsymbol{s}_j, \boldsymbol{s}_l)$, where $c_0 = (1-\phi_2)/\{(1+\phi_2)((1-\phi_2)^2 - \phi_1^2)\}$, $c_1 = \frac{\phi_1}{1-\phi_2}c_0$, and $c_d = \phi_1 c_{d-1} + \phi_2 c_{d-2}$, for $d > 1$.

8.6 In Example 8.4 discussed in Subsection 8.2.4, verify that

$$V(t_i, t_k; \boldsymbol{s}_j, \boldsymbol{s}_l) = \sigma^2 \phi_t^{n|t_i - t_k|}\rho(d_E(\boldsymbol{s}_j, \boldsymbol{s}_l)),$$

for any $t_i, t_k \in [0,1]$ and $\boldsymbol{s}_j, \boldsymbol{s}_l \in [0,1] \times [0,1]$.

8.7 Using the R package **SpTe2M** introduced in Chapter 9, reproduce the results in Example 8.5 discussed in Section 8.3.

8.8 Derive the formula for $\widetilde{\mu}_{\widehat{\varepsilon}}(t_i^*, \boldsymbol{s})$ from (8.16).

8.9 Use the R package **SpTe2M** introduced in Chapter 9 and the EWSL disease surveillance method discussed in Section 8.4 to analyze the ILI data discussed in Example 8.5. Compare the results here with those in Exercise 8.7.

9

R Package **SpTe2M** *for Nonparametric Spatio-Temporal Data Modeling and Monitoring*

9.1 Introduction

Although this book focuses on applications of spatio-temporal data analysis in disease surveillance, spatio-temporal data are actually popular in many different disciplines and areas, including agriculture, climate science, epidemiology, neuroscience, social science and more. Because of the importance of spatio-temporal data, there have been many existing methods for analyzing spatio-temporal data in the literature. Some of them have been discussed in Section 2.7 and Chapter 7. Some *R* packages have also been developed for analyzing spatio-temporal data based on these methods, including the *R* packages **SpatioTemporal**, **lgcp**, **MARSS**, **dse** and **KFAS** that are discussed in Section 2.7, and **surveillance**, **rflexscan** and **smerc** that are discussed in Chapter 7. There are some other *R* packages available for spatio-temporal modeling and prediction, including the *R* package **spTimer** (Bakar and Sahu, 2015) for hierarchical Bayesian spatio-temporal modeling, the *R* package **laGP** (Gramacy, 2016) for implementing the local approximate Gaussian process method, the *R* package **FRK** (Zammit-Mangion and Cressie, 2017) for using the fixed rank kriging method, the *R* package **BayesNSGP** (Risser and Turek, 2020) for implementing the non-stationary Gaussian process method, and the *R* package **spNNGP** (Finley et al., 2020) for using the nearest neighbor Gaussian process method.

As discussed in Chapters 7 and 8, spatio-temporal data often have complicated structure, including complex spatio-temporal variation, latent spatio-temporal correlation, and unknown data distribution, which can rarely be described properly by parametric models (cf., Yang and Qiu, 2020). However, many existing methods require various restrictive model assumptions, making their results unreliable in certain applications. In addition, the statistical methods behind most *R* packages mentioned above are designed mainly for retrospective data analysis, in which the time interval of the observed data is pre-specified. The disease surveillance problem, however, is a prospective sequential process monitoring problem in the sense that the observation time

DOI: 10.1201/9781003138150-9

of disease incidence rate keeps increasing and new observed data keep being collected over time, as discussed in Section 7.1. To overcome the major limitations of the conventional methods for handling the disease surveillance problem, some nonparametric spatio-temporal data modeling and monitoring methods have been developed and introduced in Chapter 8. In this chapter, we introduce an associated *R* package named **SpTe2M** (Yang and Qiu, 2023) for implementation of these methods, where the name of the package denotes "**Sp**atio-**Te**mporal **M**odeling and **M**onitoring".

This chapter is organized as follows. Major functions in the *R* package **SpTe2M** are first introduced in Section 9.2. Then, these functions and the related statistical methods are demonstrated using the influenza-like illness data (cf., Example 8.1) in Section 9.3.

9.2 Major Functions in the *R* Package SpTe2M

There are two ways to use the *R* Package **SpTe2M**. First, we can install it on our own computer by i) downloading the archive file **SpTe2M_1.0.0.tar.gz** from the comprehensive *R* archive network (CRAN) webpage with the following address

$$https://cran.r-project.org/web/packages/SpTe2M/index.html$$

to the current directory on our computer, and ii) installing the package by running the following commands in the *R* environment:

```
> install.packages("SpTe2M_1.0.0.tar.gz")
> library("SpTe2M")
```

Note that the sequence of numbers "1.0.0" in the archive file name **SpTe2M_1.0.0.tar.gz** represents the version of the package. Usually, the package is updated once a year. So, in order to use the latest version of the package, we need to download the archive file regularly.

Second, in the *R* environment, we can run the following command:

```
> install.packages("SpTe2M")
```

Then, a window will pop up, providing us a list of secure CRAN mirror sites. We can choose a site that is close to our physical location. After the selection, the package will be installed on our computer, and we can run the following command in order to use the related functions in the package:

```
> library("SpTe2M")
```

By comparing with the first way of package installation, we do not specify the package version in this installation. Actually, the latest version is always used in this way of package installation.

After the package is installed properly, we are ready to use its built-in functions and datasets. To have an access to the package description, use the following *R* command:

```
> help(package="SpTe2M")
```

To have an access to the description about a specific built-in function or dataset (e.g., the built-in function **SpTe_MeanEst()**), use the following *R* command:

```
> ?SpTe_MeanEst
```

All built-in functions and datasets in the *R* package **SpTe2M** are described below. Demonstration on how to use them for data analysis is given in the next section.

cv_mspe() This function is for determining the bandwidths $(h_{t,1}, h_{s,1})$ used in computing the variance and covariance estimates defined in (8.7) and (8.8) by the CV-MSPE score defined in (8.9). This function can be used in the *R* environment as follows.

```
> cv_mspe(y,st,gt=NULL,gs=NULL)
```

The arguments of the above *R* command are explained below.

y	An N-dimensional vector that contains the spatio-temporal observations $\{y(t_i, \mathbf{s}_{ij}), j = 1, 2, \ldots, m_i, i = 1, 2, \ldots, n\}$, where $N = \sum_{i=1}^{n} m_i$.
st	An $N \times 3$ matrix containing the observation locations and times $\{(\mathbf{s}'_{ij}, t_i), j = 1, 2, \ldots, m_i, i = 1, 2, \ldots, n\}$.
gt	A vector of user-specified possible values for the bandwidth in the time domain used in estimating the variance/covariance functions of Model (8.1), from which the optimal one is estimated by the CV-MSPE procedure. Its default value is NULL. In such cases, it is a vector of the sequence of values from 0 to 1 with the step 0.05.
gs	A vector of user-specified possible values for the bandwidth in the space domain used in estimating the variance/covariance functions of Model (8.1), from which the optimal one is estimated by the CV-MSPE procedure. Its default value is NULL. In such cases, it is a vector of the sequence of equally spaced values in $[0, \sqrt{2}]$.

This function returns the following values.

bandwidth	A matrix with two columns that contains all values of the bandwidths $(h_{t,1}, h_{s,1})$ considered in the bandwidth selection.
mspe	Values of the CV_MSPE score for the bandwidth values considered in the bandwidth selection.
bandwidth.opt	Selected bandwidths $(h_{t,1}, h_{s,1})$ that minimize the CV_MSPE score.
mspe.opt	Minimum value of the CV_MSPE score.

ili_dat The observed data of daily influenza-like illness (ILI) incidence rates of all 67 counties in Florida during 2012–2014 are included in the *R* Package **SpTe2M** for demonstrating the applications of the related spatio-temporal data modeling and monitoring methods. See Example 8.1 in Section 8.1 for some background introduction about this dataset. It contains the following 8 variables: County (county Name), Date (Date of the observation), Lat (latitude of the county), Long (longitude of the county), Time (standardized observation time in $[0, 1]$), Rate (observed ILI incidence rate), Temp (average air temperature) and RH (average relative humidity). This dataset can be retrieved in the *R* environment as follows.

```
> data(ili_dat)
```

Then, a data frame named "ili_dat" with 8 variables is retrieved for our use. Each variable has $N = 73,432$ spatio-temporal observations arranged by the spatial locations at each observation time. For instance, "ili_dat$Rate" denotes the long vector of the observed ILI incidence rates of all 67 counties in Florida, and

```
> ili_dat$Rate[1:67]
```

contains the observed ILI incidence rates of all 67 counties at the first observation time in the dataset.

mod_cv() This function is for selecting the bandwidths $(h_{t,0}, h_{s,0})$ used in computing the mean function estimate defined in (8.4) by the modified cross-validation (MCV) procedure defined in (8.6). It can be used in the *R* environment as follows.

```
> mod_cv(y,st,ht=NULL,hs=NULL,eps=0.1)
```

The arguments of the above *R* command are explained below.

y — An N-dimensional vector that contains the spatio-temporal observations $\{y(t_i, \mathbf{s}_{ij}), j = 1, 2, \ldots, m_i, i = 1, 2, \ldots, n\}$, where $N = \sum_{i=1}^{n} m_i$.

st — An $N \times 3$ matrix containing the observation locations and times $\{(\mathbf{s}'_{ij}, t_i), j = 1, 2, \ldots, m_i, i = 1, 2, \ldots, n\}$.

ht — A vector of user-specified candidate values for the bandwidth in the time domain used in computing the mean function estimate defined in (8.4), from which the optimal one is estimated by the MCV procedure. Its default value is NULL. In such cases, it is a vector of the sequence of values from 0 to 1 with the step 0.05.

hs — A vector of user-specified candidate values for the bandwidth in the space domain used in computing the mean function estimate defined in (8.4), from which the optimal one is estimated by the MCV procedure. Its default value is NULL. In such cases, it is a vector of the sequence of equally spaced values in $[0, \sqrt{2}]$.

eps — The constant value ϵ used in the bimodal kernel function defined in (8.5).

This function returns the following values.

bandwidth — A matrix with two columns that contains all values of the bandwidths $(h_{t,0}, h_{s,0})$ considered in the bandwidth selection.

mcv — Values of the MCV score for the bandwidth values considered in the bandwidth selection.

bandwidth.opt — Selected bandwidths $(h_{t,0}, h_{s,0})$ that minimize the MCV score.

mcv.opt — Minimum value of the MCV score.

pm25_dat The observed data of daily $PM_{2.5}$ concentration levels at 183 major cities in China during 2014–2016. This dataset was collected by the China National Environmental Monitoring Centre (CNEMC). It contains the following 6 variables: Year, Time (standardized observation time in $[0, 1]$), Long (longitude of the city), Lat (latitude of the city), City and PM2.5. This dataset can be retrieved in the *R* environment as follows.

```
> data(pm25_dat)
```

Then, a data frame named "pm25_dat" with 6 variables is retrieved for our use. Each variable has $N = 200,385$ spatio-temporal observations arranged by the spatial locations at each observation time. For instance, "pm25_dat$PM2.5" denotes the long vector of the observed $PM_{2.5}$ concentration levels of all 183 major cities in China during 2014–2016, and

```
> pm25_dat$PM2.5[1:183]
```

contains the observed $PM_{2.5}$ concentration levels of all 183 major cities in China on January 1, 2014 in the dataset.

sim_dat A simulated spatio-temporal dataset with $n = 100$ observation times and $m = 100$ time-independent spatial locations at each observation time. The data contain the following 3 variables with $N =$ 10,000 observations each: y (observed value of the response y), x (observed value of a univariate covariate x), and st (observation location $\mathbf{s} = (s_u, s_v)$ and time t). The spatio-temporal response y is generated from a model similar to the one used in Example 8.4 in Subsection 8.2.4. This simulated dataset can be retrieved in the R environment as follows.

```
> data(sim_dat)
```

Then, a data frame named "sim_dat" with 3 variables is retrieved for our use. Each variable has $N =$ 10,000 observations arranged by the spatial locations at each observation time. For instance, "sim_dat$y" denotes the long vector of the observed values of y, and

```
> sim_dat$y[1:100]
```

contains the observed y values at the 100 spatial locations at the first observation time.

spte_covest() This function is for estimating the variance and covariance functions as discussed in Subsection 8.2.3. It can be used in the R environment as follows.

```
> spte_covest(y,st,gt=NULL,gs=NULL,stE1=NULL,stE2=NULL)
```

The arguments of the above *R* command are explained below.

y	An N-dimensional vector that contains the spatio-temporal observations $\{y(t_i, \mathbf{s}_{ij}), j = 1, 2, \ldots, m_i, i = 1, 2, \ldots, n\}$, where $N = \sum_{i=1}^{n} m_i$.
st	An $N \times 3$ matrix containing the observation locations and times $\{(\mathbf{s}'_{ij}, t_i), j = 1, 2, \ldots, m_i, i = 1, 2, \ldots, n\}$.
gt	Pre-specified bandwidth in the time domain used in estimating the variance/covariance functions of Model (8.1). Its default value is NULL. In such cases, it is determined by the CV-MSPE procedure (8.9).
gs	Pre-specified bandwidth in the space domain used in estimating the variance/covariance functions of Model (8.1). Its default value is NULL. In such cases, it is determined by the CV-MSPE procedure (8.9).
stE1	An $N_1 \times 3$ matrix specifying the first set of observation locations and times for computing an $N_1 \times N_2$ covariate matrix. Its default value is NULL, in which case "stE1=st".
stE2	An $N_2 \times 3$ matrix specifying the second set of observation locations and times for computing an $N_1 \times N_2$ covariate matrix. Its default value is NULL, in which case "stE2=st".

This function returns the following values.

stE1	Same as the one in the arguments.
stE2	Same as the one in the arguments.
bandwidth	Bandwidths used in estimating the variance and covariance functions.
covhat	An $N_1 \times N_2$ estimated covariate matrix.

spte_decor() This function is for decorrelating and standardizing the observed spatio-temporal data using the estimated mean, variance and covariance functions obtained from an IC dataset, as discussed in Section 8.3. It can be used in the *R* environment as follows.

```
> spte_decor(y,st,y0,st0,T=1,ht=NULL,hs=NULL,gt=NULL,
  gs=NULL)
```

The arguments of the above *R* command are explained below.

y	An N-dimensional vector containing the spatio-temporal observations to decorrelate.
st	An $N \times 3$ matrix containing the spatial locations and times of the observations to decorrelate.
y0	An N_0-dimensional vector containing the IC observations for estimating the IC Model (8.1).
st0	An $N_0 \times 3$ matrix containing the spatial locations and times of the observations in y0.
T	Period of the periodic spatio-temporal mean and covariance functions.
ht	Pre-specified bandwidth in the time domain used in estimating the mean function of Model (8.1). Its default value is NULL. In such cases, it is determined by the MCV procedure (8.6).
hs	Pre-specified bandwidth in the space domain used in estimating the mean function of Model (8.1). Its default value is NULL. In such cases, it is determined by the MCV procedure (8.6).
gt	Pre-specified bandwidth in the time domain used in estimating the variance/covariance functions of Model (8.1). Its default value is NULL. In such cases, it is determined by the CV-MSPE procedure (8.9).
gs	Pre-specified bandwidth in the space domain used in estimating the variance/covariance functions of Model (8.1). Its default value is NULL. In such cases, it is determined by the CV-MSPE procedure (8.9).

This function returns the following values.

st	Same as the one in the arguments.
std.res	Decorrelated and standardized data

spte_meanest() This function is for estimating the mean function of the nonparametric spatio-temporal regression model (8.1) from an observed spatio-temporal dataset with or without considering the possible spatio-temporal data correlation, as discussed in Subsections 8.2.2 and 8.2.4. It can be used in the *R* environment as follows.

```
> spte_meanest(y,st,ht=NULL,hs=NULL,cor=FALSE,stE=NULL)
```

The arguments of the above *R* command are explained below.

- `y` An N-dimensional vector that contains the spatio-temporal observations $\{y(t_i, \mathbf{s}_{ij}), j = 1, 2, \ldots, m_i, i = 1, 2, \ldots, n\}$, where $N = \sum_{i=1}^{n} m_i$.
- `st` An $N \times 3$ matrix containing the observation locations and times $\{(\mathbf{s}'_{ij}, t_i), j = 1, 2, \ldots, m_i, i = 1, 2, \ldots, n\}$.
- `ht` Pre-specified bandwidth in the time domain used in estimating the mean function of Model (8.1). Its default value is NULL. In such cases, it is determined by the MCV procedure (8.6).
- `hs` Pre-specified bandwidth in the space domain used in estimating the mean function of Model (8.1). Its default value is NULL. In such cases, it is determined by the MCV procedure (8.6).
- `cor` A logical indicator. "cor=FALSE" implies that the possible spatio-temporal data correlation is ignored, and "cor=TRUE" implies that the spatio-temporal data correlation is considered. Its default value is FALSE.
- `stE` A matrix with three columns specifying the spatial locations and times for computing the mean function values. Its default value is NULL, in which case "stE=st".

This function returns the following values.

- `bandwidth` Bandwidths used in estimating the mean function.
- `stE` Same as the one in the arguments.
- `muhat` Estimated mean values at the spatial locations and times given in stE.

spte_semiparmreg() This function is for estimating the semiparametric spatio-temporal regression model (8.22) to build a functional relationship between the response y and a covariate vector $\mathbf{x}$. This function can be used in the *R* environment as follows.

```
> spte_semiparmreg(y,st,x,ht=NULL,hs=NULL,maxIter=1000,
  tol=1e-4,stE=NULL)
```

The arguments of the above R command are explained below.

y — An N-dimensional vector that contains the spatio-temporal observations $\{y(t_i, \mathbf{s}_{ij}), j = 1, 2, \ldots, m_i, i = 1, 2, \ldots, n\}$, where $N = \sum_{i=1}^{n} m_i$.

st — An $N \times 3$ matrix containing the observation locations and times $\{(\mathbf{s}'_{ij}, t_i), j = 1, 2, \ldots, m_i, i = 1, 2, \ldots, n\}$.

x — An $N \times p$ matrix containing the observed data of p covariates.

ht — User-specified bandwidth in the time domain used in estimating the nonparametric component $\mu(t, \mathbf{s})$ of Model (8.22). Its default value is NULL. In such cases, it is determined by the MCV procedure (8.6).

hs — User-specified bandwidth in the space domain used in estimating the nonparametric component $\mu(t, \mathbf{s})$ of Model (8.22). Its default value is NULL. In such cases, it is determined by the MCV procedure (8.6).

maxIter — A positive integer specifying the maximum number of iterations of the iterative algorithm for estimating Model (8.22). Its default value is 1000.

tol — A small positive number specifying the tolerance level ς of the iterative algorithm for estimating Model (8.22). Its default value is 0.0001.

stE — A matrix with three columns specifying the spatial locations and times $(\mathbf{s}', t)$ to calculate the estimated mean function $\widehat{\mu}(t, \boldsymbol{s})$. Its default value is NULL. In such cases, "stE=st".

This function returns the following values.

bandwidth — Bandwidths (h_t, h_s) used in model estimation.

stE — Same as the one in the arguments.

muhat — Estimated values of $\mu(t, \boldsymbol{s})$ at locations and times specified in stE.

beta — Estimated regression coefficient vector.

sptemnt_cusum() This function is for implementing the disease surveillance method discussed in Section 8.3. It can be used in the *R* environment as follows.

```
> sptemnt_cusum(y,st,type,ARL0=200,gamma=0.1,B=1000,bs=5,
  T=1,ht=NULL,hs=NULL,gt=NULL,gs=NULL)
```

The arguments of the above *R* command are explained below.

y	An N-dimensional vector that contains the spatio-temporal observations $\{y(t_i, \mathbf{s}_{ij}), j = 1, 2, \ldots, m_i, i = 1, 2, \ldots, n\}$, where $N = \sum_{i=1}^{n} m_i$.
st	An $N \times 3$ matrix containing the observation locations and times $\{(\mathbf{s}'_{ij}, t_i), j = 1, 2, \ldots, m_i, i = 1, 2, \ldots, n\}$.
type	An N-dimensional character vector specifying the type of each observation. Here, the type could be "IC1", "IC2" or "Mnt", where type="IC1" denotes an in-control (IC) observation for determining the control limit of the CUSUM chart (8.14)–(8.15), type="IC2" denotes an IC observation for estimating the IC model (8.1), and type="Mnt" denotes an observation for online process monitoring. If there are only observations with exactly one of the two types "IC1" and "IC2", then these observations are used for estimating the IC model and computing the control limit as well. An error message will be returned if there are no observations with either the "IC1" or the "IC2" type.
ARL0	A pre-specified value for ARL_0. Its default value is 200.
gamma	A pre-specified value for the allowance constant k. Its default value is 0.1.
B	Bootstrap sample size of the block bootstrap procedure for choosing the control limit of the CUSUM chart (8.14)–(8.15).
bs	Block size of the block bootstrap procedure.
T	Period of the periodic spatio-temporal mean and covariance functions.
ht	Pre-specified bandwidth in the time domain used in estimating the mean function of Model (8.1). Its default value is NULL. In such cases, it is determined by the MCV procedure (8.6).

hs Pre-specified bandwidth in the space domain used in estimating the mean function of Model (8.22). Its default value is NULL. In such cases, it is determined by the MCV procedure (8.6).

gt Pre-specified bandwidth in the time domain used in estimating the variance/covariance functions of Model (8.1). Its default value is NULL. In such cases, it is determined by the CV-MSPE procedure (8.9).

gs Pre-specified bandwidth in the space domain used in estimating the variance/covariance functions of Model (8.1). Its default value is NULL. In such cases, it is determined by the CV-MSPE procedure (8.9).

This function returns the following values.

ARL0 Same as the one in the arguments.

gamma Same as the one in the arguments.

cstat Values of the charting statistic for making a charting plot.

cl Control limit determined by the block bootstrap procedure.

signal_time Signal time of the CUSUM chart (8.14)–(8.15).

sptemnt_ewmac() This function is for implementing the disease surveillance method discussed in Section 8.5, which tries to use helpful information in covariates for effective detection of disease outbreaks. It can be used in the *R* environment as follows.

```
> sptemnt_ewmac(y,x,st,type,ARL0=200,ARL0.z=200,lambda=0.1,
  B=1000,bs=5,T=1,ht=NULL,hs=NULL,gt=NULL,gs=NULL)
```

The arguments of the above *R* command are explained below.

y An N-dimensional vector that contains the spatio-temporal observations $\{y(t_i, \mathbf{s}_{ij}), j = 1, 2, \ldots, m_i, i = 1, 2, \ldots, n\}$, where $N = \sum_{i=1}^{n} m_i$.

st An $N \times 3$ matrix containing the observation locations and times $\{(\mathbf{s}'_{ij}, t_i), j = 1, 2, \ldots, m_i, i = 1, 2, \ldots, n\}$.

`type` An N-dimensional character vector specifying the type of each observation. Here, the type could be "IC1", "IC2" or "Mnt", where type="IC1" denotes an in-control (IC) observation for determining the control limit of the EWMA chart (8.26)–(8.27), type="IC2" denotes an IC observation for estimating the IC model (8.22), and type="Mnt" denotes an observation for online process monitoring. If there are only observations with exactly one of the two types "IC1" and "IC2", then these observations are used for estimating the IC model and computing the control limit as well. An error message will be returned if there are no observations with either the "IC1" or the "IC2" type.

`ARL0` Pre-specified value for ARL_0. Its default value is 200.

`ARL0.z` Pre-specified value for ARL_0 of the covariate chart (8.25). Its default value is 200.

`lambda` Pre-specified value for the smoothing parameter λ of the chart (8.26)–(8.27). Its default value is 0.1.

`B` Bootstrap sample size of the block bootstrap procedure for choosing the control limits of the EWMA charts.

`bs` Block size of the block bootstrap procedure.

`T` Period of the periodic spatio-temporal mean and covariance functions.

`ht` Pre-specified bandwidth in the time domain used in estimating the mean function of Model (8.22). Its default value is NULL. In such cases, it is determined by the MCV procedure (8.6).

`hs` Pre-specified bandwidth in the space domain used in estimating the mean function of Model (8.22). Its default value is NULL. In such cases, it is determined by the MCV procedure (8.6).

`gt` Pre-specified bandwidth in the time domain used in estimating the variance/covariance functions of Model (8.22). Its default value is NULL. In such cases, it is determined by the CV-MSPE procedure (8.9).

`gs` Pre-specified bandwidth in the space domain used in estimating the variance/covariance functions of Model (8.1). Its default value is NULL. In such cases, it is determined by the CV-MSPE procedure (8.9).

This function returns the following values.

ARL0 Same as the one in the arguments.

lambda Same as the one in the arguments.

cstat Values of the charting statistic for making a charting plot.

cl Control limit determined by the block bootstrap procedure.

signal_time Signal time of the EWMA chart (8.26)–(8.27).

sptemnt_ewsl() This function is for implementing the disease surveillance method discussed in Section 8.4 which is based on the exponentially weighted spatio LASSO (EWSL) procedure. It can be used in the *R* environment as follows.

```
> sptemnt_ewsl(y,st,type,ARL0=200,lambda=0.1,B=1000,bs=5,
  T=1,ht=NULL,hs=NULL,gt=NULL,gs=NULL)
```

The arguments of the above *R* command are explained below.

y An N-dimensional vector that contains the spatio-temporal observations $\{y(t_i, \mathbf{s}_{ij}), j = 1, 2, \ldots, m_i, i = 1, 2, \ldots, n\}$, where $N = \sum_{i=1}^{n} m_i$.

st An $N \times 3$ matrix containing the observation locations and times $\{(\mathbf{s}_{ij}', t_i), j = 1, 2, \ldots, m_i, i = 1, 2, \ldots, n\}$.

type An N-dimensional character vector specifying the type of each observation. Here, the type could be "IC1", "IC2" or "Mnt", where type="IC1" denotes an in-control (IC) observation for determining the control limit of the EWSL chart (8.20)–(8.21), type="IC2" denotes an IC observation for estimating the IC model (8.1), and type="Mnt" denotes an observation for online process monitoring. If there are only observations with exactly one of the two types "IC1" and "IC2", then these observations are used for estimating the IC model and computing the control limit as well. An error message will be returned if there are no observations with either the "IC1" or the "IC2" type.

ARL0 Pre-specified value for ARL_0. Its default value is 200.

lambda Pre-specified value for the smoothing parameter λ of the chart (8.20)–(8.21). Its default value is 0.1.

B Bootstrap sample size of the block bootstrap procedure for choosing the control limit of the EWSL chart (8.20)–(8.21).

bs Block size of the block bootstrap procedure.

T Period of the periodic spatio-temporal mean and covariance functions.

ht Pre-specified bandwidth in the time domain used in estimating the mean function of Model (8.1). Its default value is NULL. In such cases, they are determined by the MCV procedure (8.6).

hs Pre-specified bandwidth in the space domain used in estimating the mean function of Model (8.22). Its default value is NULL. In such cases, it is determined by the MCV procedure (8.6).

gt Pre-specified bandwidth in the time domain used in estimating the variance/covariance functions of Model (8.1). Its default value is NULL. In such cases, it is determined by the CV-MSPE procedure (8.9).

gs Pre-specified bandwidth in the space domain used in estimating the variance/covariance functions of Model (8.1). Its default value is NULL. In such cases, it is determined by the CV-MSPE procedure (8.9).

This function returns the following values.

ARL0 Same as the one in the arguments.

lambda Same as the one in the arguments.

cstat Values of the charting statistic for making a charting plot.

cl Control limit determined by the block bootstrap procedure.

signal_time Signal time of the EWSL chart (8.20)–(8.21).

9.3 Some Demonstrations

Let us use the built-in dataset ili_dat as an example to demonstrate how to use different built-in functions in the *R* package **SpTe2M** to model and monitor spatio-temporal data. That dataset contains the observed daily influenza-like illness (ILI) incidence rates of all 67 counties in Florida during 2012–2014. A background introduction about the dataset can be found in Example 8.1 in Section 8.1. From the description about the dataset in Section 9.2, it contains the following 8 variables: County, Date, Lat, Long, Time, Rate, Temp and RH. As a demonstration, the observed ILI incidence rates of all 67 Florida counties on June 15 (a summer time) and December 15 (a winter time) in the three years 2012–2014 are presented in Figure 9.1, where darker colors denote larger values. It can be seen from the figure that the observed ILI incidence rates have seasonal patterns with larger values in the winters and smaller values in the summers, which is intuitively reasonable. In addition, they seem to have spatial patterns as well. For instance, several counties located in the northwestern part of Florida seem to have relatively large ILI incidence rates during the winter times. Furthermore, the observed ILI incidence rates of certain counties on 12/15/2014 seem unusually large, compared to the corresponding values on the same date of the previous two years.

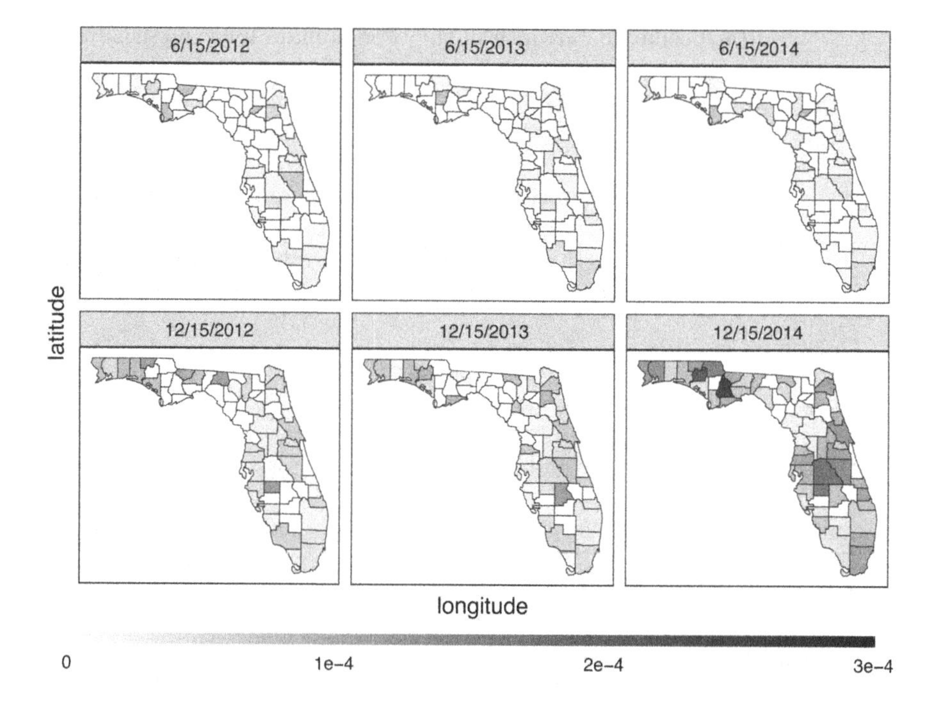

FIGURE 9.1
Observed ILI incidence rates of all 67 counties in Florida on June 15 (a summer time) and December 15 (a winter time) in the three-year period 2012–2014.

9.3.1 Spatio-Temporal Data Modeling

From Figure 9.1, the observed ILI incidence rates in the years 2012 and 2013 seem reasonably low. So, they are considered as IC data in this demonstration. Next, let us use the observed data in the year 2013 to estimate the IC nonparametric spatio-temporal regression model (8.1). To this end, the functions **spte_meanest()** and **spte_covest()** in the *R* package **SpTe2M** can be used. For instance, to estimate the mean function $\mu(t, \boldsymbol{s})$ by $\widetilde{\mu}(t, \boldsymbol{s})$ defined in (8.4), which ignores the possible spatio-temporal correlation in the observed data, the following *R* commands can be used:

```
> data(ili_dat) # Retrieve the ILI data frame
> n = 365       # Specify the number of observation times in
                # the year 2013 (i.e., 365 days)
> m = 67        # Specify the number of observation locations
                # (i.e., 67 counties)

> N1 = (1+n)*m  # Specify the number of observations in 2012
> N2 = n*m      # Specify the number of observations in 2013

> subdata = ili_dat[(N1+1):(N1+N2),] # Obtain the data in 2013
> y.sub = subdata$Rate               # Obtain y values in 2013
> # Obtain the observation locations and times in 2013
> st.sub = subdata[,c('Lat','Long','Time')]

> # Estimate the mean function by ignoring data correlation
> mu.tilde = spte_meanest(y=y.sub,st=st.sub)
```

The function **spte_meanest()** used above returns three parts of the results: bandwidth, stE and muhat, where bandwidth contains the selected bandwidth values for $(h_{t,0}, h_{s,0})$ by the MCV procedure (8.6), stE contains the observation locations and times of the original observations, and muhat contains the values of $\widetilde{\mu}(t, \boldsymbol{s})$ at the observation locations and times in stE. In this example, the selected values of $(h_{t,0}, h_{s,0})$ are $(0.100, 1.873)$, and the estimated mean values for the four counties Broward, Lake, Pinellas and Seminole are presented in Figure 9.2 by the dashed lines, along with the observed ILI incidence rates that are shown by small circles. It can be seen that the estimated spatio-temporal mean function can describe the overall longitudinal pattern of the observed ILI incidence rates quite well.

If the spatio-temporal data correlation needs to be considered, then the mean function $\mu(t, \boldsymbol{s})$ can be estimated by $\widehat{\mu}(t, \boldsymbol{s})$ defined in (8.10), which can be computed by using the following *R* command:

```
> mu.hat = spte_meanest(y=y.sub,st=st.sub,ht=0.1,
                        hs=1.873,cor=TRUE)
```

where y.sub and st.sub are defined as before. In the above command, the

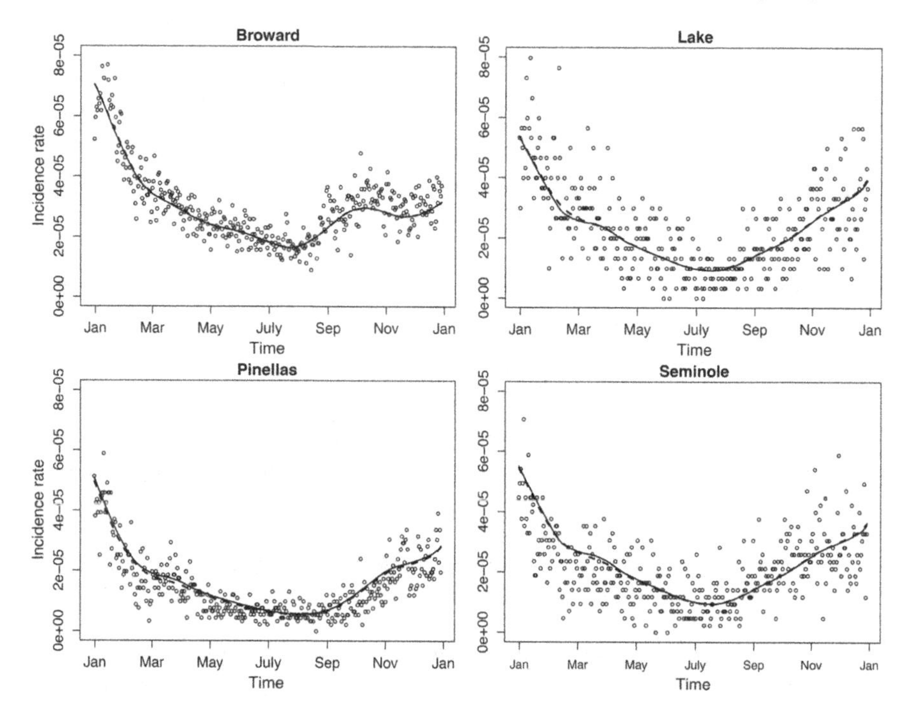

FIGURE 9.2
The observed ILI incidence rates in four Florida counties during the year 2013 (small circles) and the estimated mean functions $\widetilde{\mu}(t, \boldsymbol{s})$ defined in (8.4) (dashed lines) and $\widehat{\mu}(t, \boldsymbol{s})$ defined in (8.10) (solid lines).

bandwidths (`ht,hs`) have been pre-specified to be $(0.100, 1.873)$, which are the same as those used for computing $\widetilde{\mu}(t, \boldsymbol{s})$ above, to reduce the computing time. If they are not pre-specified, then they will be chosen by the MCV procedure (8.6), which takes a substantial amount of computing time. The estimated mean values by this approach for the four counties Broward, Lake, Pinellas and Seminole are presented in Figure 9.2 by the solid lines. It can be seen that the two estimates $\widetilde{\mu}(t, \boldsymbol{s})$ and $\widehat{\mu}(t, \boldsymbol{s})$ are almost identical in this example.

To estimate the variance function $\sigma^2(t, \boldsymbol{s})$ and the covariance function $V(t, t'; \boldsymbol{s}, \boldsymbol{s}')$ by (8.7) and (8.8), we first need to determine the bandwidths $(h_{t,1}, h_{s,1})$ used in the estimation. To this end, the CV-MSPE procedure (8.9) can be used, which can be accomplished by the following *R* command:

```
> bandwidth=cv_mspe(y=y.sub,st=st.sub)
```

From this command, the selected bandwidths are $(h_{t,1}, h_{s,1}) = (0.558, 5.244)$. Then, the estimated variance and covariance functions can be computed by the following *R* command:

```
> Cov.hat=spte_covest(y=y.sub,st=st.sub,gt=0.558,gs=5.244)
```

By the above command, the variance/covariance values for all pairs of the observation locations and times in $\{(\mathbf{s}_j, t_i), i = 1, 2, \ldots, 365, j = 1, 2, \ldots, 67\}$ have been computed. If we want to compute the variance/covariance values for some specific pairs, then we need to specify the arguments stE1 and stE2 in the above command. For instance, if we want to compute the covariance values for the Broward county only, then the following *R* commands can be used:

```
> stE1=subset(subdata,County %in% c("broward"))
      [,c('Lat','Long','Time')]
> Cov.hat=spte_covest(y=y.sub,st=st.sub,gt=0.558,gs=5.244,
                      stE1=stE1,stE2=stE1)
```

By the above command, the 365×365 estimated covariance matrix for describing the covariance of the response variable (i.e., the ILI incidence rate) at any two observation times in 2013 has been computed for the Broward county. For instance, the computed variance function estimate is shown in Figure 9.3 by the solid line.

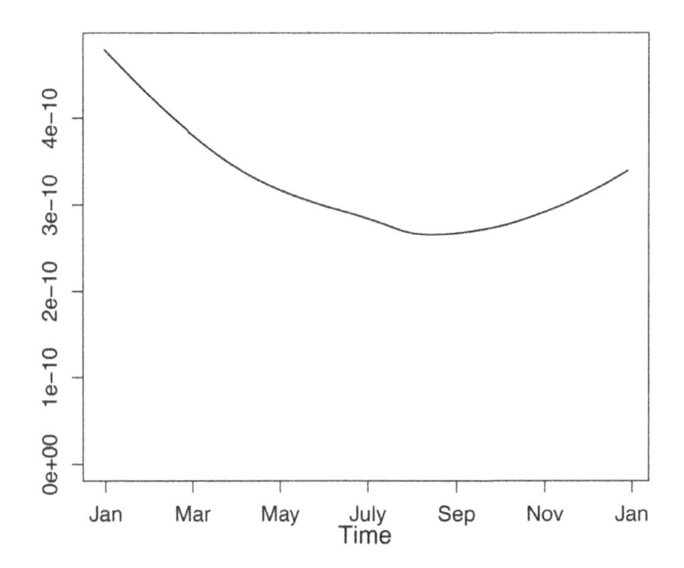

FIGURE 9.3
Estimated variance function $\widehat{\sigma}^2(t, \boldsymbol{s})$ defined in (8.7) for the observed ILI incidence rates of the Broward county in 2013.

9.3.2 Spatio-Temporal Data Monitoring

In this subsection, we demonstrate the *R* functions in the package **SpTe2M** for spatio-temporal process monitoring. First, the following *R* commands can be used for monitoring the observed ILI incidence rates of the 67 counties of Florida in 2014 by using the built-in function **sptemnt_cusum()**:

```
> data(ili_dat)
> y = ili_dat$Rate
> st = ili_dat[,c('Lat','Long','Time')]
> n = 365
> m = 67
> N1 = (1+n)*m
> N2 = n*m

> # Specifying the observed data in 2012 for determining the
> # control limit, the ones in 2013 for estimating the IC
> # model, and the ones in 2014 for online process monitoring
> type = rep(c('IC1','IC2','Mnt'),c(N1,N2,N2))

> ILI.CUSUM = sptemnt_cusum(y,st,type,ht=0.05,hs=6.5,
                             gt=0.25,gs=1.5)
```

In the above command **sptemnt_cusum()**, the bandwidths (h_t, h_s) for estimating the IC mean function and the bandwidths (g_t, g_s) for estimating the IC variance and covariance functions have been determined in advance by the MCV procedure (8.6) and the CV-MSPE procedure (8.9), respectively. In this example, their selected values are $(h_t, h_s) = (0.05, 6.50)$ and $(g_t, g_s) = (0.25, 1.50)$. The charting statistic values of the CUSUM chart (8.14)–(8.15) and its control limit corresponding to the default ARL_0 value of 200 can be accessed using ILI.CUSUM$cstat and ILI.CUSUM$cl, respectively. Based on these results, the CUSUM chart (8.14)–(8.15) is shown in the left panel of Figure 9.4. This chart gives its first signal on 10/16/2014. To better see the chart around its signal time, the chart in the time period from 09/15/2014 to 10/31/2014 is presented in the right panel of Figure 9.4.

If we want to use the EWSL chart (8.20)–(8.21) for online monitoring of the observed ILI incidence rates in 2014, then the *R* function **sptemnt_ewsl()** can be used as follows:

```
> ILI.EWSL = sptemnt_ewsl(y,st,type,ht=0.05,hs=6.5,
                           gt=0.25,gs=1.5)
```

As can be seen from the above command, the arguments of the function sptemnt_ewsl() are the same as those of the function sptemnt_cusum(). To plot the EWSL chart, the EWSL charting statistic values and the control limit saved in ILI.EWSL$cstat and ILI.EWSL$cl can be used. The resulting chart and its zoom-in part in the time period from 09/15/2014 to 10/31/2014 are shown in the left and right panels of Figure 9.5. From the plots, it can be seen that the EWSL chart gives its first signal on 10/6/2014, which is 10 days earlier than that of the CUSUM chart (8.14)–(8.15) shown in Figure 9.4.

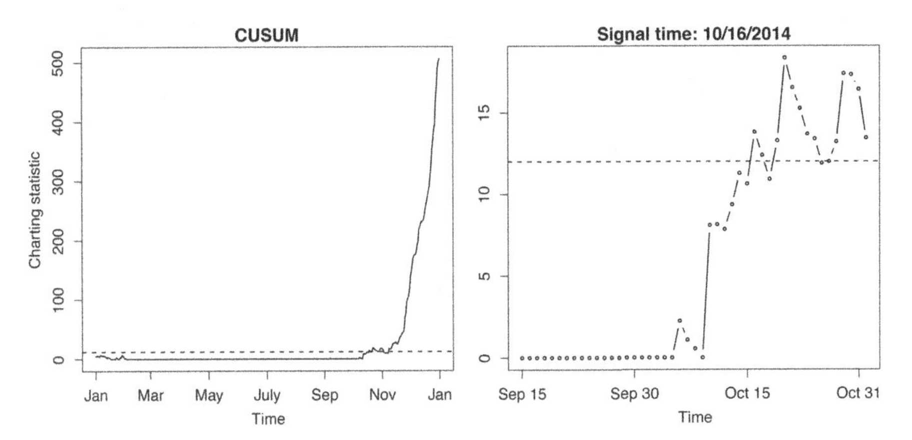

FIGURE 9.4
The CUSUM chart (8.14)–(8.15) for monitoring the ILI data in the year 2014 (left panel), and its zoom-in part in the time period from 09/15/2014 to 10/31/2014 (right panel). In each plot, the horizontal dashed line denotes the control limit of the chart.

In the ILI dataset, observed data of the two covariates "air temperature" and "relative humidity" are available. These covariates could be associated with the observed ILI incidence rates. To explore their association, the semi-parametric spatio-temporal regression model (8.22) can be considered. Estimation of this model from the IC data in the year 2013 can be accomplished by using the following *R* commands:

```
> data(ili_dat) # Retrieve the ILI data frame
> n = 365       # Specify the number of observation times in
                # the year 2013 (i.e., 365 days)
> m = 67        # Specify the number of observation locations
                # (i.e., 67 counties)

> N1 = (1+n)*m  # Specify the number of observations in 2012
> N2 = n*m      # Specify the number of observations in 2013

> subdata = ili_dat[(N1+1):(N1+N2),].  # Obtain the data in 2013
> y.sub = subdata$Rate                 # Obtain y values in 2013

> # Extract the observation locations and times in 2013
> st.sub = subdata[,c('Lat','Long','Time')]

> # Extract the observed data of the covariates in 2013
> x.sub  <- as.matrix(subdata[,c('Temp','RH')])
```

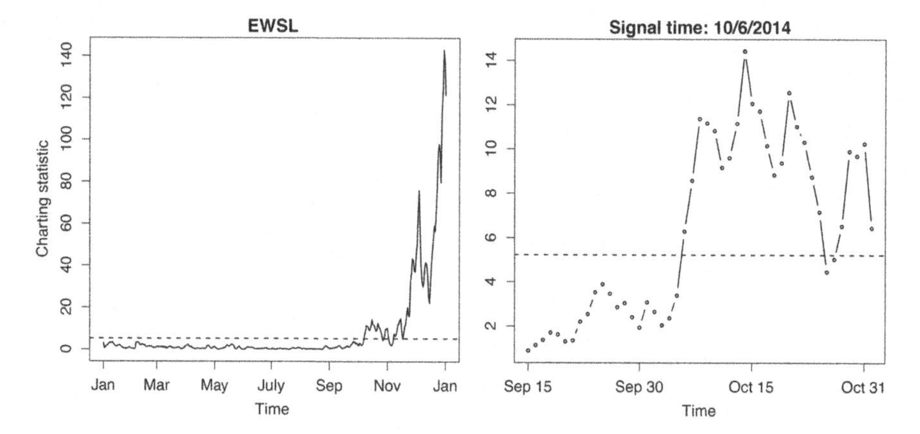

FIGURE 9.5
The EWSL chart (8.20)–(8.21) for monitoring the ILI data in the year 2014 (left panel), and its zoom-in part in the time period from 09/15/2014 to 10/31/2014 (right panel). In each plot, the horizontal dashed line denotes the control limit of the chart.

```
> # Estimate the semiparametric spatio-temporal regression model
> semi.est <- spte_semiparmreg(y=y.sub,st=st.sub,x=x.sub)
```

Then, the estimated regression coefficients in $\widehat{\boldsymbol{\beta}}$ can be obtained via semi.est$beta, from which the estimated regression coefficients of "relative humidity" and "air temperature" are -1.17×10^{-6} and -1.06×10^{-6}, respectively. Therefore, both covariates are negatively associated with the observed ILI incidence rates. This result is consistent with our intuition and with the conclusions found in the literature (cf., Pica and Bouvier, 2012).

After the semiparametric model (8.22) is estimated, the EWMA chart (8.26)–(8.27), denoted as EWMAC here, can be used to monitor the observed ILI incidence rates in the year 2014. To this end, the *R* function sptemnt_ewmac() can be used as follows:

```
> data(ili_dat)
> y = ili_dat$Rate
> st = ili_dat[,c('Lat','Long','Time')]
> n = 365
> m = 67
> N1 = (1+n)*m
> N2 = n*m

> # Specifying the observed data in 2012 for determining the
> # control limit, the ones in 2013 for estimating the IC
> # model, and the ones in 2014 for online process monitoring
> type = rep(c('IC1','IC2','Mnt'),c(N1,N2,N2))
```

```
> ILI.EWMAC <- sptemnt_ewmac(y,x,st,type,ht=0.05,hs=6.5,
                                  gt=0.25,gs=1.5)
```

The computed charting statistic values and the control limit of the EWMAC chart (8.26)–(8.27) can be obtained from ILI.EWMAC$cstat and ILI.EWMAC$cl, respectively. The resulting chart and its zoom-in part in the time period from 09/25/2014 to 10/31/2014 are shown in the left and right panels of Figure 9.6. From the plots, it can be seen that the EWMAC chart gives its first signal on 09/23/2014, which is 23 days earlier than that of the CUSUM chart (8.14)–(8.15) shown in Figure 9.4. From Figure 8.6 in Chapter 8, it can be seen that the real increase in the observed ILI incidence rates started in the middle September of 2014. Therefore, it is indeed beneficial to use the covariate information for disease surveillance in this example.

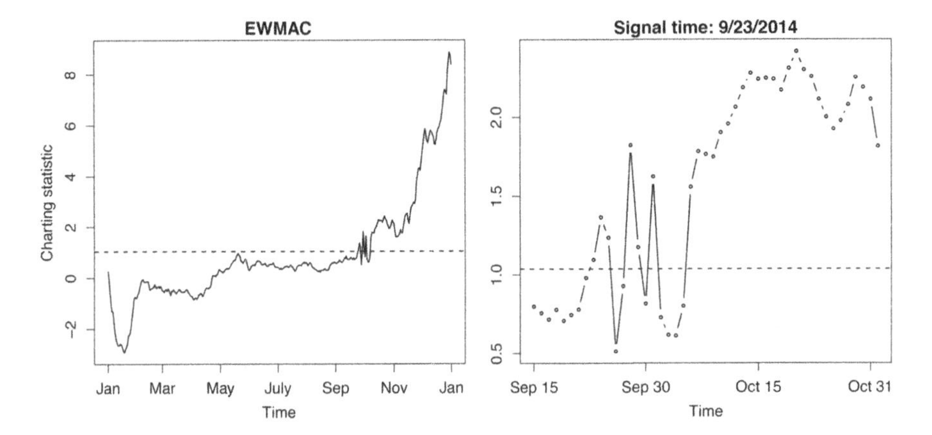

FIGURE 9.6
The EWMAC chart (8.26)–(8.27) for monitoring the ILI data in the year 2014 (left panel), and its zoom-in part in the time period from 09/25/2014 to 10/31/2014 (right panel). In each plot, the horizontal dashed line denotes the control limit of the chart.

9.4 Exercises

9.1 Use the following *R* command to read the description about the built-in function **mod_cv()**:

```
> ?mod_cv()
```

Use this function to choose the bandwidths for estimating the mean function of the observed ILI incidence rate data in 2013 by the estimate defined in (8.4). The data can be accessed using the built-in data frame ili_dat. as discussed in Subsection 9.3.1.

9.2 For the observed ILI incidence rates in Florida during 2012–2014 that are saved in the built-in data frame ili_dat, do the following analyses:

(i) Use the bandwidths calculated in Exercise 9.1 and the *R* function **spte_meanest()** to estimate the mean function $\mu(t, \boldsymbol{s})$ of the nonparametric spatio-temporal regression model (8.1) from the observed ILI data in 2013, by ignoring the possible spatio-temporal data correlation.

(ii) Use the *R* function **cv_mspe()** to choose the bandwidths for estimating the variance and covariance functions of the model (8.1) from the data mentioned in part (i).

(iii) Use the selected bandwidths in part (ii) and the *R* function **spte_covest()** to estimate the variance and covariance functions of the model (8.1) from the observed ILI data mentioned in part (i).

9.3 The simulated dataset saved in the built-in data frame sim_dat contains simulated spatio-temporal observations of a response valriable y at 100 observation times and 100 time-independent observation locations at each observation time. In this dataset, the observed data at the first 80 observation times are regarded as IC data, and those at the remaining observation times can be used for online process monitoring. For the IC data, the first half can be used for determining the control limit of a control chart and the second half can be used for estimating the IC model (8.1).

(i) For estimating the IC model (8.1), use the *R* function **mod_cv()** to determine the bandwidths for estimating the mean function $\mu(t, \boldsymbol{s})$ by the estimate defined in (8.4).

(ii) Use the selected bandwidths in part (i) and the *R* function **spte_meanest()** to estimate the mean function $\mu(t, \boldsymbol{s})$ of the model (8.1).

(iii) Use the *R* function **cv_mspe()** to choose the bandwidths for estimating the variance and covariance functions of the IC model (8.1).

(iv) Use the selected bandwidths in part (iii) and the *R* function **spte_covest()** to estimate the variance and covariance functions of the model (8.1).

9.4 For the simulated dataset discussed in Exercise 9.3,

(i) Use the *R* function **sptemnt_cusum()** and the bandwidths found in parts (i) and (iii) of Exercise 9.3 to sequentially monitor the observed data at the last 20 observation times in the dataset.

(ii) Use the *R* function **sptemnt_ewsl()** and the bandwidths found in parts (i) and (iii) of Exercise 9.3 to sequentially monitor the observed data at the last 20 observation times in the dataset. Compare the results with those in part (i).

9.5 Obtain the EWMAC chart (8.26)–(8.27) that is similar to the one shown in Figure 9.6 for monitoring the observed ILI incidence rates in the year 2014, by using "air temperature" as the only covariate.

Bibliography

A.M. Abrams, K. Kleinman, and M. Kulldorff. Gumbel based p-value approximations for spatial scan statistics. *International Journal of Health Geographics*, 61:https://doi.org/10.1186/1476–072X–9–61, 2010.

C.C. Aggarwal. *Neural Networks and Deep Learning.* Springer: New York, NY, USA, 2018.

A. Agresti. *Categorical Data Analysis.* John Wiley & Sons: New York, NY, USA, 2nd edition, 2002.

H.S. Ahn, H.J. Kim, and H.G. Welch. Korea's thyroid-cancer "epidemic" – screening and overdiagnosis. *New England Journal of Medicine*, 371:1765–1767, 2014.

H. Akaike. Information theory and an extension of the maximum likelihood principle. *Second International Symposium on Information Theory Proceeding*, 1:610–624, 1992.

D. Allen. The relationship between variable selection and data augmentation and a method for prediction. *Technometrics*, 16:125–127, 1974.

J.A. Alloway, Jr., and M. Raghavachari. Control chart based on the Hodges-Lehmann estimator. *Journal of Quality Technology*, 23:336–347, 1991.

N.S. Altman. Kernel smoothing of data with correlated errors. *Journal of the American Statistical Association*, 85:749–759, 1990.

R. Amin, M.R. Reynolds, Jr., and S.T. Bakir. Nonparametric quality control charts based on the sign statistic. *Communications in Statistics - Theory and Methods*, 24:1597–1623, 1995.

D.W. Apley and J. Shi. The GLRT for statistical process control of autocorrelated processes. *IIE Transactions*, 31:1123–1134, 1999.

D.W. Apley and F. Tsung. The autoregressive T^2 chart for monitoring univariate autocorrelated processes. *Journal of Quality Technology*, 34:80–96, 2002.

R.B. Ash. *Real Analysis and Probability.* Academic Press: San Diego, CA, USA, 1972.

P.C. Austin, D.S. Lee, and J.P. Fine. Introduction to the analysis of survival data in the presence of competing risks. *Circulation*, 133:601–609, 2016.

K.S. Bakar and S.K. Sahu. spTimer: spatio-temporal Bayesian modeling using R. *Journal of Statistical Software*, 63:1–32, 2015.

R.D. Baker. A modified Knox test of space-time clustering. *Journal of Applied Statistics*, 31:457–463, 2004.

S.T. Bakir. A distribution-free Shewhart quality control chart based on signed-ranks. *Quality Engineering*, 16:611–621, 2004.

S.T. Bakir and M.R. Reynolds, Jr. A nonparametric procedure for process control based on within group ranking. *Technometrics*, 21:175–183, 1979.

D.E. Barton and F.N. David. The random intersection of two graphs. In *Research Papers in Statistics, Festschrift for J. Neyman (edited by David, F.N.)*, pages 445–459. John Wiley & Sons, Inc.: Hoboken, New Jersey, USA, 2006.

D. Bates, M. Maechler, B. Bolker, S. Walker, R.H.B. Christensen, H. Singmann, B. Dai, F. Scheipl, G. Grothendieck, P. Green, J. Fox, A. Bauer, and P.N. Krivitsky. *Linear Mixed-Effects Models using 'Eigen' and S4*. https://github.com/lme4/lme4/, 2020.

J. Besag, J. York, and A. Mollié. Bayesian image restoration, with two applications in spatial statistics (with discussion). *Annals of the Institute of Statistical Mathematics*, 43:1–20, 1991.

N.G. Best, S. Richardson, and A. Thomson. A comparison of bayesian spatial models for disease mapping. *Statistical Methods in Medical Research*, 14: 35–59, 2005.

J.M. Boone and S. Chakraborti. Two simple Shewhart-type multivariate nonparametric control charts. *Applied Stochastic Models in Business and Industry*, 28:130–140, 2012.

K.D. Brabanter, J.D. Brabanter, J.A.K. Suykens, and B.D. Moor. Kernel regression in the presence of correlated errors. *Journal of Machine Learning Research*, 12:1955–1976, 2011.

L. Breiman. Random forests. *Machine Learning*, 45:5–32, 2010.

A. Brix and P.J. Diggle. Spatiotemporal prediction for log-Gaussian Cox processes. *Journal of the Royal Statistical Society (Series B)*, 63:823–841, 2001.

H.M. Bush, P. Chongfuangprinya, V.C.P. Chen, T. Sukchotrat, and S.B. Kim. Nonparametric multivariate control charts based on a linkage ranking algorithm. *Quality and Reliability Engineering International*, 26:663–675, 2010.

Z. Cai and Y. Sun. Local linear estimation for time-dependent coefficients in Cox's regression models. *Scandinavian Journal of Statistics*, 30:93–111, 2003.

P. Campolucci, A. Uncini, F. Piazza, and B.D. Rao. On-line learning algorithms for locally recurrent neural networks. *IEEE Transactions on Neural Networks*, 10:253–271, 1999.

G. Capizzi. Recent advances in process monitoring: nonparametric and variable-selection methods for phase I and phase II. *Quality Engineering*, 27:44–67, 2015.

G. Capizzi and G. Masarotto. An adaptive exponentially weighted moving average control chart. *Technometrics*, 45:199–207, 2003.

G. Capizzi and G. Masarotto. Practical design of generalized likelihood ratio control charts for autocorrelated data. *Technometrics*, 50:357–370, 2008.

G. Capizzi and G. Masarotto. Phase I distribution-free analysis of univariate data. *Journal of Quality Technology*, 45:273–284, 2013.

G. Capizzi and G. Masarotto. Efficient control chart calibration by simulated stochastic approximation. *IIE Transactions*, 48:57–65, 2016.

J. Carpenter and M.G. Kenward. *Multiple Imputation and Its Application.* John Wiley & Sons, Inc.: Hoboken, New Jersey, USA, 2013.

T.P. Carvalhoa, F. Soares, R. Vita, R. Francisco, J.P. Basto, and S.G.S. Alcala. A systematic literature review of machine learning methods applied to predictive maintenance. *Computers & Industrial Engineering*, 137:106024, 2019.

G. Casella and R.L. Berger. *Statistical Inference.* Duxbury Press: Pacific Grove, CA, USA, 2nd edition, 2002.

P. Castagliola and P.E. Maravelakis. A CUSUM control chart for monitoring the variance when parameters are estimated. *Journal of Statistical Planning and Inference*, 141:1463–1478, 2011.

CDC. *The Community Guide to Preventive Services: Systematic Reviews and Evidence-Based Recommendations.* Centers for Disease Control and Prevention: Atlanta, GA, 2005.

S. Chakraborti and S. Eryilmaz. A nonparametric Shewhart-type signed-rank control chart based on runs. *Communications in Statistics - Simulation and Computation*, 36:335–356, 2007.

S. Chakraborti and M. Graham. *Nonparametric Statistical Process Control.* John Wiley & Sons, Inc.: Hoboken, New Jersey, USA, 2019.

S. Chakraborti, P. van der Laan, and S.T. Bakir. Nonparametric control charts: an overview and some results. *Journal of Quality Technology*, 33: 304–315, 2001.

S. Chakraborti, P. Qiu, and A. Mukherjee. Editorial to the special issue: Nonparametric statistical process control charts. *Quality and Reliability Engineering International*, 31:1–2, 2015.

S. Chatterjee and P. Qiu. Distribution-free cumulative sum control charts using bootstrap-based control limits. *Annals of Applied Statistics*, 3:349–369, 2009.

H. Chen, D. Zeng, and P. Yan. *Infectious Disease Informatics*. Springer: New York, NY, USA, 2009.

J.H. Chen and S.M. Asch. Machine learning and prediction in medicine – Beyond the peak of inflated expectations. *New England Journal of Medicine*, 376:2507–2509, 2017.

K. Chen and Z. Jin. Local polynomial regression analysis of clustered data. *Biometrika*, 92:59–74, 2005.

N. Chen, X. Zi, and C. Zou. A distribution-free multivariate control chart. *Technometrics*, 58:448–459, 2016.

S. Chen and F.D. Bowman. A novel support vector classifier for longitudinal high dimensional data. *Statistical Analysis and Data Mining*, 4:604–611, 2011.

I. Choi, B. Li, and X. Wang. Nonparametric estimation of spatial and space-time covariance function. *Journal of Agricultural, Biological, and Environmental Statistics*, 18:611–630, 2013.

S.W. Choi and I.B. Lee. Nonlinear dynamic process monitoring based on dynamic kernel PCA. *Chemical Engineering Science*, 59:5897–5908, 2004.

K.L. Chung. *A Course in Probability Theory*. Academic Press: San Diego, CA, USA, 3rd edition, 2001.

W.G. Cochran. *Sampling Techniques: Probability and Mathematical Statistics*. John Wiley & Sons: New York, NY, USA, 2nd edition, 1977.

C. Cortes and V.N. Vapnik. Support-vector networks. *Machine Learning*, 20: 273–297, 1995.

D.R. Cox. Regression models and life-tables (with discussions). *Journal of the Royal Statistical Society (Series B)*, 34:187–220, 1972.

N. Cressie and H.C. Huang. Classes of nonseparable, spatio-temporal stationary covariance functions. *Journal of the American Statistical Association*, 94:1330–1340, 1999.

N. Cressie and C.K. Wikle. *Statistics for Spatio-Temporal Data.* John Wiley & Sons, Inc.: Hoboken, New Jersey, USA, 2011.

S.V. Crowder. Design of exponentially weighted moving average schemes. *Journal of Quality Technology*, 21:155–162, 1989.

L.A. Cupples, H.T. Arruda, E.J. Benjamin, et al. The Framingham Heart Study 100K SNP genome-wide association study resource: overview of 17 phenotype working group reports. *BMC Medical Genetics*, 8:(Suppl 1): S1, 2007.

M. Davidian and D.M. Giltinan. *Nonlinear Models for Repeated Measurement Data.* Chapman & Hall/CRC: Boca Raton, FL, USA, 1995.

A.P. Dempster, N.M. Laird, and D.B. Rubin. Maximum likelihood from incomplete data via the EM algorithm. *Journal of the Royal Statistical Society (Series B)*, 39:1–38, 1977.

J.L. Devore. *Probability and Statistics for Engineering and the Sciences.* Duxbury Press: Pacific Grove, CA, USA, 8th edition, 2011.

P. Diggle, B. Rowlingson, and T.L. Su. Point process methodology for on-line spatio-temporal disease surveillance. *Environmetrics*, 16:423–434, 2005.

P.J. Diggle. *Statistical Analysis of Spatial and Spatio-Temporal Point Patterns.* Chapman & Hall/CRC: Boca Raton, FL, USA, 3rd edition, 2014.

P.J. Diggle, P. Heagerty, K.-Y. Liang, and S.L. Zeger. *Analysis of Longitudinal Data.* Oxford University Press: Oxford, UK, 2nd edition, 2002.

W.J. Dixon and F.J. Massey. *Introduction to Statistical Analysis.* McGraw-Hill Book Company: New York, NY, USA, 3rd edition, 1969.

S. Dupond. A thorough review on the current advance of neural network structures. *Annual Reviews in Control*, 41:200–230, 2019.

J.F. Dupuy, I. Grama, and M. Mesbah. Asymptotic theory for the Cox model with missing time-dependent covariate. *Annals of Statistics*, 34:903–924, 2006.

M. Dwass. Modified randomization tests for nonparametric hypotheses. *Annals of Mathematical Statistics*, 28:181–187, 1957.

B. Efron. Bootstrap methods: another look at the jackknife. *The Annals of Statistics*, 7:1–26, 1979.

B. Efron and R. Tibshirani. *An Introduction to the Bootstrap.* Chapman & Hall/CRC: Boca Raton, FL, USA, 1993.

V.A. Epanechnikov. Non-parametric estimation of a multivariate probability density. *Theory of Probability and Its Applications*, 14:153–158, 1969.

J. Fan and I. Gijbels. Data-driven bandwidth selection in local polynomial fitting: variable bandwidth and spatial adaptation. *Journal of the Royal Statistical Society (Series B)*, 57:371–394, 1995.

J. Fan and I. Gijbels. *Local Polynomial Modelling and Its Applications*. Chapman & Hall/CRC: Boca Raton, FL, USA, 1996.

J. Fan and R. Li. Variable selection via nonconcave penalized likelihood and its oracle properties. *Journal of the American Statistical Association*, 96: 1348–1360, 2001.

J. Fan, Q. Yao, and H. Tong. Estimation of conditional densities and sensitivity measures in nonlinear dynamical systems. *Biometrika*, 83:189–206, 1996.

B.A. Ference, M.S. Chauhan, and S. Izumo. Will genetics revolutionize medicine? *New England Journal of Medicine*, 343:1497–1498, 2000.

J.P. Fine and R.J. Gray. A proportional hazards model for the subdistribution of a competing risk. *Journal of the American Statistical Association*, 94: 496–509, 1999.

A.O. Finley, S. Banerjee, and A. Gelfand. SpBayes for large univariate and multivariate point-referenced spatio-temporal data models. *Journal of Statistical Software*, 63:1–28, 2020.

A.E. Fiore, T.M. Uyeki, K. Broder, L. Finelli, G.L. Euler, J.A. Singleton, J.K. Iskander, P.M. Wortley, D.K. Shay, J.S. Bresee, and N.J. Cox. Prevention and control of influenza with vaccines: recommendations of the advisory committee on immunization practices (acip). *MMWR Recommendations and Reports*, 59:1–62, 2010.

G.M. Fitzmaurice, N.M. Laird, and J.H. Ware. *Applied Longitudinal Analysis*. McGraw-Hill Book Company: New York, NY, USA, 2nd edition, 2011.

V. Francois-Lavet, P. Henderson, R. Islam, M.G. Bellemare, and J. Pineau. An introduction to deep reinforcement learning. *Foundations and Trends in Machine Learning*, 11:219–354, 2018.

J. Friedman, T. Hastie, H. Höfling, and R. Tibshirani. Pathwise coordinate optimization. *Annals of Applied Statistics*, 1:302–332, 2007.

E.D. Frohlich and P.J. Quinlan. Coronary heart disease risk factors: public impact of initial and later-announced risks. *The Ochsner Journal*, 14:532–537, 2014.

M. Fuentes, P. Guttorp, and P.D. Sampson. Using transforms to analyze space-time processes. In *Statistical Methods for Spatio-Temporal Systems (edited by Finkenstädt, B., Held, L., and Isham, V.)*, pages 77–150. Chapman & Hall/CRC: Boca Raton, FL, USA, 2006.

F.F. Gan. Joint monitoring of process mean and variance using exponentially weighted moving average control charts. *Technometrics*, 37:446–453, 1995.

M.G. Genton. Separable approximations of space-time covariance matrices. *Environmetrics*, 18:681–695, 2007.

J.D. Gibbons and S. Chakraborti. *Nonparametric Statistical Inference.* Marcel Dekker, Inc.: New York, NY, USA, 4th edition, 2003.

T. Gneiting. Nonseparable stationary covariance functions for space-time data. *Journal of the American Statistical Association*, 97:590–600, 2002.

V. Gómez-Rubio, P. Moraga, and B. Rowlingson. DClusterm: model-based detection of disease clusters. *R package version 0.2-3*, pages https://CRAN.R-project.org/package=DClusterm, 2019.

P.I. Good. *Permutation, Parametric and Bootstrap Tests of Hypotheses.* Springer: New York, NY, USA, 3rd edition, 2005.

M.A. Graham, S. Chakraborti, and S.W. Human. A nonparametric exponentially weighted moving average signed-rank chart for monitoring location. *Computational Statistics and Data Analysis*, 55:2490–2503, 2011.

R.B. Gramacy. laGP: large-scale spatial modeling via local approximate Gaussian processes in R. *Journal of Statistical Software*, 72:1–46, 2016.

C. Gygi, B. Williams, and N. DeCarlo. *Six Sigma For Dummies.* John Wiley & Sons: New York, NY, USA, 2nd edition, 2012.

P. Hackl and J. Ledolter. A control chart based on ranks. *Journal of Quality Technology*, 23:117–124, 1991.

P. Hall, N.I. Fisher, and B. Hoffmann. On the nonparametric estimation of covariance functions. *Annals of Statistics*, 22:2115–2134, 1994.

W. Härdle, P. Hall, and J.S. Marron. Regression smoothing parameters that are not far from their optimal. *Journal of the American Statistical Association*, 87:227–233, 1992.

T.J. Harris and W.H. Ross. Statistical process control procedures for autocorrelated observations. *Canadian Journal of Chemical Engineering*, 69:48–57, 1991.

T. Hastie and R. Tibshirani. Varying-coefficient models. *Journal of the Royal Statistical Society (Series B)*, 55:757–796, 1993.

T. Hastie, R. Tibshirani, and J. Friedman. *The Elements of Statistical Learning – Data Mining, Inference, and Prediction.* Springer: New York, NY, USA, 2001.

D.M. Hawkins. On the distribution and power of a test for a single outlier. *South African Statistical Journal*, 3:9–15, 1969.

D.M. Hawkins. Self-starting cusums for location and scale. *The Statistician*, 36:299–315, 1987.

D.M. Hawkins and Q. Deng. A nonparametric change-point control chart. *Journal of Quality Technology*, 42:165–173, 2010.

D.M. Hawkins and E.M. Maboudou-Tchao. Self-starting multivariate exponentially weighted moving average control charting. *Technometrics*, 49: 199–209, 2007.

D.M. Hawkins and D.H. Olwell. *Cumulative Sum Charts and Charting for Quality Improvement.* Springer: New York, NY, USA, 1998.

D.M. Hawkins, P. Qiu, and C.W. Kang. The changepoint model for statistical process control. *Journal of Quality Technology*, 35:355–366, 2003.

S.H. Heisterkamp, A.L.M. Dekkers, and J.C.M. Heijne. Automated detection of infectious disease outbreaks: hierarchical time series models. *Statistics in Medicine*, 25:4179–4196, 2006.

N.J. Higham. Computing a nearest symmetric positive semidefinite matrix. *Linear Algebra and Its Applications*, 103:103–118, 1988.

A. Hohl, E.M. Delmelle, M.R. Desjardins, and Y. Lan. Daily surveillance of COVID-19 using the prospective space-time scan statistic in the United States. *Spatial and Spatio-Temporal Epidemiology*, 34: https://doi.org/10.1016/j.sste.2020.100354, 2020.

M.D. Holland and D.M. Hawkins. A control chart based on a nonparametric multivariate change-point model. *Journal of Quality Technology*, 46:63–77, 2014.

M. Hollander and D.A. Wolfe. *Nonparametric Statistical Methods.* John Wiley & Sons: New York, NY, USA, 2nd edition, 1999.

D.R. Hoover, J.A. Rice, C.O. Wu, and L.P. Yang. Nonparametric smoothing estimates of time-varying coefficient models with longitudinal data. *Biometrika*, 85:809–822, 1998.

N.J. Hsu, Y.M. Chang, and H.C. Huang. A group lasso approach for non-stationary spatial-temporal covariance estimation. *Environmetrics*, 23:12–23, 2012.

G.M. Jacquez. *Stat!: Statistical Software for the Clustering of Health Events.* BioMedware: Ann Arbor, Michigan, 1994.

G.M. Jacquez. A k nearest neighbor test for spacetime interaction. *Statistics in Medicine*, 15:1935–1949, 1996.

W.A. Jensen, L.A. Jones-Farmer, C.W. Champ, and W.H. Woodall. Effects of parameter estimation on control chart properties: a literature review. *Journal of Quality Technology*, 38:349–364, 2006.

F. Jiang, Y. Jiang, H. Zhi, Y. Dong, H. Li, S. Ma, Y. Wang, Q. Dong, H. Shen, and Y. Wang. Artificial intelligence in healthcare: Past, present and future. *Stroke and Vascular Neurology*, 2:230–243, 2017.

N.L. Johnson, A.W. Kemp, and S. Kotz. *Univariate Discrete Distributions.* John Wiley & Sons: New York, NY, USA, 2nd edition, 1992.

N.L. Johnson, S. Kotz, and N. Balakrishnan. *Continuous Univariate Distributions (Volume 1).* John Wiley & Sons: New York, NY, USA, 2nd edition, 1994.

N.L. Johnson, S. Kotz, and N. Balakrishnan. *Continuous Univariate Distributions (Volume 2).* John Wiley & Sons: New York, NY, USA, 2nd edition, 1995.

R.A. Johnson and M. Bagshaw. The effect of serial correlation on the performance of CUSUM tests. *Technometrics*, 16:103–112, 1974.

L.A. Jones, C.W. Champ, and S.E. Rigdon. The run length distribution of the CUSUM with estimated parameters. *Industrial Quality Control*, 36:95–108, 2004.

L.A. Jones-Farmer, V. Jordan, and C.W. Champ. Distribution-free phase I control charts for subgroup location. *Journal of Quality Technology*, 41: 304–317, 2009.

L.A. Jones-Farmer, W.H. Woodall, S.H. Steiner, and C.W. Champ. An overview of Phase I analysis for process improvement and monitoring. *Journal of Quality Technology*, 46:265–280, 2014.

I. Jung. A generalized linear models approach to spatial scan statistics for covariate adjustment. *Statistics in Medicine*, 28:1131–1143, 2009.

I. Jung and G. Park. p-value approximations for spatial scan statistics using extreme value distributions. *Statistics in Medicine*, 34:504–514, 2015.

K. Kafadar. Smoothing geographical data, particularly rates of disease. *Statistics in Medicine*, 15:2539–2560, 1996.

J. Kim, J. Hong, and H. Park. Prospects of deep learning for medical imaging. *Precision and Future Medicine*, 2:37–52, 2018.

A. Kite-Powell, A. Ofori-Addo, and J. Hamilton. *ESSENCE User Guide (Version 1.0).* Florida Department of Health, Bureau of Epidemiology, Tallahassee, FL, USA, 2010.

J.P. Klein and M.L. Moeschberger. *Survival Analysis: Techniques for Censored and Truncated Data.* Springer: New York, NY, USA, 2nd edition, 2003.

K. Kleinman, R. Lazarus, and R. Platt. A generalized linear mixed models approach for detecting incident clusters of disease in small areas, with an application to biological terrorism. *American Journal of Epidemiology*, 159: 217–224, 2004.

E. Knox and M. Bartlett. The detection of space-time interactions. *Journal of the Royal Statistical Society (Series C)*, 13:25–30, 1964.

K. Koehler. Goodness-of-fit tests for loglinear models in sparse contingency tables. *Journal of the American Statistical Association*, 81:483–493, 1986.

K. Koehler and K. Larntz. An empirical investigation of goodness-of-fit statistics for sparse multinomials. *Journal of the American Statistical Association*, 75:336–344, 1980.

M. Kulldorff. A spatial scan statistic. *Communications in Statistics-Theory and Methods*, 26:1481–1496, 1997.

M. Kulldorff. Prospective time periodic geographical disease surveillance using a scan statistic. *Journal of the Royal Statistical Society (Series A)*, 164:61–72, 2001.

M. Kulldorff and U. Hjalmars. The knox method and other tests for spacetime interaction. *Biometrics*, 55:544–552, 1999.

M. Kulldorff, L. Huang, L.W. Pickle, and L. Duczmal. An elliptic spatial scan statistic. *Statistics in Medicine*, 25:3929–3943, 2006.

P.H. Kvam and B. Vidakovic. *Nonparametric Statistics with Applications to Science and Engineering.* John Wiley & Sons: New York, NY, USA, 2007.

S.N. Lahiri. *Resampling Methods for Dependent Data.* Springer-Verlag: New York, NY, USA, 2003.

A.B. Lawson, A.B. Biggeri, D. Boehning, E. Lesaffre, J.-F. Viel, A. Clark, P. Schlattmann, and F. Divino. Disease mapping models: an empirical evaluation. *Statistics in Medicine*, 19:2217–2241, 2000.

E.L. Lehmann and G. Casella. *Theory of Point Estimation.* Springer-Verlag: New York, NY, USA, 2nd edition, 1998.

E.L. Lehmann and J.P. Romano. *Testing Statistical Hypotheses.* Springer-Verlag: New York, NY, USA, 3rd edition, 2005.

J. Li and P. Qiu. Nonparametric dynamic screening system for monitoring correlated longitudinal data. *IIE Transactions*, 48:772–786, 2016.

J. Li and P. Qiu. Construction of an efficient multivariate dynamic screening system. *Quality and Reliability Engineering International*, 33:1969–1981, 2017.

J. Li, X. Zhang, and D.R. Jeske. Nonparametric multivariate CUSUM control charts for location and scale changes. *Journal of Nonparametric Statistics*, 25:1–20, 2013.

J. Li, K. Liu, and X. Xian. Causation-based process monitoring and diagnosis for multivariate categorical processes. *IISE Transactions*, 49:332–343, 2017.

S.Y. Li, L.C. Tang, and S.H. Ng. Nonparametric CUSUM and EWMA control charts for detecting mean shifts. *Journal of Quality Technology*, 42:209–226, 2010.

W. Li and P. Qiu. A general charting scheme for monitoring serially correlated data with short-memory dependence and nonparametric distributions. *IISE Transactions*, 52:61–74, 2020.

Y. Li. Efficient semiparametric regression for longitudinal data with nonparametric covariance estimation. *Biometrika*, 98:355–370, 2011.

K.Y. Liang and S.L. Zeger. Longitudinal data analysis using generalized linear models. *Biometrika*, 73:13–22, 1986.

D.Y. Lin and Z. Ying. Cox regression with incomplete covariate measurements. *Journal of the American Statistical Association*, 88:1341–1349, 1993.

P.S. Lin, Y.H. Kung, and M. Clayton. Spatial scan statistics for detection of multiple clusters with arbitrary shapes. *Biometrics*, 72:1226–1234, 2016.

X. Lin and R.J. Carroll. Nonparametric function estimation for clustered data when the predictor is measured without/with error. *Journal of the American Statistical Association*, 95:520–534, 2000.

X. Lin and R.J. Carroll. Semiparametric regression for clustered data using generalized estimating equations. *Journal of the American Statistical Association*, 96:1045–1056, 2001.

J. Lindström, A.A. Szpiro, P.D. Sampson, A.P. Oron, M. Richards, T.V. Larson, and L. Sheppard. A flexible spatio-temporal model for air pollution with spatial and spatio-temporal covariates. *Environmental and Ecological Statistics*, 21:411–433, 2014.

J. Lindström, A.A. Szpiro, P.D. Sampson, S. Bergen, and L. Sheppard. SpatioTemporal: an R package for spatio-temporal modelling of air-pollution. *https://cran.r-project.org/web/packages/SpatioTemporal/index.html*, 2015.

L. Liu, F. Tsung, and J. Zhang. Adaptive nonparametric CUSUM scheme for detecting unknown shifts in location. *International Journal of Production Research*, 52:1592–1606, 2014.

C.R. Loader. Large-deviation approximation to the distribution of scan statistics. *Advances in Applied Probability*, 23:751–771, 1991.

C.R. Loader. Bandwidth selection: classical or plug-in? *The Annals of Statistics*, 27:415–438, 1999.

C.A. Lowry, W.H. Woodall, C.W. Champ, and S.E. Rigdon. Multivariate exponentially weighted moving average control chart. *Technometrics*, 34: 46–53, 1992.

C.W. Lu and M.R. Reynolds, Jr. Control charts for monitoring an autocorrelated process. *Journal of Quality Technology*, 33:316–334, 2001.

S.L. Lu. An extended nonparametric exponentially weighted moving average sign control chart. *Quality and Reliability Engineering International*, 31: 3–13, 2015.

J.M. Lucas and M.S. Saccucci. Exponentially weighted moving average control schemes: properties and enhancements (with discussions). *Technometrics*, 32:1–29, 1990.

R.A. Maller, G. Müller, and A. Szimayer. GARCH modelling in continuous time for irregularly spaced time series data. *Bernoulli*, 14:519–542, 2008.

C.L. Mallows. Some comments on C_p. *Technometrics*, 15:661–675, 1973.

V. Mante, D. Sussillo, K.V. Shenoy, and W.T. Newsome. Context-dependent computation by recurrent dynamics in prefrontal cortex. *Nature*, 503:78–84, 2013.

N. Mantel. The detection of disease clustering and a generalized regression approach. *Cancer Research*, 27:209–220, 1967.

J.B. Marshall, D.J. Spitzner, and W.H. Woodall. Use of the local Knox statistic for the prospective monitoring of disease occurrences in space and time. *Statistics in Medicine*, 26:1579–1593, 2007.

R.J. Marshall. A review of methods for the statistical analysis of spatial patterns of disease. *Journal of the Royal Statistical Society (Series A)*, 154: 421–441, 1991.

P. McCullagh and J.A. Nelder. *Generalized Linear Models*. Chapman & Hall/CRC: Boca Raton, FL, USA, 2nd edition, 1992.

V. Mnih, K. Kavukcuoglu, D. Silver, A.A. Rusu, J. Veness, M.G. Bellemare, A. Graves, M.A. Riedmiller, A.K. Fidjeland, G. Ostrovski, S. Petersen, C. Beattie, A. Sadik, I. Antonoglou, H. King, D. Kumaran, D. Wierstra, S. Legg, and D. Hassabis. Human-level control through deep reinforcement learning. *Nature*, 518:529–533, 2015.

D.C. Montgomery. *Introduction to Statistical Quality Control.* John Wiley & Sons: New York, NY, USA, 7th edition, 2012.

D.C. Montgomery and C.M. Mastrangelo. Some statistical process control methods for autocorrelated data. *Journal of Quality Technology*, 23:179–204, 1991.

A.S. Morrison. *Screening in Chronic Disease.* Oxford University Press, Inc.: New York, NY, USA, 2nd edition, 1992.

G.V. Moustakides. Optimal stopping times for detecting changes in distributions. *The Annals of Statistics*, 14:1379–1387, 1986.

E.A. Nadaraya. On estimating regression. *Theory of Probability and Its Applications*, 9:141–142, 1964.

J.I. Naus. The distribution of the size of the maximum cluster of points on the line. *Journal of the American Statistical Association*, 60:532–538, 1965.

L. Ngo, I.B. Tager, and D. Hadley. Application of exponential smoothing for nosocomial infection surveillance. *American Journal of Epidemiology*, 143: 637–647, 1996.

C. Ngufor, H.V. Houten, B.S. Caffo, N.D. Shah, and R.G. McCoy. Mixed effect machine learning: A framework for predicting longitudinal change in hemoglobin a1c. *Journal of Biomedical Informatics*, 89:56–67, 2019.

W. Ning, A.B. Yeh, X. Wu, and B. Wang. A nonparametric phase I control chart for individual observations based on empirical likelihood ratio. *Quality and Reliability Engineering International*, 31:37–55, 2015.

M. Noordzij, F.W. Dekker, C. Zoccali, and K.J. Jager. Measures of disease frequency: prevalence and incidence. *Nephron Clinical Practice*, 115:c17–c20, 2010.

N.A. Obuchowski. Receiver operating characteristic curves and their use in radiology. *Radiology*, 229:3–8, 2003.

P.P. Odiowei and Y. Cao. Nonlinear dynamic process monitoring using canonical variate analysis and kernel density estimations. *IEEE Transactions on Industrial Informatics*, 6:36–45, 2010.

H. Oja. *Multivariate Nonparametric Methods with R.* Springer-Verlag, New York, NY, USA, 2010.

J. Opsomer, Y. Wang, and Y. Yang. Nonparametric regression with correlated errors. *Statistical Science*, 16:134–153, 2001.

J. Ostmeyer and L. Cowell. Machine learning on sequential data using a recurrent weighted average. *Neurocomputing*, 331:281–288, 2019.

E.S. Page. Continuous inspection scheme. *Biometrika*, 41:100–115, 1954.

M.C. Paik and W.Y. Tsai. On using the Cox proportional hazards model with missing covariates. *Biometrika*, 84:579–593, 1997.

K.Y. Park and P. Qiu. Model selection and diagnostics for joint modeling of survival and longitudinal data with crossing hazard rate functions. *Statistics in Medicine*, 33:4532–4546, 2014.

E. Parzen. On estimation of a probability density function and mode. *Annals of Mathematical Statistics*, 33:1065–1076, 1962.

M. Parzen, S. Ghosh, S. Lipsitz, D. Sinha, G.M. Fitzmaurice, B K. Mallick, and J.G. Ibrahim. A generalized linear mixed model for longitudinal binary data with a marginal logit link function. *Annals of Applied Statistics*, 5: 449–467, 2011.

K. Pearson. On the criterion that a given system of deviations from the probable in the case of a correlated system of variables is such that it can be reasonably supposed to have arisen from random sampling. *Philosophical Magazine*, 50:157–175, 1900.

C. Pelat, P.-Y. Boëlle, B. J. Cowling, F. Carrat, A. Flahault, and S. Ansart. Online detection and quantification of epidemics. *BMC Medical Informatics and Decision Making*, 7:article 29, 2007.

M.J. Pencina, A.M. Navar, D. Wojdyla, R.J. Sanchez, I. Khan, J. Elassal, R.M. D'Agostino Sr, E.D. Peterson, and A.D. Sniderman. Quantifying importance of major risk factors for coronary heart disease. *Circulation*, 139:1603–1611, 2019.

M.S. Pepe. *The Statistical Evaluation of Medical Tests for Classification and Prediction.* Oxford University Press: New York, NY, USA, 2003.

N. Pica and N.M. Bouvier. Environmental factors affecting the transmission of respiratory viruses. *Current Opinion in Virology*, 2:90–95, 2012.

P. Qiu. *Image Processing and Jump Regression Analysis.* John Wiley & Sons, Inc.: Hoboken, New Jersey, USA, 2005.

P. Qiu. Distribution-free multivariate process control based on log-linear modeling. *IIE Transactions*, 40:664–677, 2008.

P. Qiu. *Introduction to Statistical Process Control.* Chapman & Hall/CRC: Boca Raton, FL, USA, 2014.

P. Qiu. Some perspectives on nonparametric statistical process control. *Journal of Quality Technology*, 50:49–65, 2018a.

P. Qiu. Jump regression, image processing and quality control (with discussions). *Quality Engineering*, 30:137–153, 2018b.

P. Qiu and D.M. Hawkins. A rank based multivariate CUSUM procedure. *Technometrics*, 43:120–132, 2001.

P. Qiu and D.M. Hawkins. A nonparametric multivariate CUSUM procedure for detecting shifts in all directions. *Journal of the Royal Statistical Society (Series D) - The Statistician*, 52:151–164, 2003.

P. Qiu and C. Le. ROC curve estimation based on local smoothing. *Journal of Statistical Computation and Simulation*, 70:55–69, 2001.

P. Qiu and Z. Li. On nonparametric statistical process control of univariate processes. *Technometrics*, 53:390–405, 2011a.

P. Qiu and Z. Li. Distribution-free monitoring of univariate processes. *Statistics and Probability Letters*, 81:1833–1840, 2011b.

P. Qiu and D. Xiang. Univariate dynamic screening system: an approach for identifying individuals with irregular longitudinal behavior. *Technometrics*, 56:248–260, 2014.

P. Qiu and D. Xiang. Surveillance of cardiovascular diseases using a multivariate dynamic screening system. *Statistics in Medicine*, 34:2204–2221, 2015.

P. Qiu and X. Xie. Transparent sequential learning for statistical process control of serially correlated data. *Technometrics*, 64:487–501, 2022.

P. Qiu and K. Yang. Effective disease surveillance by using covariate information. *Statistics in Medicine*, 40:5725–5745, 2021.

P. Qiu and K. Yang. Spatio-temporal process monitoring using exponentially weighted spatial LASSO. *Journal of Quality Technology*, 55:163–180, 2023.

P. Qiu and L. You. Dynamic disease screening by joint modeling of survival and longitudinal data. *Journal of the Royal Statistical Society (Series C)*, 71:1158–1180, 2022.

P. Qiu, C. Zou, and Z. Wang. Nonparametric profile monitoring by mixed effects modeling (with discussions). *Technometrics*, 52:265–277, 2010.

P. Qiu, X. Zi, and C. Zou. Nonparametric dynamic curve monitoring. *Technometrics*, 60:386–397, 2018.

P. Qiu, W. Li, and J. Li. A new process control chart for monitoring short-range serially correlated data. *Technometrics*, 62:71–83, 2020a.

P. Qiu, Z. Xia, and L. You. Process monitoring ROC curve for evaluating dynamic screening methods. *Technometrics*, 62:236–248, 2020b.

H. Rao, X. Shi, and X. Zhang. Using the Kulldorff's scan statistical analysis to detect spatio-temporal clusters of tuberculosis in Qinghai Province, China, 2009–2016. *BMC Infectious Diseases*, 17:https://doi.org/10.1186/s12879-017-2643-y, 2017.

B.Y. Reis and K.D. Mandl. Time series modeling for syndromic surveillance. *BMC Medical Informatics and Decision Making*, 3:article 2, 2003.

J. Rice and C.O. Wu. Nonparametric mixed effects models for unequally sampled noisy curves. *Biometrics*, 57:253–259, 2001.

M.D. Risser and D. Turek. Bayesian inference for high-dimensional nonstationary Gaussian processes. *Journal of Statistical Computation and Simulation*, 90:2902–2928, 2020.

S.V. Roberts. Control chart tests based on geometric moving averages. *Technometrics*, 1:239–250, 1959.

P.A. Rogerson. Monitoring point patterns for the development of space-time clusters. *Journal of the Royal Statistical Society (Series A)*, 164:87–96, 2001.

M. Rosenblatt. Remarks on some nonparametric estimates of a density function. *Annals of Mathematical Statistics*, 27:832—-837, 1956.

D. Rubin. *Multiple Imputation for Nonresponse in Surveys.* John Wiley & Sons: New York, NY, USA, 1987.

G.C. Runger and T.R. Willemain. Model-based and model-free control of autocorrelated processes. *Journal of Quality Technology*, 27:283–292, 1995.

D. Ruppert, S.J. Sheather, and M.P. Wand. An efficient bandwidth selector for local least squares regression. *Journal of the American Statistical Association*, 90:1257–1270, 1995.

D.V. Samarov, J. Hwang, and M. Litorja. The spatial LASSO with applications to unmixing hyperspectral biomedical images. *Technometrics*, 57: 503–513, 2015.

P.D. Sampson, A.A. Szpiro, L. Sheppard, J. Lindström, and J.D. Kaufman. Pragmatic estimation of a spatio-temporal air quality model with irregular monitoring data. *Atmospheric Environment*, 45:6593–6606, 2011.

G. Schwarz. Estimating the dimension of a model. *The Annals of Statistics*, 6:461–464, 1978.

L. Shand and B. Li. Modeling nonstationarity in space and time. *Biometrics*, 73:759–768, 2017.

S.S. Shantharam, M. Mahalingam, A. Rasool, J.A. Reynolds, A.R. Bhuiya, T.D. Satchell, J.M. Chapel, N.A. Hawkins, C.D. Jones, V. Jacob, and D.P. Hopkins. Systematic review of self-measured blood pressure monitoring with support: intervention effectiveness and cost. *American Journal of Preventive Medicine*, 62:285–298, 2022.

W.A. Shewhart. *Economic Control of Quality of Manufactured Product.* D. Van Nostrand Company: New York, NY, USA, 1931.

M. Shi, Weiss R.E., and J.M.G. Taylor. An analysis of paediatric CD4 counts for acquired immune deficiency syndrome using flexible random curves. *Applied Statistics*, 45:151–163, 1996.

L. Shu and W. Jiang. A Markov chain model for the adaptive CUSUM control chart. *Journal of Quality Technology*, 38:135–147, 2006.

B.W. Silverman. *Density Estimation For Statistics and Data Analysis.* Chapman & Hall/CRC: Boca Raton, FL, USA, 1986.

N. Simon, J. Friedman, T. Hastie, and R. Tibshirani. Regularization paths for Cox's proportional hazards model via coordinate descent. *Journal of Statistical Software*, 39:1–13, 2011.

I.N. Soyiri and D.D. Reidpath. An overview of health forecasting. *Environmental Health and Preventive Medicine*, 18:1–9, 2013.

R.S. Sparks. CUSUM charts for signalling varying location shifts. *Journal of Quality Technology*, 32:157–171, 2000.

P. Speckman. Kernel smoothing in partial linear models. *Journal of the Royal Stattistical Society (Series B)*, 50:413–436, 1988.

L. Stern and D. Lightfoot. Automated outbreak detection: a quantitative retrospective analysis. *Epidemiology and Infection*, 122:103–110, 1999.

J.R. Stroud, P. Müller, and B. Sansó. Dynamic models for spatiotemporal data. *Journal of the Royal Statistical Society (Series B)*, 63:673–689, 2001.

D. Stroup, M. Wharton, K. Kafadar, and A. Dean. Evaluation of a method for detecting aberrations in public health surveillance data. *American Journal of Epidemiology*, 137:373–380, 1999.

J.H. Sullivan and L.A. Jones. A self-starting control chart for multivariate individual observations. *Technometrics*, 44:24–33, 2002.

Y. Sun, J.D. Hart, and M.G. Genton. Nonparametric inference for periodic sequences. *Technometrics*, 54:83–96, 2012.

B.C. Sutradhar. *Longitudinal Categorical Data Analysis.* Springer: New York, NY, USA, 2014.

A.A. Szpiro, P.D. Sampson, L. Sheppard, T. Lumley, S. Adar, and J.D. Kaufman. Predicting intra-urban variation in air pollution concentrations with complex spatio-temporal dependencies. *Environmetrics*, 21:606–631, 2010.

K. Takahashi, M. Kulldorff, T. Tango, and K. Yih. A flexibly shaped space-time scan statistic for disease outbreak detection and monitoring. *International Journal of Health Geographics*, 7:14, 2008.

T. Tango. *Statistical Methods for Disease Clustering.* Springer: New York, NY, USA, 2010.

T. Tango and K. Takahashi. A flexibly shaped spatial scan statistic for detecting clusters. *International Journal of Health Geographics*, 4:Article Number: 11, 2005.

B.M. Taylor, T.M. Davies, B.S. Rowlingson, and P.J. Diggle. lgcp: an R package for inference with spatial and spatio-temporal log-Gaussian Cox processes. *Journal of Statistical Software*, 52:http://www.jstatsoft.org/, 2013.

L. Tian, D. Zucker, and L.J. Wei. On the Cox model with time-varying regression coefficients. *Journal of the American Statistical Association*, 100: 172–183, 2005.

R. Tibshirani. Regression shrinkage and selection via the lasso. *Journal of the Royal Statistical Society (Series B)*, 58:267–288, 1996.

R. Tibshirani. The LASSO method for variable selection in the Cox model. *Statistics in Medicine*, 16:385–395, 1997.

R. Tibshirani and J. Taylor. The solution path of the generalized LASSO. *The Annals of Statistics*, 39:1335–1371, 2011.

B.W. Turnbull, E.J. Iwano, W.S. Burnett, H.L. Howe, and L.C. Clark. Monitoring for clusters of disease: application to leukemia incidence in upstate New York. *American Journal of Epidemiology*, 132:S136–S143, 1990.

D.E. Tyler. A distribution-free M-estimator of multivariate scatter. *Annals of Statistics*, 15:234–251, 1987.

USDOH. *The Power of Prevention, Steps to a Healthier US: A Program and Policy Perspective.* US Department of Health and Human Services: Washington, DC, 2003.

S. van Buuren. *Flexible Imputation of Missing Data.* Chapman & Hall/CRC: Boca Raton, FL, USA, 2nd edition, 2018.

S. van Buuren and K. Groothuis-Oudshoorn. mice: Multivariate imputation by chained equations in R. *Journal of Statistical Software*, 45:1–67, 2011.

V.V. Vityazev. Time series analysis of unequally spaced data: the statistical properties of the Schuster periodogram. *Astronomical and Astrophysical Transactions*, 11:159–173, 1996.

M. Vogt and O. Linton. Nonparametric estimation of a periodic sequence in the presence of a smooth trend. *Biometrika*, 101:121–140, 2014.

H.M. Wadsworth, K.S. Stephens, and A.B. Godfrey. *Modern Methods for Quality Control and Improvement.* John Wiley & Sons: New York, NY, USA, 2002.

L.A. Waller and C.A. Gotway. *Applied Spatial Statistics for Public Health Data.* John Wiley & Sons: New York, NY, USA, 2005.

M.P. Wand and M.C. Jones. *Kernel Smoothing.* Chapman & Hall/CRC: Boca Raton, FL, USA, 3rd edition, 1995.

K. Wang and W. Jiang. High-dimensional process monitoring and fault isolation via variable selection. *Journal of Quality Technology*, 41:247–258, 2009.

D.G. Wardell, H. Moskowitz, and R.D. Plante. Run length distributions of special-cause control charts for correlated processes. *Technometrics*, 36: 3–17, 1994.

M. Warren. The approach to predictive medicine that is taking genomics research by storm. *Nature*, 562:181–183, 2018.

G.S. Watson. Smooth regression analysis. *Sankhya (Series A)*, 26:359–372, 1964.

M.A. Weinstock. A generalised scan statistic test for the detection of clusters. *Internationally Journal of Epidemiology*, 10:289–293, 1981.

C.K. Wikle, A. Zammit-Mangion, and N. Cressie. *Spatio-Temporal Statistics with R.* Chapman & Hall/CRC: Boca Raton, FL, USA, 2019.

F. Wilcoxon, S.K. Katti, and R.A. Wilcox. Critical values and probability levels for the Wilcoxon rank sum test and the Wilcoxon signed rank test. In *Selected Tables in Mathematical Statistics*, volume 1, pages 171–259. American Mathematical Society, Providence, RI, USA, 1972.

S.S. Wilks. The large-sample distribution of the likelihood ratio for testing composite hypotheses. *The Annals of Mathematical Statistics*, 9:60–62, 1938.

J.M.G. Wilson and G. Jungner. Principles and practice of screening for disease. *WHO Chronicle*, 22:281–393, 1968.

W.H. Woodall, J.B. Marshall, Jr Joner, M.D., S.E. Fraker, and A.S.G. Abdel-Salam. On the use and evaluation of prospective scan methods for health-related surveillance. *Journal of the Royal Statistical Society (Series A)*, 171: 223–237, 2008.

D.J. Wright. Forecasting data published at irregular time intervals using an extension of Holt's method. *Management Science*, 32:499–510, 1986.

H. Wu and J. Zhang. Local polynomial mixed-effects models for longitudinal data. *Journal of the American Statistical Association*, 97:883–897, 2002.

W.B. Wu. Asymptotic theory for stationary processes. *Statistics and Its Interface*, 4:207–226, 2011.

M.S. Wulfsohn and A.A. Tsiatis. A joint model for survival and longitudinal data measured with error. *Biometrics*, 53:330–339, 1997.

X. Xian, J. Li, and K. Liu. Causation-based monitoring and diagnosis for multivariate categorical processes with ordinal information. *IEEE Transactions on Automation Science and Engineering*, 16:886–897, 2019.

D. Xiang, P. Qiu, and X. Pu. Nonparametric regression analysis of multivariate longitudinal data. *Statistica Sinica*, 23:769–789, 2013.

X. Xie and P. Qiu. Control chart for dynamic process monitoring with an application to air pollution surveillance. *Annals of Applied Statistics*, 17: 47–66, 2023a.

X. Xie and P. Qiu. A general framework for robust monitoring of multivariate correlated processes. *Technometrics*, DOI: 10.1080/00401706.2023.2224411, 2023b.

L. Xue and P. Qiu. A nonparametric CUSUM chart for monitoring multivariate serially correlated processes. *Journal of Quality Technology*, 53:396–409, 2021.

H. Yan, K. Paynabar, and J. Shi. Real-time monitoring of high-dimensional functional data streams via spatio-temporal smooth sparse decomposition. *Technometrics*, 60:181–197, 2018.

K. Yang and P. Qiu. Spatiotemporal incidence rate data analysis by nonparametric regression. *Statistics in Medicine*, 37:2094–2107, 2018.

K. Yang and P. Qiu. Nonparametric estimation of the spatio-temporal covariance structure. *Statistics in Medicine*, 38:4555–4565, 2019.

K. Yang and P. Qiu. Online sequential monitoring of spatio-temporal disease incidence rates. *IISE Transactions*, 52:1218–1233, 2020.

K. Yang and P. Qiu. Adaptive process monitoring using covariate information. *Technometrics*, 63:313–328, 2021.

K. Yang and P. Qiu. A three-step local smoothing approach for estimating the mean and covariance functions of spatio-temporal data. *Annals of the Institute of Statistical Mathematics*, 74:49–68, 2022.

K. Yang and P. Qiu. SpTe2M: An *R* package for nonparametric modeling and monitoring of spatio-temporal data. *Journal of Quality Technology*, in press, 2023.

Y. Yang. Can the strengths of AIC and BIC be shared? A conflict between model identification and regression estimation. *Biometrika*, 92:937–950, 2005.

A.B. Yeh, D.K.J. Lin, and C. Venkataramani. Unified CUSUM charts for monitoring process mean and variability. *Quality Technology and Quantitative Management*, 1:65–86, 2004.

A.B. Yeh, L. Huwang, R.N. McGrath, and Z. Zhang. On monitoring process variance with individual observations. *Quality and Reliability Engineering International*, 26:631–641, 2010.

L. You and P. Qiu. Fast computing for dynamic screening systems when analyzing correlated data. *Journal of Statistical Computation and Simulation*, 89:379–394, 2019.

L. You and P. Qiu. An effective method for online disease risk monitoring. *Technometrics*, 62:249–264, 2020a.

L. You and P. Qiu. A nonparametric control chart for dynamic disease risk monitoring. In *Distribution-Free Methods for Statistical Process Monitoring and Control*, pages 243–257. Springer-Verlag: New York, NY, USA, 2020b.

L. You and P. Qiu. A robust dynamic screening system by estimation of the longitudinal data distribution. *Journal of Quality Technology*, 53:383–395, 2021a.

L. You and P. Qiu. Joint modeling of multivariate nonparametric longitudinal data and survival data – a local smoothing approach. *Statistics in Medicine*, 40:6689–6706, 2021b.

L. You and P. Qiu. *DySS: Dynamic Screening System*. https://cran.r-project.org/web/packages/DySS/index.html, 2022.

L. You, P. Qiu, B. Huang, and P. Qiu. Early detection of severe juvenile idiopathic arthritis by sequential monitoring of patients' health-related quality of life scores. *Biometrical Journal*, 62:1343–1356, 2020.

K. Yu and M. Jones. Local linear quantile regression. *Journal of the American Statistical Association*, 93:228–237, 1998.

Z. Yu and X. Lin. Semiparametric regression with time-dependent coefficients for failure time data analysis. *Statistica Sinica*, 20:853–869, 2010.

A. Zammit-Mangion and N. Cressie. FRK: an R package for spatial and spatio-temporal prediction with large datasets. *Journal of Statistical Software*, 98: 1–48, 2017.

J. Zhang, Y. Kang, Y. Yang, and P. Qiu. Statistical monitoring of the hand, foot, and mouth disease in China. *Biometrics*, 71:841–850, 2015.

T. Zhang and G. Lin. Spatial scan statistics in loglinear models. *Computational Statistics and Data Analysis*, 53:2851–2858, 2009.

Y. Zhao, D. Zeng, A.H. Herring, A. Ising, A. Waller, D. Richardson, and M.R. Kosorok. Detecting disease outbreaks using local spatiotemporal methods. *Biometrics*, 67:1508–1517, 2011.

H. Zhou and A. B. Lawson. EWMA smoothing and Bayesian spatial modeling for health surveillance. *Statistics in Medicine*, 27:5907–5928, 2008.

Q. Zhou and P. Qiu. Phase I monitoring of serially correlated nonparametric profiles by mixed-effects modeling. *Quality and Reliability Engineering International*, 38:134–152, 2022.

X.H. Zhou, N.A. Obuchowski, and D.K. McClish. *Statistical Methods in Diagnostic Medicine*. John Wiley & Sons, Inc.: Hoboken, New Jersey, USA, 2002.

C. Zou and P. Qiu. Multivariate statistical process control using LASSO. *Journal of the American Statistical Association*, 104:1586–1596, 2009.

C. Zou and F. Tsung. Likelihood ratio-based distribution-free EWMA control charts. *Journal of Quality Technology*, 42:1–23, 2010.

C. Zou and F. Tsung. A multivariate sign EWMA control chart. *Technometrics*, 53:84–97, 2011.

C. Zou, X. Ning, and F. Tsung. LASSO-based multivariate linear profile monitoring. *Annals of Operations Research*, 192:3–19, 2012a.

C. Zou, Z. Wang, and F. Tsung. A spatial rank-based multivariate EWMA control chart. *Naval Research Logistics*, 59:91–110, 2012b.

H. Zou. The adaptive LASSO and its oracle properties. *Journal of the American Statistical Association*, 101:1418–1429, 2006.

H. Zou and T. Hastie. Regularization and variable selection via the elastic net. *Journal of the Royal Statistical Society (Series B)*, 67:301–320, 2005.

D.M. Zucker and A.F. Karr. Nonparametric survival analysis with time-dependent covariate effects: a penalized partial likelihood approach. *Annals of Statistics*, 18:329–353, 1990.

Index

Printed in the United States
by Baker & Taylor Publisher Services